Clinical Challenges in the Biopsychosocial Interface

Advances in Psychosomatic Medicine

Vol. 34

Series Editor

T.N. Wise Falls Church, Va.

Editors

R. Balon Detroit, Mich.
G.A. Fava Bologna
I. Fukunishi Tokyo
M.B. Rosenthal Cleveland, Ohio

Clinical Challenges in the Biopsychosocial Interface

Update on Psychosomatics for the 21st Century

Volume Editors

R. Balon Detroit, Mich.

T.N. Wise Falls Church, Va.

9 Figures, 16 tables, 2015

KARGER

Basel · Freiburg · Paris · London · New York · Chennai · New Delhi · Bangkok · Beijing · Shanghai · Tokyo · Kuala Lumpur · Singapore · Sydney

Advances in Psychosomatic Medicine

Founded 1960 by
F. Deutsch (Cambridge, Mass.)
A. Jores (Hamburg)
B. Stockvis (Leiden)

Continued 1972–1982 by
F. Reichsman (Brooklyn, N.Y.)

Library of Congress Cataloging-in-Publication Data

Clinical challenges in the biopsychosocial interface : update on psychosomatics for the 21st century / volume editors, R. Balon, T.N. Wise.
p. ; cm. -- (Advances in psychosomatic medicine, ISSN 0065-3268 ; vol. 34)
Includes bibliographical references and indexes.
ISBN 978-3-318-02966-6 (hard cover : alk. paper) -- ISBN 978-3-318-02967-3 (electronic version)
I. Balon, Richard, editor. II. Wise, Thomas N., editor. III. Series: Advances in psychosomatic medicine ; v. 34. 0065-3268
[DNLM: 1. Psychosomatic Medicine--methods. W1 AD81 v.34 2015 / WM 90]
RC49
616.08--dc23
2015002067

Bibliographic Indices. This publication is listed in bibliographic services, including Current Contents® and Index Medicus.

Disclaimer. The statements, opinions and data contained in this publication are solely those of the individual authors and contributors and not of the publisher and the editor(s). The appearance of advertisements in the book is not a warranty, endorsement, or approval of the products or services advertised or of their effectiveness, quality or safety. The publisher and the editor(s) disclaim responsibility for any injury to persons or property resulting from any ideas, methods, instructions or products referred to in the content or advertisements.

Drug Dosage. The authors and the publisher have exerted every effort to ensure that drug selection and dosage set forth in this text are in accord with current recommendations and practice at the time of publication. However, in view of ongoing research, changes in government regulations, and the constant flow of information relating to drug therapy and drug reactions, the reader is urged to check the package insert for each drug for any change in indications and dosage and for added warnings and precautions. This is particularly important when the recommended agent is a new and/or infrequently employed drug.

www.karger.com
Printed in Germany on acid-free and non-aging paper (ISO 9706) by Kraft Druck, Ettlingen
ISSN 0065–3268
e-ISSN 1622–2855
ISBN 978–3–318–02966–6
e-ISBN 978–3–318–02967–3

KARGER 125 YEARS

Contents

Preface

Medicine has always been a changing field in terms of explanations of disease states, the appearance of new disorders, and therapeutic interventions. Psychiatry and psychosomatic medicine are in a dramatic state of change if one takes a decades-long perspective. Only a century ago, therapeutic options were almost nonexistent for the major psychoses. Within two decades, convulsive therapies offered an option for psychotic depressions. A few decades later, the advent of neuroleptics offered hope to those with schizophrenia who previously languished in isolated hospital wards. More recently, newer antidepressants have minimized side effects and allowed primary care physicians to effectively treat uncomplicated mood and anxiety disorders.

However, as time moves forward, problems both persist in the limited access of patients with psychiatric disorders to care and arise with new challenges, such as the reduced length of stay demanded by third-party payors and the ever-increasing prices of both new and old treatments. Another challenge is the high comorbidity of chronic mental illnesses and various chronic physical illnesses, such as diabetes mellitus, obesity, and cardiovascular disease, which significantly contributes to the shortened lifespan of people with chronic mental illness. Finally, the stigmas of mental illness, substance abuse, and some physical illnesses present yet another challenge, as they constitute yet another barrier in access to health care, especially in patients with multiple stigmatizing conditions.

The rise of population medicine, with special attention to preventive measures and to the importance of treating psychiatric disorders, substance abuse, and comorbid illnesses, may offer better treatments and increased access to care.

Psychosomatic medicine is considered to be one of the leading approaches to treating comorbid disorders and conditions, such as distress in the patient with cancer, demoralization and depression in the dermatological patient, or anxiety in the patient awaiting surgery. This volume addresses new, *psychosomatic* views on such conditions and approaches. It crisscrosses psychosomatic medicine, from basic sciences to clinical medicine, and discusses areas previously covered rarely, if at all, such as telomeres and mental illness, communication with seriously ill patients, fibromyalgia, psychiatric symptomatology in Huntington's disease, grieving in prostate cancer patients, and dimensional psychopharmacology. We hope that this volume offers new ideas and increased recognition of the advances of contemporary psychosomatic medicine.

Richard Balon, MD
Thomas N. Wise, MD

Balon R, Wise TN (eds): Clinical Challenges in the Biopsychosocial Interface. Update on Psychosomatics for the 21st Century. Adv Psychosom Med. Basel, Karger, 2015, vol 34, pp 1–9 (DOI: 10.1159/000369043)

Psychosomatic Medicine in the 21st Century: Understanding Mechanisms and Barriers to Utilization

Thomas N. Wise[a] · Richard Balon[b]

[a]Departments of Psychiatry at Inova Fairfax Hospital, Johns Hopkins University, George Washington University, and Virginia Commonwealth University, Falls Church, Va., and [b]Departments of Psychiatry and Behavioral Neurosciences and Anesthesiology, Wayne State University, Detroit, Mich., USA

Abstract

The psychosomatic approach arose in antiquity as mankind looked for explanations for illness and death. With the rise of modern medicine, the links between emotions and medical conditions, such as cardiac disease and diabetes, were described by astute clinical observers, but the mechanisms for these conditions were based on correlation from observations rather than on experimental design. Psychoanalytic theory was often utilized to explain many common diseases. For example, peptic ulcer disease was blamed upon anger and stress, but scientific methodology discovered *Helicobacter pylori* to be the significant causal factor of this disease and resulted in the development of more effective treatments. Nevertheless emotional factors are still linked to disease states and morbidity; for example, depression is a risk factor for mortality following myocardial infarction. Advances in neuroscience demonstrate that the reduction of telomere length by anxiety and stress leads to more rapid aging and potential disease vulnerability. Thus, neuroscientific probes may allow for the elucidation of psychosomatic mechanisms. Sadly, clinical barriers, in terms of time pressure upon physicians and the current separation of mental health services from primary care settings, continue the dualistic treatment of many conditions where psychological factors are important. It is not clear whether a mandate for the integration of behavioral health into primary care will remedy this partition and finally maximize a psychosomatic approach to medical care.

The psychosomatic approach, which links emotional factors to 'organic' disease states, has been an enduring theme in explaining the genesis and maintenance of disease states since antiquity [1, 2]. Ancient man looked for explanations to diseases and death and connected emotions to such events [2]. The term 'psychosomatic' was first utilized by Coleridge in a poem about opium dreams (though the reversed term 'somapsyche' occurs in the New Testament). In 1818, Johann Heinroth first utilized the term 'psycho-somatic' from a medical viewpoint – he believed that each mental illness could cause a somatic illness. Even as the Enlightenment fostered a more rigorous scientific

An earlier version of this text was published as: Wise NT: Psychosomatics: past present, and future. Psychother Psychosom 2014; 83: 65–69.

method in medicine, physicians continued to report the role of emotions in disease states. Thus, in the 17th century, Sir Thomas Willis observed that sorrow brings on the sweet urine (diabetes). This underscores the problem that has plagued psychosomatics, *observation*, such as Willis's aphorism, in the absence of *experimentation*, which is required to confidently link such emotions to disease genesis or comorbidity [3]. The sorrow that he observed may well have been a confounding factor of the fatigue that is inherent in the diabetic state. On the other hand, advances in physiology and molecular biology led physicians to ignore psychiatric/emotional issues, which may play a contributory or even etiological role, and even today few laboratory tests exist that confirm a diagnosis/etiology and allow mind-body linkages [4]. Nevertheless, the psychosomatic paradigm has endured. This introductory chapter will primarily focus upon the development of psychosomatics during the last 100 years (the excellent work from Europe has been recently reviewed by Schuffel [5]), with a closing discussion of the challenges that the field of psychosomatics will face in the future.

While ancient medicine utilized the four humors – black bile, yellow bile, blood and phlegm – to elucidate psychosomatic mechanisms and describe the first rudimental, yet fundamental, personality types (melancholic, choleric, sanguine and phlegmatic), contemporary psychosomatics arose with the psychoanalytic revolution (work of Sigmund Freud and Joseph Breuer) to explain the genesis of many diseases. Concurrently, stress research has incorporated the basic physiology of fear and flight to explain how emotional factors are interrelated in disease states. The limitation of early psychoanalytic reports was that the observations were deductive, that is, top-down reasoning with psychoanalytic theory that is considered as the general and only truth, which led to conclusions that were biased by such all-encompassing beliefs [6]. The psychoanalysts postulated that unconscious factors were important for the genesis of disease states [7]. Franz Alexander popularized mind-body themes for the lay public by conceptualizing specific disease states, such as peptic ulcer disease, to have specific unconscious conflicts that, once combined with constitutional factors, could produce such disorders [8]. Even so, some psychoanalysts attempted to utilize more rigorous qualitative and quantitative strategies. Michael Balint qualitatively studied primary care physicians' interactions to explain how they understood psychological problems [9]. He began groups for general practitioners to discuss psychodynamic factors related to their patients and their problems. Arthur Mirsky, an internist, physiologist and psychoanalyst, developed seminal research on the biopsychosocial aspects of peptic ulcer disease, utilizing urinary pepsinogen as a biological marker and projective tests to ascertain psychological issues in candidates undergoing the stressful Army induction process [10]. He found that certain psychological themes interacted with biological vulnerability to produce the duodenal ulcers that were found in those with the biological vulnerability [11]. However, *Helicobacter pylori* is currently considered to be a necessary pathogenic agent in peptic ulcer disease, yet the presence of this bacterium is not sufficient for the disease in itself, since 50% of the population is infected (*Helicobacter pylori* infects the upper gastrointestinal tract) and because 80% of those who are infected are asymptomatic (do not have the ulcer disease). Consistent with a psychosomatic model, Levenstein [12] warns against reductionism. He views *Helicobacter pylori* as one of several risk factors for ulcers, similar to high cholesterol being a risk factor but not a cause of myocardial infarction. He [12] postulates that *Helicobacter pylori* is one of many factors, including gastric acid hypersecretion, smoking, psychological stress and genetic predisposition, that play roles in ulcer formation, even when *Helicobacter pylori* is directly implicated. This example illustrates the complexity of the intertwined factors that are considered in psychosomatic concepts of various diseases. Concurrent with such provocative concepts, stress physiologists, such as I. P. Pavlov, Hans Selye (father of the term 'stress response') and Walter Cannon (who first described the fight-or-flight response), utilized their laboratories to demonstrate the role of the autonomic nervous system in the reaction to stress. Phenomenon such as 'Voodoo death' have been explained by stress-induced physiology that promotes fear and a profound bradycardia with escape arrhythmias; others opine that the victims of voodoo become hopeless and dehydrated, which leads to their demise [13–15]. Nevertheless, the profound seriousness of emotions leading to bad medical outcomes is reified. Modern molecular biology may not only expand our knowledge of disease and health but also reaffirm psychosomatic concepts, as suggested decades ago by Weiner [16, 17].

As medicine evolved to a true science that utilized the scientific method to understand pathology, diagnosis and treatment, many physicians abandoned psychosocial factors and focused primarily on the objective and quantitative elements of a disease process. This does not, however, suggest that the physicians were ignoring patient suffering, but they instead tended to minimize the scientific importance of that suffering. Roy Grinker coined the term *biopsychosocial* to urge psychiatrists to incorporate such advances, rather than to rely purely on psychoanalytic dogma [18] (interestingly, Grinker was one of the last of Freud's analysands). Years before this call for attention to biological issues, psychiatrists began to recognize external organic elements (toxic states) that foster delirium (e.g., [19]). Delirious states were often discussed by 19th century physicians as specific case histories, which eventually led Karl Bonhoffer to categorize them as 'exogenous psychoses' [20], but such observations appeared predominantly in the European and British literature and in North American delirium studies focused on alcohol withdrawal phenomena [21]. Lipowski combined such literature with his remarkable scholarship [22], and his influence over DSM III and IV led to the broad category of organic mental disorders [23]. He then regularly updated the research on delirium in classic review articles [24]. In contradistinction to Grinker [18], who urged more attention to biology, George Engel (Grinker's contemporary), an internist and psychoanalyst, began to advocate a more comprehensive approach that concentrated on the patient rather than completely focused upon the molecular biologic systems [25, 26]. The 'biopsychosocial' approach was widely disseminated in his classic article, 'The Need for a new medical model: a challenge for biomedicine' [27]. Engel contrasted the biopsychosocial model to 'biomedical reductionism', an approach that is unfortunately still seen too frequently. His work reaffirmed Osler's aphorism that it is essential to know '*who* the patient is' as well as '*what* disease they have'. Engel began his career with biologically focused research on delirium, and his concept of delirium 'as a syndrome of cerebral insufficiency' taught the general medical audience, not just psychiatrists, a clinically useful approach to identify and manage acute organic brain syndromes [28]. Engel then shifted from delirium to the role of affective states in an infant, Monica, with a gastric fistula [29, 30]. His most enduring contribution, however, was in medical education, where he taught students to appreciate the psychosocial issues in medical patients. He emphasized the importance of looking at each person as their own unique control to better understand the life setting in which the patient became ill [31, 32]. Often, individuals were found to have problems when separated from important people, which were termed 'vicarious objects', or to experience feelings of helplessness and hopelessness, all of which led Engel, Schmale and others to develop and expand the concept of conservation-withdrawal syndrome [33–37]. Although much of their work was observational, they developed interview techniques that utilized open-ended questions that became important vehicles for understanding patients. It is not by accident that the father of modern psychoneuroimmunology, Robert Ader, worked at Rochester, N.Y., and was a regular participant in Engel's seminars at the University of Rochester [38, 39]. Engel's work, however, is not without its critics. Nassir Ghaemi, in his provocative book *'The Rise and Fall of the Biopsychosocial Model'* [40] challenges Engel's biopsychosocial construct. His critique asserts that Engel did not outline a method to study the tripartite biopsychosocial elements of each individual. Such critiques have also been voiced by others who emphasize the methodological differences between the *'Erklären'* method of explanation, which denotes a more empirically based approach, versus those of *'Verstehen'*, which require empathy and understanding [41, 42]. Earlier, Schwartz [43] voiced similar critiques. A published symposium entitled *'Biopsychosocial Medicine'* also discussed the benefits and challenges of the biopsychosocial model, but in a less polemical manner [44]. Despite such criticisms, Engel's legacy endures as a clinical compass to the patient encounter [45].

Social factors have long been understood as important elements in understanding health and disease [46]. Low socioeconomic status can be a major variable in elevating the risk of infectious disease as well as other disease states, such as coronary vascular disease (and some mental disorders). Conversely, animal and human studies demonstrate that social support provides a buffer against disease states. Some investigators estimate that the lack of social support is equivalent to hypertension, smoking or obesity as a health risk factor [47]. Hinkle [48] found a clustering effect indicating that a subset of individuals within a larger population utilize more health care services, irrespective of their actual physical health status. He hypothesized that, for such individuals, the social environment was threatening or lacked support [48]. Hinkle also urged paying more attention to the individual-social system nexus in disease and health. He termed this focus upon the social environment *human ecology*. His prescient ideas on social support and cohesion were reaffirmed in a longitudinal study by his colleague, Stewart Wolf, at Cornell. Wolf, an internist, and his colleagues explored the anomalous finding of very low rates of cardiovascular disease in a small Pennsylvania town, Roseto, in comparison with neighboring towns composed of similar Italian immigrants [49]. He found that as individuals in this town moved to suburbs, the rates of cardiovascular disease rose to levels equivalent to those of their neighbors. He and his colleagues concluded that social support, solidarity and cohesion were the preeminent factors in such risk disparity [50–52]. We can see a clear line of thinking that connects the soma and psyche throughout the history of medicine and psychiatry.

Today and Tomorrow: Challenges and Opportunities

With the growth of experimental approaches in Mind-Body research, we can begin to link psychiatric syndromes to pathophysiology in other systems within the body, rather than only observing psychosomatic relationships in a clinical setting. Animal models that induce chronic stress, alter neurotrophic levels and foster changes in brain morphology have begun to explain psychosomatic phenomena [53]. This has led stress researchers to conceptualize the phenomenon of 'allostatic' load, which denotes the physiologic processes that allow an organism to maintain internal stability despite external changes [54]. This is, in essence, a sophisticated approach to Bernard's homeostasis. McEwen has developed this concept and includes stress from cognitive elements such as symbolic meanings of external events [55, 56]. Recent research suggest that secretion of cortisol is not only stimulated by the outcomes of cognitive transaction but also feeds back and contributes positively to the cognitive adaptation that is a feature of stress resilience [54]. The true 'psychosomatic loop' from CNS to periphery and back!

From a clinical perspective, consultation liaison psychiatry has been the clinical derivative of psychosomatic medicine. This subspecialty of psychiatry is currently moving from hospital-based settings to the ambulatory sector [57, 58]. Although such outpatient endeavors have been termed 'integration', this should be more accurately labeled 'collaboration'. Collaborative care models have been more successful in closed panel health care systems rather than in open fee for service systems [59, 60]. However, how to utilize psychosocial principles in both resource-rich, developed countries and in those with less robust health systems in a cost-effective and clinically meaningful manner remains to be answered.

A significant challenge in psychosomatic medicine has been whether any psychosocial interventions can really modify the course of disease once it has presented. The case in point is cardiovascular disease. The impetus for interest in psychosocial intervention in cardiovascular diseases was the observations by both Osler in 1912 and later by Meyer Friedman, which found that a type A personality, which is characterized by being ambitious, rigidly organized, sensitive, truthful, and impatient, as well as one who worries over time and work pressures and has hostile cynicism, is a risk factor for cardiovascular disease [61, 62]. Sirri et al. [63] carefully reviewed the current conceptualization of this construct [63]. In their fairly large study, they found that Type A behavior occurred in about a third of patients with cardiovascular disease, which was significantly higher than for other medical illnesses (36.1% vs. 10.8%). Interestingly, only a limited number of patients suffered from depression. There is clear data that behavioral therapy as well as medication, such as buspirone, can change elements of a type A personality, but the long-term outcomes from such interventions are not known [64–66]. As depression occurs frequently in patients with acute coronary syndrome and constitutes an independent risk factor for morbidity and mortality, several studies have been conducted to see whether treatment of depression could reduce this increased risk. The Sertraline Antidepressant Heart Randomized Trial study [67] found that sertraline was a safe and effective treatment for recurrent depression in patients with recent myocardial infarction or unstable angina, and the Enhancing Recovery in Coronary Heart Disease study [68] used cognitive behavioral therapy supplemented with a selective serotonin reuptake inhibitor, when indicated, for cardiac patients who were depressed and had low perceived social support. The intervention improved the depression symptoms and social isolation, but did not increase event-free survival. As Ziegelstein [69] wrote, based on the results of these studies, 'it is not clear whether depression treatment improves cardiac outcomes. It is also not clear whether improving depression comes first and reduced cardiac events follows or whether the depression of patients whose cardiac status improves also improves' [69]. Thus, Rafanelli et al. [70], when discussing data from a variety of similar studies, suggested that investigators were perhaps looking at the wrong variables (i.e., depression) for such outcomes and may wish to consider personality factors such as Type A characteristics. For another disease status, breast cancer, psychological interventions appear to be effective in improving survival at 12 months but not at longer-term follow-up, and these interventions are effective in reducing psychological symptoms of only some of the outcomes that were assessed in women with metastatic breast cancer [71]. Thus, questions regarding psychosocial treatments modifying disease outcomes remain to be answered.

The future of psychosomatic research is definitely promising. However, the 'black box' that connects psychosocial factors to biology is becoming less opaque. Epigenetics may explain how environmental elements, both psychological and social, relate to disease vulnerability [72]. However, molecular biological data indicate that fear and anxiety may directly promote gene activation via histone acetylation and that demethylation can modify chromatin remodeling [73, 74]. These factors can result in a variety of health outcomes that include neoplastic, autoimmune and psychiatric disorders.

Neuroscience is beginning to study the role of telomeres, which are protective caps that reflect the functional age of a chromosome. Investigators have found that chronic stress reduces telomerase length and thus, in essence, promotes functional aging and potential disease onset in stressed individuals [75, 76]. Such data may explicate allostasis in the relationships between stress and disease genesis. These findings, however, have to be translated into clinical care, and whether such biopsychosocial care should be utilized remains to be seen, given the caveats below.

Despite advances, the field of psychosomatics will encounter multiple challenges in the coming decades. There is a practical mandate to demonstrate that consultation psychiatry, whether in the collaborative-care setting or through other arrangements, can lower costs and improve quality, and our current atmosphere to control health care costs will not abate. To date, studies are not clear as to whether the psychosomatic approach can lower costs, but this approach may very well improve the quality of care.

Two significant issues must be discussed among the psychosomatic 'community': What is the effect of electronic medical records (EMRs) on a comprehensive evaluation that includes a biopsychosocial perspective; and second, how does the role of evidence-based medicine function for psychosomatic advocates, i.e., what constitutes real clinical evidence?

EMRs are increasingly being utilized in developed countries. These records promise (but do not yet fulfill) better communication between heath care providers in different systems of care that can expedite care and reduce redundancy. Research has generally found that patients and physicians positively endorse this digital record keeping, and reviews suggest that the data in EMRs have been generally accurate and consistent with reasonable physician acceptance of the use of computers for data input and review [77]. Others have questioned the accuracy of such databases for secondary analyses, which may indicate that the EMRs could have flawed data that could potentially become repeated in successive episodes of chart review [78]. This is especially important for psychiatry, whose diagnoses in general medical charts are often imprecise and do not use standard measures of outcome. The greatest challenge for EMR and biopsychosocial evaluations is the loss of the narrative. The life history of patients, with their triumphs and tragedies, is an essential feature of medicine, in general, and of psychiatry, specifically. Discrete digital data points that are inherent in the EMR may loosen the woven fabric of the individual's biography and miss important elements [79]. Psychiatrists at Johns Hopkins University are some of the few who have challenged the EMR on this basis [80]. One of the essential features of the patient's biography is the acceptance of the person as a unique human being with subjective reactions to life events, and an EMR may catalogue events but cannot confidently give meaning to them. Psychosomatic evaluations will have to be more than a digital record of such data points. As Fava [81] suggests, clinical judgments are essential for patient care, and such judgments must include a coherent life history.

An additional challenge encountering the use of EMRs is the existence of numerous EMR systems and the lack of if not impossibility of communication among EMR systems. In addition, psychiatric EMRs are, at times, required to be separate from the rest of EMRs within one health care system for confidentiality reasons. Thus, many important pieces of information may get lost due to the lack of communication between various EMR systems.

The second great challenge to psychosomatic medicine as well as to the biopsychosocial model is the demand to utilize evidence-based medicine, whose 'gold standard' is the randomized controlled trial (RTC). Certainly medicine must be evidence-based rather than based on art- or theory-based deductive methods, such as astrology, whose general premise lacks validity. Gupta [82] and Gupta and Upshur [83], however, have cogently questioned the role of evidence-based medicine in psychiatric practice. They review two basic issues that may limit generalization of the role of RTCs in producing evidence. First are the limits of many RTCs, which utilize patients whose diagnoses are not the same as those in clinical practice. Thus, the therapeutic efficacy of treatments in such trials, frequently pharmacological treatments, cannot easily be generalized to 'real world' practice. In other terms, we have a good number of so-called efficacy trials, but a lesser number of effectiveness trials that are closer to clinical reality. Second, it has been noted that psychiatric practice is often dependent upon the narrative of the patient and on the 'meaningfulness of personal experience', which are rarely considered reliable enough to measure. Therefore, in many RTCs, the results are statistically significant but not clinically meaningful. The RTCs in psychiatry also use outcome measures, which are too complex or too plentiful. The complexity of these outcome measures, coupled with a lack of consensus on their use, suggest that it is the researchers who primarily benefit from using them, and not the clinicians or the public [84]. In psychiatry and in psychosomatics, it is time to bring mortality, health care utilization, functioning, quality of life and other simple and meaningful measures back into treatment trials of mental illness. These issues create obstacles for psychosomatic approaches to patient care, which brings us back to Osler's requirement of knowing the patient as well as what disease(s) they have. The offset to these problems is that EMRs and evidence-based approaches help in research, which could give clinicians the data to require a psychosomatic approach.

In conclusion, psychosomatic medicine has a proud past but an exciting future that will begin to 'document' the importance of psychosocial factors in clinical assessments. The historic role of clinical observation has generated hypotheses that can guide experimental approaches to integrate biopsychosocial constructs; however, no rigorous, 'evidence-based' study can now ignore psychosocial variables [82, 83]. A truly psychosomatic approach will help us elucidate the questions raised in our current unitary approaches that ignore the biopsychosocial approach to disease genesis and treatment [85].

References

1 Steinberg H, Herrmann-Lingen C, Himmerich H: Johann Christian August Heinroth: psychosomatic medicine eighty years before Freud. Psychiatr Danub 2013;25:11–16.
2 Ackerknecht EH: The history of psychosomatic medicine. Psychol Med 1982;12: 17–24.
3 Rothman KJ, Greenland S: Causation and causal inference in epidemiology. Am J Public Health 2005;95(suppl 1): S144–S150.
4 Balint M: The crisis of medical practice. Am J Psychoanal 2002;62:7–15.
5 Schuffel W: Continuing friendship in the face of European destruction and European construction: the European conference on psychosomatic research. Psychother Psychosom 2013;82:273–278.
6 Sperling M: Psychosomatic Disorders in Childhood. New York, Jason Aronson, 1977.
7 Schur M: Comments on the metapsychology of somatization. Psychoanalytic Study of the Child 1955;10:119–164.
8 Alexander F: The development of psychosomatic medicine. Psychosom Med 1962;24:13–24.
9 Balint M: The doctor, his patient, and the illness. Lancet 1955;268:683–688.
10 Mirsky IA: Physiologic, psychologic, and social determinants in the etiology of duodenal ulcer. Am J Dig Dis 1958;3: 285–314.
11 Mirsky IA: Physiologic, psychologic and social determinants of psychosomatic disorders. Dis Nerv Syst 1960;21(suppl): 50–56.

12 Levenstein S: Helicobacter pylori and ulcers. Against reductionism. BMJ 2009; 339:b3855.
13 Cannon WB: Voodoo death. Psychosom Med 1957;19:182–190.
14 Samuels MA: Voodood death revisited: The modern lesson of neurocardiology. Cleve Clin J Med 2007;74(suppl 1):S8–S16
15 Lester D: Voodoo death. Omega (Westport) 2009;59:1–18.
16 Weiner H: The dynamics of the organism: implications of recent biological thought for psychosomatic theory and research. Psychosom Med 1989;51:608–635.
17 Weiner H: Praise be to psychosomatic medicine. Psychosom Med 1999;61: 259–262.
18 Grinker RR: Psychiatry rides madly in all directions. Arch Gen Psychiatry 1964; 10:228–237.
19 Griffith W: Convulsions during delirium ebriosum. Prov Med J Retrosp Med Sci 1843;5:428.
20 Bonhoffer K: Exogenous psychoses; in Sheperd M, Hirsch S (eds): Themes and Variations in European Psychiatry. Charlottesville, University of Virginia, 1974, pp 47–52.
21 Victor M: 33. The pathophysiology of alcoholic epilepsy. Res Publ Assoc Res Nerv Ment Dis 1968;46:431–454.
22 Lipowski ZJ: Delirium: how its concept has developed. Int Psychogeriatr 1991;3: 115–120.
23 Lipowski ZJ: Organic mental disorders and DSM-IV. Am J Psychiatry 1990;147: 947.
24 Lipowski ZJ: Update on delirium. Psychiatr Clin North Am 1992;15:335–346.
25 Engel GL: How much longer must medicine's science be bound by a seventeenth century world view? Psychother Psychosom 1992;57:3–16.
26 Engel GL: Physician-scientists and scientific physicians. Resolving the humanism-science dichotomy. Am J Med 1987; 82:107–111.
27 Engel GL: The need for a new medical model: a challenge for biomedicine. Science 1977;196:129–136.
28 Engel GL, Romano J: Delirium, a syndrome of cerebral insufficiency. 1959. J Neuropsychiatry Clin Neurosci 2004;16: 526–538.
29 Engel GL, Frader M, Barry C, Morrow G: Sadness evoked by a film on grief: an experimental study. Int J Psychiatry Med 1984;14:1–30.
30 Reichsman F, Engel GL, Harway V, Escalona S: Monica, an infant with gastric fistula and depression; an interim report on her development to the age four years. Psychiatr Res Rep Am Psychiatr Assoc 1957;135:12–27.
31 Engel GL: Sounding board. The biopsychosocial model and medical education. Who are to be the teachers? N Engl J Med 1982;306:802–805.
32 Reichsman F: Teaching psychosomatic medicine to medical students, residents and postgraduate fellows. Int J Psychiatry Med 1975;6:307–316.
33 Greene WA Jr: Role of a vicarious object in the adaptation to object loss. II. Vicissitudes in the role of the vicarious object. Psychosom Med 1959;21:438–447.
34 Greene WA Jr: Role of a vicarious object in the adaptation to object loss. I. Use of a vicarious object as a means of adjustment to separation from a significant person. Psychosom Med 1958;20:344–350.
35 Schmale AH: Giving up as a final common pathway to changes in health. Adv Psychosom Med 1972;8:20–40.
36 Engel GL: A life setting conducive to illness. The giving-up-given-up complex. Bull Menninger Clin 1968;32:355–365.
37 Schmale AH, Iker H: Hopelessness as a predictor of cervical cancer. Soc Sci Med 1971;5:95–100.
38 Ader R: Psychoneuroimmunology. ILAR J 1998;39:27–29.
39 Ader R: Conditioned immunomodulation: research needs and directions. Brain Behav Immun 2003;17(suppl 1): S51–S57.
40 Ghaemi SN: The Rise and Fall of the Biopsychosocial Model. Baltimore, Johns Hopkins, 2010.
41 Garnar A, Hardcastle VG: Neurobiological model, an unnecessary divide-neural models in psychiatry; in Radden J (ed): The Philosophy of Psychiatry. International Perspectives on Philosophy and Psychiatry. New York, New York, Oxford University Press, 2004, pp 366–380.
42 Schwartz M, Wiggins O: Phenomenological: hermeneutics, understanding and interpretation in psychiatry; in Radden J (ed): The Philosophy of Psychiatry. International Perspectives on Philosophy and Psychiatry. New York, New York, Oxford University Press, 2004, pp 351–363.
43 Schwartz MA, Wiggins OP: Systems and the structuring of meaning: contributions to a biopsychosocial medicine. Am J Psychiatry 1986;143:1213–1221.
44 White P (ed): Biopsychosocial Medicine. An Integrated Approach to Understanding Illness. Oxford, United Kingdom, Oxford University, 2005.
45 Novack DH, Cameron O, Epel E, Ader R, Waldstein SR, Levenstein S, Antoni MH, Wainer AR: Psychosomatic medicine: the scientific foundation of the biopsychosocial model. Acad Psychiatry 2007; 31:388–401.
46 Eisenberger NI: Social ties and health: a social neuroscience perspective. Curr Opin Neurobiol 2013;23:407–413.
47 Eisenberger NI: An empirical review of the neural underpinnings of receiving and giving social support: implications for health. Psychosom Med 2013;75: 545–556.
48 Hinkle LE Jr: Human ecology and psychosomatic medicine. Psychosom Med 1967;29:391–395.
49 Wolf S: Mortality from myocardial infarction in Roseto. JAMA 1966;195:186.
50 Egolf B, Lasker J, Wolf S, Potvin L: The Roseto effect: a 50-year comparison of mortality rates. Am J Public Health 1992;82:1089–1092.
51 Lasker JN, Egolf BP, Wolf S: Community social change and mortality. Soc Sci Med 1994;39:53–62.
52 Wolf S, Herrenkohl RC, Lasker J, Egolf B, Philips BU, Bruhn JG: Roseto, Pennsylvania 25 years later – highlights of a medical and sociological survey. Trans Am Clin Climatol Assoc 1989;100:57–67.
53 Iio W, Matsukawa N, Tsukahara T, Kohari D, Toyoda A: Effects of chronic social defeat stress on MAP kinase cascade. Neurosci Lett 2011;504:281–284.
54 McVicar A, Ravalier JM, Greenwood C: Biology of stress revisited: intracellular mechanisms and the conceptualization of stress. Stress Health 2014;30:272–279.
55 Karatsoreos IN, McEwen BS: Psychobiological allostasis: resistance, resilience and vulnerability. Trends Cogn Sci 2011; 15:576–584.
56 Puterman E, Epel E: An intricate dance: Life experience, multisystem resiliency, and rate of telomere decline throughout the lifespan. Soc Personal Psychol Compass 2012;6:807–825.

57 Vickers KS, Ridgeway JL, Hathaway JC, Egginton JS, Kaderlik AB, Katzelnick DJ: Integration of mental health resources in a primary care setting leads to increased provider satisfaction and patient access. Gen Hosp Psychiatry 2013;35:461–467.
58 Kupfer DJ, Kuhl EA, Wulsin L: Psychiatry's integration with medicine: the role of DSM-5. Annu Rev Med 2013;64:385–392.
59 Walker S, Walker J, Richardson G, Palmer S, Wu Q, Gilbody S, Martin P, Hansen CH, Sawhney A, Murray G, Sculpher M, Sharpe M: Cost-effectiveness of combining systematic identification and treatment of co-morbid major depression for people with chronic diseases: the example of cancer. Psychol Med 2014;44:1451–1460.
60 Archer J, Bower P, Gilbody S, Lovell K, Richards D, Gask L, Dickens C, Coventry P: Collaborative care for depression and anxiety problems. Cochrane Database Syst Rev 2012;10:CD006525.
61 Osler W: An address on high blood pressure. BMJ 1912;2:1–12.
62 Weisse AB, Friedland GW: Meyer Friedman. Clin Cardiol 2004;27:308–309.
63 Sirri L, Fava GA, Guidi J, Porcelli P, Rafanelli C, Bellomo A, Grandi S, Grassi L, Pasquini P, Picardi A, Quartesan R, Rigatelli M, Sonino N: Type A behaviour: a reappraisal of its characteristics in cardiovascular disease. Int J Clin Pract 2012;66:854–861.
64 Fava M, Littman A, Halperin P, Pratt E, Drews FR, Oleshansky M, Knapik J, Thompson C, Bielenda C: Psychological and behavioral benefits of a stress/type A behavior reduction program for healthy middle-aged army officers. Psychosomatics 1991;32:337–342.
65 Littman AB, Fava M, Halperin P, Lamon-Fava S, Drews FR, Oleshansky MA, Bielenda CC, MacLaughlin RA: Physiologic benefits of a stress reduction program for healthy middle-aged Army officers. J Psychosom Res 1993;37:345–354.
66 Littman AB, Fava M, McKool K, Lamon-Fava S, Pegg E: Buspirone therapy for Type A behavior, hostility, and perceived stress in cardiac patients. Psychother Psychosom 1993;59:107–110.
67 Glassman AH, O'Connor CM, Califf RM, Swedberg K, Schwartz P, Bigger JT Jr, Krishnan KR, va Zyl LT, Swenson JR, Finkel MS, Landau C, Shapiro PA, Pepine CJ, Mardekian J, Harrison WM, Barton D, McIvor M; Sertraline Antidepressant Heart Randomized Trial (SADHEART) Group: Sertraline treatment of major depression in patients with acute MI or unstable angina. JAMA 2001;288:701–709.
68 Berkman LF, Blumenthal J, Burg M, Carney RM, Catellier D, Cowan MJ, Czajkowski SM, DeBusk R, Hisking J, Jaffe A, Kaufman PG, Mitchell P, Norman J, Powell LH, Raczynski JM, Schneiderman N; Enhancing Recovery in Coronary Heart Disease Patient Investigators (EMRICHD): Effects of treating depression and low perceived social support on clinical events after myocardial infarction: the Enhancing Recovery in Coronary Heart Disease Patients (ENRICHD) randomized trial. JAMA 2003;298:3106–3116.
69 Ziegelstein RC: Improving depression and reducing cardiac events: which is the chicken and which is the egg? J Psychosom Res 2013;74:454–457.
70 Rafanelli C, Sirri L, Grandi S, Fava GA: Is depression the wrong treatment target for improving outcome in coronary artery disease? Psychother Psychosom 2013;82:285–291.
71 Mustafa M, Carson-Stevens A, Gillespie D, Edwards AG: Psychological interventions for women with metastatic breast cancer. Cochrane Database Syst Rev 2013;6:CD004253.
72 Karatsoreos IN, McEwen BS: Annual research review: the neurobiology and physiology of resilience and adaptation across the life course. J Child Psychol Psychiatry 2013;54:337–347.
73 Wong CC, Caspi A, Williams B, Craig IW, Houts R, Ambler A, Moffitt TE, Mill J: A longitudinal study of epigenetic variation in twins. Epigenetics 2010;5:516–526.
74 Stahl SM: Epigenetics and methylomics in psychiatry. J Clin Psychiatry 2009;70:1204–1205.
75 Wolkowitz OM, Mellon SH, Epel ES, Lin J, Dhabhar FS, Su Y, Reus VI, Rosser R, Burke HM, Kupferman E, Compagnone M, Nelson JC, Blackburn EH: Leukocyte telomere length in major depression: correlations with chronicity, inflammation and oxidative stress – preliminary findings. PLoS One 2011;6:e17837.
76 Epel ES, Lin J, Dhabhar FS, Wolkowitz OM, Puterman E, Karan L, Blackburn EH: Dynamics of telomerase activity in response to acute psychological stress. Brain Behav Immun 2010;24:531–539.
77 Hayrinen K, Saranto K, Nykanen P: Definition, structure, content, use and impacts of electronic health records: a review of the research literature. Int J Med Inform 2008;77:291–304.
78 Botsis T, Hartvigsen G, Chen F, Weng C: Secondary use of EHR: data quality issues and informatics opportunities. AMIA Jt Summits Transl Sci Proc 2010; 2010:1–5.
79 Treisman GJ, McHugh PS: Life story as the focus of psychotherapy: the Johns Hopkins conceptual and didactic perspectives; in Alarcon RD, Frank JB (eds): The Psychotherapy of Hope. The Legacy of Persuasion and Healing. Baltimore, Johns Hopkins, 2012, pp 22–33.
80 Safeguarding 'the Phipps History' patient examination. Hopkins Brain Wise, 2013;Summer:3.
81 Fava GA: Clinical judgment in psychiatry. Requiem or reveille? Nord J Psychiatry 2013;67:1–10.
82 Gupta M: Does evidence-based medicine apply to psychiatry? Theor Med Bioeth 2007;28:103–120.
83 Gupta M, Upshur R: Critical thinking in clinical medicine: what is it? J Eval Clin Pract 2012;18:938–944.
84 Arfken CL, Balon R: Another look at outcomes and outcome measures in psychiatry: cui bono? Psychother Psycosom 2014;83:6–9.
85 Fava GA, Sonino N: Psychosomatic medicine. Int J Clin Pract 2010;64:1155–1161.

Thomas N. Wise, MD
Department of Psychiatry, Inova Fairfax Hospital
3300 Gallows Rd.
Falls Church, VA 22042 (USA)
E-Mail Thomas.Wise@inova.org

Balon R, Wise TN (eds): Clinical Challenges in the Biopsychosocial Interface. Update on Psychosomatics for the 21st Century. Adv Psychosom Med. Basel, Karger, 2015, vol 34, pp 10–23 (DOI: 10.1159/000369050)

Communication with Patients Suffering from Serious Physical Illness

Luigi Grassi[a, b] • Rosangela Caruso[a] • Anna Costantini[c]

[a]Institute of Psychiatry, Department of Biomedical and Specialty Surgical Sciences, School of Medicine, University of Ferrara, Ferrara, [b]University Hospital Psychiatry Unit, Psycho-Oncology and Psychiatry in Palliative Care Program, Integrated Department of Mental Health, University S. Anna Hospital and Local Health Authorities, Ferrara, [c]Psycho-Oncology Departmental Unit, Sant'Andrea Hospital, Faculty of Medicine and Psychology, La Sapienza University of Rome, Rome, Italy

Abstract

Communication is the corner stone of the relationship with the patient in all medical settings with the main aims of creating a good inter-personal relationship, exchanging information, and making treatment-related decisions. In a rapidly changing cultural and social context, the paternalistic approach of doctors knowing the best and deciding what should be done for a patient has been replaced by a shared decision-making approach, with patients being advised to educate themselves, ask questions and influence the course of the discussion with their doctors. Thus, a need for an improvement in the communication skills of physicians is extremely important for patients affected by serious physical illness (e.g. cancer, HIV infection, multiple sclerosis, amyotrophic lateral sclerosis). Certain attitudes, behaviour and skills (e.g. capacity to impart confidence, being empathetic, providing a 'human touch', relating on a personal level, being forthright, being respectful, and being thorough) are part of effective communication. However, some specific aspects influencing doctor-patient communication and relationships, such as personality variables, coping and attachment styles, as well as cultural factors, should also be taken in to account. The development of training curricula to help doctors acquire proper skills in communication is mandatory, since research has shown that training in communication may facilitate the effectiveness of a doctor-patient relationship and the patient's satisfaction with care and give a general sense of humanity, which is easily lost in a biotechnologically oriented medicine.

Introduction

Communication is the corner stone of the relationship with the patient in all medical settings with the main aims of creating a good inter-personal relationship, exchanging information, and making treatment-related decisions [1]. Communication is in fact the most important component of good medical practice and of patient-centred care, which has been defined as 'a moral philosophy, which values considering patients' needs, wants and perspectives, offers patients opportunities to provide input into and participate in their care, and enhances partnership and understanding in the doctor-patient relationship' [2]. As some authors have underlined, in a rapidly changing cultural and social context, the paternalistic approach of doctors knowing best and deciding what should be done for a patient has been replaced by a shared decision-making approach, with patients being advised to educate themselves, ask questions and influence the course of the discussion with their doctors [3].

This change clearly stresses the need for an improvement in the communication skills of physicians, making the centrality of communication even more poignant. This area has been particularly studied for patients affected by serious physical illness (e.g. cancer, HIV infection, multiple sclerosis, amyotrophic lateral sclerosis), with accumulating data showing how the development of curricula to help doctors acquire proper communication skills may facilitate the effectiveness of their relationship with their patients and the patient's satisfaction with care as well as a general sense of humanity, which is easily lost in biotechnologically oriented medicine.

However, the literature over the last 30 years has shown that doctor-patient relationships are often poor or incomplete and extremely technical, with a marked split between 'curing' (as a technical action dealing with the physical disease as an object in a material body – *Körper*) and 'caring' (as a holistic process dealing with the person as a subject in a lived body – *Leib*) [4]. It is a fact that new paradigms in medicine (e.g. holistic, humanistic, narrative and narrative-evidence-based medicine, medical cosmology, and patient-centred medicine) have been repeatedly proposed as a way to combat modern biotechnological reductionism and to put the person, in all her dimensions, at the centre of the therapeutic encounter [5]. Textbooks, guidelines and a huge body of psychosocial literature currently exist on the topic of communication. In this chapter, we will discuss some of the main aspects of communication for patients affected by serious illness, including cancer and palliative care settings, as well as the essential role of training to improve communication in medical settings.

The Problem of Communication with Physically Ill Patients

Patients affected by physical illness, particularly life-threatening and/or chronic illnesses, have significant needs that should be part of a doctor-patient communication interchange. Among those needs are non-medical symptomatic areas, specifically interpersonal, psychological and/or spiritual needs, that are often unmet in medical settings [6]. In a study of patients in advanced stages of medical disease, Moadel et al. [7] showed that a number of needs were reported, including being helped with overcoming their fears (51%), finding hope (42%), finding meaning in life (40%), finding spiritual resources (39%), or finding someone to talk to about finding peace of mind (43%). Likewise, Chochinov et al. [8] found that a very high percentage of patients, also in an advanced stage of illness, presented spiritual and interpersonal problems that needed to be taken into account, such as the feeling of being a burden to others (87.1%), feeling of not making a meaningful and/or lasting contribution in one's own life (83.7%), and not feeling worthwhile or valued (81.4%). Thus, health care professionals (HCPs) should be aware that good communication is an essential ingredient for providing the best quality of health care and that they have a special responsibility of responding to each patient's needs as a way to improve his/her experience and increase satisfaction with health care [9].

Besides spiritual and existential needs, a huge amount of psychosocial literature in medicine has indicated that at least 30–40% of patients with serious medical illness present symptoms of emotional distress, with anxiety, depression, dis-

Table 1. Some possible barriers to doctor-patient communication (adapted and modified from [19])

Barriers due to patients and families
Alignment to the cultural tendency of expecting to speak about physical rather than psychological issues.
Feeling that one's own emotional problems are not interesting or not important in medical settings.
Misunderstanding of illness, treatment options and prognosis.
Possible stigma (e.g. shame in not being able to react, fear of being criticised as not strong enough)
Lack of support; lack of coping mechanisms.
Physical and emotional depletion.
Fear of losing control if emotions are expressed.
Barriers due to health care providers
Perception that curing is not caring and that the role of the doctor is to cure the body and the disease, not the mind.
Perception that there is a lack of time and that the job is overwhelming.
Fear of giving wrong answers, of not being able to answer difficult questions, or of not being able to sustain a difficult conversation.
Fear of being enmeshed with a psychological discussion and being overwhelmed by emotions.
Personal experiences of illness and death.
Physical, emotional and psychological stress and depletion.
Lack of training and poor role models.
Fears of appearing weak or unprofessional when displaying emotions.

orders secondary to stress (stress-related and adjustment disorders), and other psychosocial conditions reported to affect medically ill patients (e.g. demoralisation, health anxiety), irrespective of the disease and the medical setting (inpatient, outpatient, day-hospital services) [10–12].

A specific issue with this is that, although a physician's ability to treat physical and stress symptoms has improved much over the last years, the knowledge base and skill set that is necessary to recognise, assess, and compassionately address the psychosocial, existential, and spiritual aspects of serious physical illness still remains less developed in medical settings. This lack of knowledge and skill has occurred for several reasons, as discussed in the next paragraph.

Barriers to Communication in Medical Settings

Many common communication challenges should be dealt with by doctors when relating with patients affected by serious physical illnesses, including breaking bad news when making the diagnosis, bad test results, recurrence or worsening of the disease, information about prognosis, discussing treatment failure, and transition from curative to palliative care. However, several barriers and obstacles to the doctor-patient relationship have been described and have shown how these obstacles can undermine communication and the recognition of psychosocial problems and existential issues in medical settings.

As reported in table 1, these barriers can be both related to the patient and his/her way of dealing with the illness and to the physician and his/her way of dealing with his/her patient [13, 14]. In palliative settings, where the prognosis is a specific communication challenge, the literature indicates that HCPs report discomfort at having to bring up the topic of life expectancy and prognosis, with the tendency to withhold information or not disclose prognosis. In these cases, reasons for this discomfort include perceived lack of training, stress, no time to attend to the patient's emotional needs, fear of a negative impact on the patient, uncertainty about prognostication, requests from family members to withhold information and a feeling of inadequacy or hopelessness regarding the unavailability of further curative treatment [15]. In other cases, physicians may find it uncomfortable to delve into a patient's feelings (e.g. depression and suicidal ideation among cancer patients) or behaviour (e.g. sexual history of patients with HIV infection) because they are concerned about intrusion or about the idea that emotional symptoms, once elicited, would be too difficult to manage. As a reaction, it may be tempting, for instance, to adopt a paternalistic attitude by avoiding discussions with an emotional focus, offering inappropriately early reassurance, using ambiguous terms, or giving in to the temptation of communicating false hope. In other cases, patients may evoke in clinicians frustrating emotions, such as sadness, anger, boredom and sense of failure. For these reasons, knowledge of the most important components of effective communication and of ways to develop interpersonal doctor-patient relationships are the most important issues to be addressed in medical settings.

Characteristics of Effective Communication

The fact that patients and their caregivers prefer a trusted health professional who shows empathy and honesty, encourages questions, and clarifies an individual's information needs and level of understanding has been repeatedly reported [16], and this fact should guide physicians in moulding their attitude and behaviour within a honest communication framework. In fact, patients usually prefer to have interested, empathic and available doctors rather than non-interested, cold, and highly technical doctors. Data from palliative care literature also show that patients prefer honesty from their professional team, with benefits associated with realistic awareness including enhanced control and end-of-life planning, which have been seen to engender hope. It has been indicated that for some patients, hope and realism are irreconcilable when presented with detailed or unequivocal information, underlying the need for professionals to respect the specific needs of their patients, including the maintenance of some ambiguity about the future, if that is a patient's wish [17]. However, a recent, large, population-based, cross-national telephone survey in seven European countries, including Italy, showed that among 9,344 healthy subjects, 73.9% of respondents endorsed the view of always being informed when in the scenario of having a serious illness with less than 1 year to live [18].

As confirmation, studies have shown that some specific attitudes and behaviours of the physician are preferred and reinforce hope; in contrast, other attitudes and behaviours have been reported to increase the sense of abandonment and hopelessness in patients with serious medical illness. The former includes the tendency to establish eye contact at the beginning of the consultation and maintain it at reasonable intervals, to show interest by using 'active listening' and open questions, to focus attention on the person and ask about psychosocial and existential needs, to discuss treatment options, and to give support. The latter includes the tendency to attend to only the physical aspects of the disease, to offer advice and reassurance before the main problems have been identified, to switch topics, to use medical jargon and to be technical and detached [19, 20]. A main series of ingredients, which are considered the key communication skills in medicine, especially for physicians working with patients affected by serious illnesses, such as cancer, have been reported [21]. These factors that should be part of every medical encounter, include the capacity to impart confidence (e.g. greeting the patient with warmth, making eye contact, encouraging patient queries), being empathetic (e.g. eliciting a patient's concerns, acknowledging distress, and recognising and being sensitive to emotions), providing a 'human touch' (e.g. using appropriate physical contact, being attentive and present to the patient and the situation, showing interest and compassion), relating on a personal level (e.g. asking the patient about his/her life, acknowledging a pa-

Table 2. Communication issues that improve the dignity of patients affected by serious physical illness (adapted from [19])

A = Attitude, that is, the physicians' examinations of their own attitudes and assumptions towards patients, including asking questions about themselves (e.g. How would I be feeling in this patient's situation? Could my attitude towards the patient be based on my own experiences, anxieties, or fears?).
B = Behaviour, acknowledging that certain communication behaviours (e.g. contact, respect, seating at a comfortable distance for conversation, at the patient's eye level when possible, and small acts of kindness, like getting the patient a glass of water) enhance the trust and connection between patients and their healthcare providers.
C = Compassion, referring to a deep awareness of the suffering of another, coupled with the wish to relieve it, can be conveyed by any form of communication – spoken or unspoken – that shows some recognition of the human stories that accompany illness.
D = Dialogue, as a critical element of dignity-conserving care, must acknowledge personhood beyond the illness itself and recognise the emotional impact that accompanies illness. It should also be used to acquaint the healthcare provider with aspects of the patient's life that must be known to provide the best care possible.

tient's family, and remembering details about the patient's life from visit to visit), being forthright (e.g. being honest and not withholding information, asking the patient to recap the conversation to ensure understanding), being respectful (e.g. listening carefully and not interrupting, taking care of the dignity of the patient), and being thorough (e.g. providing detailed explanations, giving instructions in writing, following up in a timely manner). These elements are the main tools that, by favouring the promotion of reciprocal trust and consolidating therapeutic alliance, allow the achievement of early detection and treatment of possible psychosocial problems and foster shared decision making, particularly in difficult consultations [22]. This, in turn, improves the quality of care and enhances the well-being and satisfaction of both the physicians, as human beings and professionals, and of their patients [23]. From a similar perspective, Chochinov [24, 25], by stressing the notion that, in medicine, a main role of the physician, besides curing, is caring in the sense of preserving the dignity of their patients, has proposed an easily remembered core framework of dignity conserving care, expressed as A, B, C, and D, that can guide physicians to better relate and communicate with their patients (table 2).

Specific Aspects Influencing Doctor-Patient Communication and Relationships

Other significant elements should be taken into account by a physician when communicating with patients, specifically, the patients' personality and coping repertoire, attachment styles and cultural variables.

Personality and Coping Styles
The first specific issue regards the *personality characteristics* of the patient and her way of coping with stressful events *(coping styles).* For example, Steptoe et al. [26] showed that some patients need to know all of the details about their situation, as a way of coping with the event ('monitors'), while others tend to adopt an avoidant style by passing the management of their own situation to family members or supportive figures ('blunters'). Sardell and Trierweiler [27] have shown that patients with fighting coping styles tend to perceive communication that centres on how to deal with the situation as hopeful, while patients with fatalistic or stoic coping tend to regard a paternalistic communication style that is based on physician-centred decision-making as more hopeful. These aspects should be taken into account, and communication should be adapted

Table 3. Coping styles, defence mechanisms and attachment styles that can be problematic in doctor-patient communication (adapted from [68])

Maladaptive coping

Hopelessness: the tendency to give up and to feel at a loss about one's own physical disease, with the inability to react and to return to life.

Anxious preoccupation: the tendency to be extremely worried about one's own illness and its implications, allowing the disease to dominate life; attention-focused on the body.

Defence mechanisms

Neurotic defences

- Conversion: expression of unacknowledged emotional distress in the guise of a physical symptom.
- Control: tendency to control the environment to avoid or reduce anxiety, loss of control causes anxiety.

Immature defences

- Passive aggression: indirect and passive expression of anger.
- Acting out: direct expression of impulse or wish.
- Projection: attribution of unacceptable impulse or ideas to others.
- Devaluation: depreciation of others.
- Denial: refusal to acknowledge painful relatives.

Psychotic defences

- (Pathological) Denial: refusal to confront reality (e.g. cancer that is completely obliterated).
- (Delusional) Projection: externalisation of conflicts and distress in reality (reality testing is minimal or absent).

Attachment styles

Preoccupied attachment: dependency; amplified expressiveness and need to maintain emotional and physical closeness to attachment figures (e.g. family members, health care staff); sense of personal fragility and hypervigilance for threat caused by cancer; high levels of perceived stress.

Dismissing attachment: proximity seeking is reduced; attachment figures are considered unimportant; signs of personal vulnerability or distress are suppressed, with symptoms minimised or reported too late; possible interference with collaboration with health care staff (e.g. mistrust or impatience with professionals).

Fearful attachment: high attachment anxiety (characteristic of the preoccupied pattern) and high attachment avoidance (characteristic of the dismissing pattern), with an untenable combination of distress and avoidance of medical help; ambivalence towards health care staff.

accordingly. In fact, coping, as the pattern of thoughts, beliefs and behaviours in response to stressful events, may not only influence communication but also adjustment to illness, with data showing that certain styles of coping are dysfunctional and associated with maladaptive psychological responses. Furthermore, in advanced phases of medical illness, the needs and wishes of the patient may change over time, and physicians should be sensitive to adapting to these needs, rather than following their own agenda [28].

Defence mechanisms, such as automatic, intrapsychic psychological processes by which the mind deals with psychological threats or conflicts between wishes and reality, can also inform the physician about that particular patient, explaining his/her emotional and behavioural response to the disease (table 3).

Attachment Styles

A second issue that has attracted attention in medical settings is the *attachment style,* which is how relations between a patient and caregiving figures in the past relates to the current view of herself and to the expectation she has from the health care provider (or health care system). Maunder and Hunter [29, 30] have described, in medical settings, four possible patterns of attachment that are related to both health care relationships and communication as well as to the patient's illness behaviour and health outcomes, namely secure, preoccupied, dismissing and fearful patterns [31] (table 3). Tan et al. [32] have described the importance of attachment processes as critically important determinants of therapeutic relationships in the setting of palliative care, particularly when the aims of the clinicians are to improve the quality of life of the patients and to address the suffering that encompasses the physical, psychosocial and spiritual realms of the individuals' and families' experiences with terminal illness.

Cultural Issues

Another important issue regarding communication in medical settings is the need to acknowledge the patient's culture. In fact, culture moulds the patients' and communities' trust in HCPs and institutions, their views on human experimentation, as well as the cognitive, emotional and behavioural responses to the disease. A patient's attitudes towards the concepts of illness and suffering, decisions about treatment, and the whole of care are in fact framed by cultural factors. For example, as Surbone [33] states, cultural perceptions and reactions to cancer, suffering and dying, are different in the health care systems of different cultures, and these differences, in turn, influence the provision and effectiveness of care. For these reasons, data have accumulated regarding the specific role of cultural competence as a set of congruent behaviours, attitudes, and policies among professionals and in a system or agency that enables effective work in cross-cultural situations [34, 35]. Thus, both knowledge of the different cultural values and having compassion and cultural sensitivity are extremely important in the communication process when relating to patients affected by serious medical illnesses. For example, in cancer settings, the role of cultural factors in influencing coping has emerged as an important issue, with data showing that psychosocial concerns related to worry about children and burdening the family, body image and sexual health concerns, beliefs about illness, gender role, family obligations (e.g. self-sacrifice), as well as language barriers among breast cancer survivors of different backgrounds (i.e., African American, Asian American, Latina, and Caucasian) were significantly different among the different cultural groups [36]. In another study, immigrant Chinese breast cancer survivors expressed symptoms in a culturally unique way (e.g. hot-cold imbalances) and were also at higher risk for emotional distress compared with US-born Chinese and non-Hispanic breast cancer survivors because of cultural norms that influence the tendency to express one's own needs to physicians or to challenge physicians when one's own needs are not met [37].

All these data confirm the need for cultural sensitivity and competence of both HCPs and, in general, of the whole health system. According to Anderson et al. [38], a culturally competent healthcare setting should include a culturally diverse staff that reflects the communities served, health care providers or translators who speak the patients' languages, training for providers on the culture and language of the people they serve, signage and instructional literature in the patients' languages that are consistent with their cultural norms, and culturally specific health care settings. Therefore, interventions to improve cultural competence in health care systems, such as programmes to recruit and retain staff members who reflect the cultural diversity of the community served, use of interpreter services or bilingual providers, cultural competency training for healthcare providers, use of linguistically and culturally appropriate health education materials, and culturally specific healthcare settings (e.g. neighbourhood clinics for immigrant populations), are necessary (table 4) [39].

Training in Communication

From the immense number of studies that have been collected over the last years, it is clear that professional communication is a skill that, like

Table 4. The SPIKES protocol as a model to improve communication (adapted from [48])

SPIKES protocol
1. Step 1 **S** = Setting up the interview (arrange for some privacy, involve significant others, sit down, make a connection with the patient, manage time constraints and interruptions).
2. Step 2 **P** = Assessing patient's Perception (before you tell, ask thorough, open-ended questions to create a reasonably accurate picture of how the patient perceives the medical situation – what it is and whether it is serious or not).
3. Step 3 **I** = Obtaining the patient's Invitation (determine the way in which the patient wants to receive the information, e.g. a global picture or the details).
4. Step 4 **K** = Giving Knowledge and information (give the information by starting at the level of comprehension and vocabulary of the patient: try to use non-technical words, avoid excessive bluntness, give information in small chunks, and periodically check the patient's understanding).
5. Step 5 **E** = Addressing the patient's Emotions (look for any emotion on the part of the patient; identify the emotion experienced by the patient by naming it to oneself; identify the reason for the emotion; let the patient know that you have connected the emotion with the reason for the emotion by making a connecting statement).
6. Step 6 **S** = Strategy and Summary (ask patients if they are ready at that time for such a discussion; share the responsibility for decision-making with the patient; check for misunderstanding of the discussion by the patient).

any skill, can and must be learned, since being a nice person does not automatically correspond to good and effective communication with patients suffering from medical illness and their families. For these reasons, guidelines for improving doctor-patient communication within the realm of serious diseases, such as cancer, chronic kidney disease, haematology, neurology and palliative care, have been developed and proposed for application in specific training curricula courses. Specific communication skills training (CST) courses have been applied, with interesting results, across the several medical disciplines and have included physicians [40–42] as well as residents and medical students [43].

The objectives of CST courses are usually to develop the main components of effective communication when dealing with seriously ill patients and their families. For example, these components could include demonstrating empathy and caring using verbal and non-verbal language, being able to break bad news, listening and responding to the needs (informational and emotional) of patients and their families, honestly addressing, in clear language, the concerns of the patient and his/her family and ensuring their comprehension of any imparted information, being able to communicate and not destroy hope or provide false hope, recognising situations in which HCPs will have difficulty in interacting with the patient and/or family and developing communication skills to overcome these difficulties (in a way that is sensitive to culture and religious issues), and in palliative care settings, being able to communicate and discuss end-of-life decisions. Empathy, as the process of understanding an individual's subjective experiences by vicariously sharing that experience while maintaining an observant stance, is considered one of the key elements that should be taught since it provides the physician with a more personalised view of the patient and because it provides the patient

Table 5. Ten tasks of communication curricula in emergency medicine (adapted from [57])

- Demonstrate the ability to respectfully, effectively, and efficiently develop a therapeutic relationship with patients and their families.
- Demonstrate respect for diversity and cultural, ethnic, spiritual, emotional, and age-specific differences in patients and other members of the health care team.
- Demonstrate effective listening skills and the ability to elicit and provide information using verbal, non-verbal, written, and technological skills.
- Demonstrate the ability to develop flexible communication strategies and to adjust them based on the clinical situation.
- Demonstrate effective participation in and leadership of the health care team.
- Demonstrate the ability to elicit a patient's motivation for seeking health care.
- Demonstrate the ability to negotiate as well as resolve conflicts. Demonstrate effective written communication skills with other providers and the ability to effectively summarise for the patient upon discharge.
- Demonstrate the ability to effectively use the feedback provided by others.
- Demonstrate the ability to handle situations unique to emergency medicine (e.g. DNR/end-of-life decisions, high-risk-refusal-of-care patients, disaster medicine).

with a sense of connectedness to the physician that may allow the patient herself to more freely express her emotional distress [44]. According to Larson and Yao [45], physicians should be able to engage in an emotional tuning with their patients, both in terms of what they call 'surface acting' (i.e., forging empathic behaviours towards the patient, absence of consistent emotional and cognitive reactions) and 'deep acting' (i.e., generating empathy-consistent emotional and cognitive reactions before and during empathic interactions with the patient).

In oncology, consensus exists regarding the fact that learner-centred courses that meet individual and group needs must be run by trained and competent facilitators, that role playing with structured/constructive feedback on communication skills is essential, and that specific goals (e.g. relationship building, emotion handling, discussing complex information) might be achieved via group discussion, role playing and/or didactic material, including prepared videos with patients or actors [46]. A number of CST interventions have been developed with respect to this in several countries [47]. The SPIKES model [48] (table 5) is an example of a protocol that has been introduced as a part of intensive CST workshops in the USA and has been subsequently adapted and applied in different cultural contexts, such as in Japan [49], Italy [50, 51] and Southern European countries [52], with interesting results. In general, it has been reported that CSTs have a role in improving communication in cancer settings [53] but also that the individual and psychological characteristics of the physicians have a role in the effectiveness of CST courses, as described above [54]. Furthermore, CSTs should consider cultural issues as an important variable for identifying and negotiating different styles of communication, decision-making preferences, the roles of family, sexual and gender issues, and issues of mistrust, prejudice, and racism, according to the patient's cultural background [55].

Other significant experiences in communication have been developed in palliative care settings that consider that physicians can convey their caring and empathy for patients at the end of life and provide good quality care only through good communication. Many examples, such as the Project to Educate Physicians on End-of-life Care from the Institute for Ethics at the American Medical Association, which consists of specific modules, some of which follow the strategies de-

Table 6. Culturally competent communication skills that can be useful in multicultural settings (adapted from [39])

- Non-verbal behaviours: reflect the physician's respect, concern and interest in the patient's well-being (active listening, focusing on the patient, and moderating culturally variable aspects of the interaction, such as eye contact, touch, physical space, facial expressiveness, and the use of gestures).
- Verbal behaviour skills: asking about and assessing the patient's problems; showing understanding; and acknowledging, reflecting, and calibrating emotions to help form a connection.
- Recognition and exploration of potential cultural differences: evaluation of the patient's community and family, of the skills and abilities that aid the patient and his/her family in dealing with the illness, of factors that contribute to understanding health issues (e.g. education, mental acuity, familiarity with disease), of aspects of the patient's environment that influence his/her ability to care for him/herself (e.g. socio-economic factors, structural environment, stressors), and of the emotional implications of illness.
- Incorporation of and adaptation to cultural knowledge: integrating a patient's cultural values or beliefs into the encounter; having awareness of and the ability to adapt communication behaviours to maximise the patient's comfort; reconciling misunderstandings; and being responsive to the patient's values.
- Negotiation and collaboration: operating with awareness and adaptability to negotiate a shared understanding with the patient; reaching an agreement as to how the patient's symptoms will be prioritised, diagnosed, and treated; and discussing the meaning of screening and assessment and the risks and benefits of different treatment options in ways that are individualised to the patient's socio-cultural and biomedical context.

veloped in oncology settings, such as the SPIKES protocol, exist. The Education for Physicians on End-of-life Care curriculum [56], which was developed in the USA in 1997 and was subsequently adapted to expand the scope and range of palliative care to include the entire spectrum of illnesses, including Oncology, Emergency Medicine, Geriatrics and Long-term Care, has focused attention on several areas related to doctor-patient communication (e.g. communicating bad news, depression, anxiety and delirium, withdrawing/withholding treatment, medical futility, physician-assisted suicide, and psychosocial issues). Important steps in this direction have also been taken in emergency medicine, where education and the assessment of communication and interpersonal skills are considered critical components of all training programmes and are a requirement of the Accreditation Council for Graduate Medical Education Outcome Project [57], where several specific communication competencies and assessment techniques used to evaluate skills and competencies have been defined (table 6).

An important issue that should be taken into account when discussing communication and CST courses is the importance of doctors paying attention to their own emotions. It is important to underline the fact that communication with seriously physically ill patients is founded on cooperation, and the clinician has to be aware that what originates from the relationship with the patient is the result of the co-participation of two active counterparts. Unlike during simple information exchange, paying attention to his/her emotions encompasses a therapeutic value and requires from the clinician the ability to reflect about him/herself and about his/her relational styles and personal emotions. It has been reported that a physician's response to the patient's needs and emotions may result in a sense of failure frustration when the possibility of 'rescuing' their patients cannot be realised. Feelings of powerlessness and grief and the fear of becoming ill oneself can affect the quality of medical care as well as the physician's own sense of well-being [58]. These issues are related to the importance of reducing the risk of burn-out, which is a well-known complication of the art of medicine and on which immense literature has been presented over the last years, particularly for HCPs working with seriously ill patients [59–62]. Oncology burnout has been reported to be one of the most common manifestations of distress, with studies suggesting a prevalence of 35% among medical oncologists, 38% among radiation oncologists, and 28–36% among surgical oncologists, resulting in a negative impact on the quality of care as well as on the physicians' quality of life [63]. Thus, models aimed at increasing a physician's self-awareness, identifying their own emotions, and providing other interventions (e.g. psychoeducation, cognitive-behavioural interventions, interpersonal communication, mindfulness, and meditation) have been developed and proposed in medical curricula, with data showing a decrease in burnout among physicians [64, 65].

Conclusions

Compassionate, individually tailored, and effective responses to the mounting vulnerability and increasingly difficult physical, psychosocial, and spiritual challenges facing persons with serious physical illness in the medical encounter should be constantly explored. If it is true that communication challenges raised by patients with severe physical illnesses are many and complex (e.g. recurrence or worsening of the disease, information about prognosis, transition from curative to palliative care, end-of-life care), proper training in communication may help to improve the scenario and change the long-lasting biotechnological and objectifying approach to a more humane and subjectifying approach. In a recent meta-analysis in oncology, CST courses have been shown to be effective in improving some types of communication skills related to information gathering and supportive skills, but more data are necessary regarding the maintenance of the effects over time, whether consolidation sessions are necessary, and which types of CST programmes are most likely to work [66]. On the other hand, it has been confirmed that training healthcare providers in patient-centred approaches positively impacts patient satisfaction with care and that interventions that transfer patient-centred skills to providers to promote patient-centred care within clinical consultations are effective across studies [67].

However, more research is necessary to understand the correct application and efficacy of communication and CST courses for HCPs in medical settings and to understand the effect of communication on significant variables, other than the patient's satisfaction, including outcome of the disease and change in the organisation of the health care system.

Acknowledgements

The authors would like to thank the University of Ferrara for sustaining research in psychosocial oncology and psychiatry in palliative care.

Appendix 1

Clinical vignette	
Jennifer is at an outpatient clinic, waiting for the doctor, to receive the results of the exams (lump biopsy) she had undergone a few days back. She is alone, nervous and worried. Doctor G. sees and greets her, asks her to come into the room, looks her in her eyes, shakes her hand and makes her comfortable, offering for her to have a seat.	Preparation of the setting (S in SPIKES protocol)

Appendix 1 Continued

Clinical vignette	
Doctor (D): 'Well, how are you, and how have you been in the last week since we met?' Jennifer (J): 'You can imagine, doctor, tense and extremely worried to understand what is going on with me'.	Open question
D.: 'I see, yes, it should have been difficult, this waiting time'. J.: 'Yes very difficult'.	Recognition of emotion, empathic response
D.: 'What have been your thoughts and worries?' J.: 'I had bad feelings... I did not sleep well at night.... with bad dreams...'	Exploration
D.: '... Bad dreams?' J. 'Yes, bad dreams about my situation; they told me I had cancer... and when I woke up, I knew it was the reality'.	Reflective questioning, more exploration
D.: '...I understand that your mind was very concentrated on the biopsy you had and that this created a lot of anxiety and tension... Is that the perception you have about the lump?'	Recognition of emotions and empathic response (Perception in the SPIKES protocol)
J.: 'Exactly... you know... and I am here to have the results of the biopsy...' D.: 'Yes, in fact, regarding the biopsy and tests, we have the results now... Do you want me to explain what we have?' J.: 'Yes, please, I need to know'.	(Invitation in the SPIKES protocol)
Doctor G. informs Jennifer about her cancer, using a gentle and delicate tone, monitoring her reactions...	(Knowledge in the SPIKES protocol)
D.: 'I am sorry to have these bad news...' Jennifer starts crying... D.: 'I know it is difficult... I am sorry... Tell me...' J.: '...Sorry, I was thinking about my children...' D.: '...Please, go on...'	Doctor is close to Jennifer and empathic, explores the emotions (Empathy and Exploration of Emotion in SPIKES protocol)
Jennifer expresses her worries about the children seeing herself bald and weak, worrying about the trouble of being a good mother. D.: 'Well, I see there are many fears, understandable fears, and many anxieties about the future... I know' – doctor offers tissue to Jennifer – 'Do you want me to wait a little...' Jennifer, after a while, asks the doctor to give some practical information about what to do now.	Jennifer is opening up Recognition and naming of the emotions, normalisation and validation. Doctor is close to Jennifer and asks permission to proceed or stop, following Jennifer's pace.
Doctor G. summarises the procedures and the following medical steps, offers reassurance in a honest way, checks if Jennifer has understood, if she has questions or doubts, and if she wants to have an additional meeting with her husband.	(Summary and Strategy of the SPIKES protocol)

References

1 Ong LM, de Haes JC, Hoos AM, Lammes FB: Doctor-patient communication: a review of the literature. Soc Sci Med 1995;40:903–918.

2 Epstein RM, Franks P, Fiscella K, Shields CG, Meldrum SC, Kravitz RL, Duberstein PR: Measuring patient-centered communication in patient-physician consultations: theoretical and practical issues. Soc Sci Med 2005;61:1516–1528.

3 Teutsch C: Patient-doctor communication. Med Clin North Am 2003;87:1115–1145.

4 Grassi L: Quam bene vivas referre: curing and caring in psycho-oncology. Psychooncology 2013;22:1679–1687.

5 Miles A: On a medicine of the whole person: away from scientistic reductionism and towards the embrace of the complex in clinical practice. J Eval Clin Pract 2009;15:941–949.

6 Sanson-Fisher R, Girgis A, Boyes A, Bonevski B, Burton L, Cook P: The unmet supportive care needs of patients with cancer. Supportive Care Review Group. Cancer 2000;88:226–237.
7 Moadel A, Morgan C, Fatone A, Grennan J, Carter J, Laruffa G, Skummy A, Dutcher J: Seeking meaning and hope: self-reported spiritual and existential needs among an ethnically-diverse cancer patient population. Psychooncology 1999;8:378–385.
8 Chochinov HM, Krisjanson LJ, Hack TF, Hassard T, McClement S, Harlos M: Dignity in the terminally ill: revisited. J Palliat Med 2006;9:666–672.
9 Chochinov HM: Dying, dignity, and new horizons in palliative end-of-life care. CA Cancer J Clin 2006;56:84–103; quiz 104–105.
10 Fava GA, Mangelli L, Ruini C: Assessment of psychological distress in the setting of medical disease. Psychother Psychosom 2001;70:171–175.
11 Fabbri S, Fava GA, Sirri L, Wise TN: Development of a new assessment strategy in psychosomatic medicine: the diagnostic criteria for psychosomatic research. Adv Psychosom Med 2007;28: 1–20.
12 Sirri L, Fava GA, Wise TN: Psychiatric classification in the setting of medical disease: comparing the clinical value of different proposals J Psychosom Res 2011;70:493–495.
13 Buckman R: Breaking bad news: why is it still so difficult? Lancet 1984;288: 1597–1599.
14 Ptacek JT, Eberhardt TL: Breaking bad news. A review of the literature. JAMA 1996;276:496–502.
15 Hancock K, Clayton JM, Parker SM, Wal der S, Butow PN, Carrick S, Currow D, Ghersi D, Glare P, Hagerty R, Tattersall MH: Truth-telling in discussing prognosis in advanced life-limiting illnesses: a systematic review. Palliat Med 2007;21: 507–517.
16 Parker SM, Clayton JM, Hancock K, Walder S, Butow PN, Carrick S, Currow D, Ghersi D, Glare P, Hagerty R, Tattersall MH: A systematic review of prognostic/end-of-life communication with adults in the advanced stages of a life-limiting illness: patient/caregiver preferences for the content, style, and timing of information. J Pain Symptom Manage 2007;34:81–93.
17 Innes S, Payne S: Advanced cancer patients' prognostic information preferences: a review. Palliat Med 2009;23: 29–39.
18 Harding R, Simms V, Calanzani N, Higginson IJ, Hall S, Gysels M, Meñaca A, Bausewein C, Deliens L, Ferreira P, Toscani F, Daveson BA, Ceulemans L, Gomes B, on behalf of PRISMA: If you had less than a year to live, would you want to know? A seven-country European population survey of public preferences for disclosure of poor prognosis. Psychooncology DOI: 10.1002/pon.3283.
19 Maguire P, Pitceathly C: Key communication skills and how to acquire them. BMJ 2002;325:697–700.
20 Fallowfield L, Jenkins V: Communicating sad, bad, and difficult news in medicine. Lancet 2004;363:312–319.
21 Baile W, Costantini A: Communicating with cancer patients and their families; in Wise T, Biondi M, Costantini A (eds): Psycho-Oncology. Arlington, American Psychiatric Publishing, 2013, pp 57–90.
22 Maguire P, Pitceathly C: Managing the difficult consultation. Clin Med 2003;3: 532–537.
23 Bub B: The patient's lament: hidden key to effective communication: how to recognise and transform. Med Humanit 2004;30:63–69.
24 Chochinov HM: Dignity-conserving care–a new model for palliative care: helping the patient feel valued. JAMA 2002;287:2253–2260.
25 Chochinov HM: Dignity and the essence of medicine: the A, B, C, and D of dignity conserving care. BMJ 2007;335: 184–187.
26 Steptoe A, Sutcliffe I, Allen B, Coombes C: Satisfaction with communication, medical knowledge, and coping style in patients with metastatic cancer. Soc Sci Med 1991;32:627–632.
27 Sardell AN, Trierweiler SJ: Disclosing the cancer diagnosis. Procedures that influence patient hopefulness. Cancer 1993;72:3355–3365.
28 Fallowfield LJ, Jenkins VA, Beveridge HA: Truth may hurt but deceit hurts more: communication in palliative care. Palliat Med 2002;16:297–303.
29 Maunder RG, Hunter JJ: Assessing patterns of adult attachment in medical patients. Gen Hosp Psychiatry 2009;31: 123–130.
30 Maunder RG, Hunter JJ: A prototype-based model of adult attachment for clinicians. Psychodyn Psychiatry 2012; 40:549–573.
31 Hunter JJ, Maunder RG: Using attachment theory to understand illness behavior. Gen Hosp Psychiatry 2001;23: 177–182.
32 Tan A, Zimmermann C, Rodin G: Interpersonal processes in palliative care: an attachment perspective on the patient/clinician relationship. Palliat Med 2005; 19:143–150.
33 Surbone A: Bioethical challenges: understanding cultural differences and reducing health disparities; in Grassi L, Riba M (eds): Clinical Psycho-Oncology: An International Perspective. Chichester, Wiley, 2012, pp 199–210.
34 Seeleman C, Suurmond J, Stronks K: Cultural competence: a conceptual framework for teaching and learning. Med Educ 2009;43:229–237.
35 Surbone A: Cultural competence: why? Ann Oncol 2004;15:697–699.
36 Ashing-Giwa KT, Padilla G, Tejero J, Kraemer J, Wright K, Coscarelli A, Clayton S, Williams I, Hills D: Understanding the breast cancer experience of women: a qualitative study of African American, Asian American, Latina and Caucasian cancer survivors. Psychooncology 2004;13:408–428.
37 Wang JH, Adams I, Huang E, Ashing-Giwa K, Gomez SL, Allen L: Physical distress and cancer care experiences among Chinese-American and non-Hispanic White breast cancer survivors. Gynecol Oncol 2012;124:383–388.
38 Anderson LM, Scrimshaw SC, Fullilove MT, Fielding JE, Normand J, the Task Force on Community Preventive Services: Culturally competent healthcare systems. A systematic review. Am J Prev Med 2003;24:68–79.
39 Teal CR, Street RL: Critical elements of culturally competent communication in the medical encounter: a review and model. Soc Sci Med 2009;68:533–543.
40 Michel DM, Moss AH: Communicating prognosis in the dialysis consent process: a patient-centered, guideline-supported approach. Adv Chronic Kidney Dis 2005;12:196–201.
41 Lee SJ, Back AL, Block SD, Stewart SK: Enhancing physician-patient communication. Hematology Am Soc Hematol Educ Program 2002:464–483.

42 Borasio GD, Sloan R, Pongratz DE: Breaking the news in amyotrophic lateral sclerosis. J Neurol Sci 1998; 160(suppl 1):S127–S133.
43 Rosenbaum ME, Ferguson KJ, Lobas JG: Teaching medical students and residents skills for delivering bad news: a review of strategies. Acad Med 2004;79: 107–117.
44 Zinn W: The empathic physician. Arch Intern Med 1993;153:306–312.
45 Larson EB, Yao X: Clinical empathy as emotional labor in the patient-physician relationship. JAMA 2005;293:1100–1106.
46 Stiefel F, Barth J, Bensing J, Fallowfield L, Jost L, Razavi D, Kiss A; participants. Communication skills training in oncology: a position paper based on a consensus meeting among European experts in 2009. Ann Oncol 2010;21:204–207.
47 Kissane DW, Bylund CL, Banerjee SC, Bialer PA, Levin TT, Maloney EK, D'Agostino TA: Communication skills training for oncology professionals. J Clin Oncol 2012;30:1242–1247.
48 Baile WF, Buckman R, Lenzi R, Glober G, Beale EA, Kudelka AP: SPIKES-a six-step protocol for delivering bad news: application to the patient with cancer. Oncologist 2000;5:302–311.
49 Fujimori M, Oba A, Koike M, Okamura M, Akizuki N, Kamiya M, Akechi T, Sakano Y, Uchitomi Y: Communication skills training for Japanese oncologists on how to break bad news J Cancer Educ 2003;18:194–201.
50 Costantini A, Baile WF, Lenzi R, Costantini M, Ziparo V, Marchetti P, Grassi L: Overcoming cultural barriers to giving bad news: feasibility of training to promote truth-telling to cancer patients. J Cancer Educ 2009;24:180–185.
51 Lenzi R, Baile WF, Costantini A, Grassi L, Parker PA: Communication training in oncology: results of intensive communication workshops for Italian oncologists. Eur J Cancer Care (Engl) 2011; 20:196–203.
52 Grassi L, Travado L, Gil F, Campos R, Lluch P, Baile W: A communication intervention for training southern European oncologists to recognize psychosocial morbidity in cancer. I – development of the model and preliminary results on physicians' satisfaction. J Cancer Educ 2005;20:79–84.
53 Barth J, Lannen P: Efficacy of communication skills training courses in oncology: a systematic review and meta-analysis. Ann Oncol 2011;22:1030–1040.
54 De Vries AM, de Roten Y, Meystre C, Passchier J, Despland JN, Stiefel F: Clinician characteristics, communication, and patient outcome in oncology: a systematic review. Psychooncology 2014; 23:375–381.
55 Epner DE, Baile WF: Patient-centered care: the key to cultural competence. Ann Oncol 2012;23(suppl 3):33–42.
56 Emanuel LL, von Gunten CF, Ferris FD: The Education for Physicians on End-of-life Care (EPEC) curriculum, 1999. www.epec.net (accessed December 12, 2014).
57 Hobgood CD, Riviello RJ, Jouriles N, Hamilton G: Assessment of communication and interpersonal skills competencies Acad Emerg Med 2002;9:1257–1269.
58 Meier DE, Back AL, Morrison RS: The inner life of physicians and care of the seriously ill. JAMA 2001;286:3007–3014.
59 Böhmert M, Kuhnert S, Nienhaus A: Psychological stress and strain in dialysis staff: a systematic review. J Ren Care 2011;37:178–189.
60 Nyssen AS, Hansez I: Stress and burnout in anaesthesia. Curr Opin Anaesthesiol 2008;21:406–411.
61 Pereira SM, Fonseca AM, Carvalho AS: Burnout in palliative care: a systematic review. Nurs Ethics 2011;18:317–326.
62 Balch CM, Freischlag JA, Shanafelt TD: Stress and burnout among surgeons: understanding and managing the syndrome and avoiding the adverse consequences. Arch Surg 2009;144:371–376.
63 Shanafelt T, Dyrbye L: Oncologist burnout: causes, consequences, and responses. J Clin Oncol 2012;30:1235–1241.
64 Awa WL, Plaumann M, Walter U: Burnout prevention: a review of intervention programs. Patient Educ Couns 2010;78: 184–190.
65 Regehr C, Glancy D, Pitts A, LeBlanc VR: Interventions to reduce the consequences of stress in physicians: a review and meta-analysis. J Nerv Ment Dis 2014;202:353–359.
66 Moore PM, Rivera Mercado S, Grez Artigues M, Lawrie TA: Communication skills training for healthcare professionals working with people who have cancer Cochrane Database Syst Rev 2013;3: CD003751.
67 Dwamena F, Holmes-Rovner M, Gaulden CM, Jorgenson S, Sadigh G, Sikorskii A, Lewin S, Smith RC, Coffey J, Olomu A: Interventions for providers to promote a patient-centred approach in clinical consultations Cochrane Database Syst Rev 2012;12:CD003267.
68 Grassi L, Riba M: Diagnostic issues; in Grassi L, Riba M (eds): Psychopharmacology in Oncology and Palliative Care. Berlin, Springer, 2014, pp 31–48.

Luigi Grassi, MD
Institute of Psychiatry, Department of Biomedical and Specialty Surgical Sciences, University of Ferrara
Corso Giovecca 203
IT–44121 Ferrara (Italy)
E-Mail luigi.grassi@unife.it

Balon R, Wise TN (eds): Clinical Challenges in the Biopsychosocial Interface. Update on Psychosomatics for the 21st Century. Adv Psychosom Med. Basel, Karger, 2015, vol 34, pp 24–35 (DOI: 10.1159/000369082)

Dimensional Psychopharmacology in Somatising Patients

Massimo Biondi • Massimo Pasquini

Department of Neurology and Psychiatry, SAPIENZA University of Rome, Rome, Italy

Abstract

Despite the recent DSM-5 review of somatoform disorders, which are now called somatic symptom and related disorders, the categorical definitions of these syndromes have inherent limitations because their causal mechanism or presumed aetiologies are still unknown. These limitations may affect everyday clinical practice and decision-making abilities. As a result, physicians have limited information at their disposal to treat these patients. Furthermore, the clinical presentations of somatic disorders may vary a lot. The purpose of this chapter is to illustrate a psychopathological dimensional approach to the somatising patient. This approach is constantly unconsciously applied in clinical practice using continuous variables, such as rating scales. Moreover, treatment strategies might be improved by adding a dimensional approach, simply recognising the prominent components of the presenting psychopathology of a given patient and addressing them with drugs according to their different mechanisms, targeting circuits and neurotransmitters. Some authors have proposed a shift from the nosological to functional application of psychotropic drugs, in which functional psychopharmacology will be dysfunction oriented and therefore inevitably geared towards utilising drug combinations. Here, we present a summary of the advantages of functional/dimensional psychopharmacology for the treatment of somatic symptoms and related disorders.

Introduction

Somatisation is the tendency to experience, communicate, and amplify psychological and interpersonal distress in the form of somatic distress and medically unexplained symptoms [1]. The DSM-5 [2] contains a review of somatoform disorders, which are now called somatic symptom and related disorders, stressing the relevance of abnormal thoughts, feelings, and behaviours in response to these somatic symptoms rather than highlighting the absence of a medical explanation for them. In this perspective, the ways patients present and interpret somatic symptoms are of essential importance. This is particularly true for the diagnoses of somatic symptom disorder and illness anxiety disorder, while the diagnoses of conversion disorder (functional neurological symptom disorder) and psychological factors affecting other medical conditions are more composite. The diagnosis of psychological factors affecting other medical conditions implies the presence of an organic disease, and a functional neurological symptom disorder is often present in patients suffering from neurological disorders. A common feature of the diagnosis of this class is the referral of affected patients to a primary care physician, neurologist or other medical doctor.

Given that all mental disorders are still considered syndromes and not diseases, in this class, which is different from other mental disorders, such as bipolar disorder and schizophrenia, the boundaries between normalcy and pathology are very close. In this way, diagnoses of somatic and related disorders are formulated based on the magnitude of suffering or on quantitative rather than qualitative criteria. All individuals have experienced the somatic equivalent of anxiety on many occasions, but few have experienced auditory hallucinations or delusions. For this reason, categorical approaches to these diagnoses leave some uncertainty or approximation. Recently, Regier has highlighted the need to incorporate the dimensional approach into the DSM-5 [3]. In particular, Hudziak et al. [4] have stressed the limitations of the DSM-IV, such as its multiple sources of variance, including gender, age, and informant comorbidity. Moreover, Slade and Andrews, using taxonometric analysis, have highlighted that depression is a continuously distributed syndrome rather than a discrete diagnosis [5].

However, translation of these concepts into research fields remains difficult. Thus, the dimensional approach is constantly applied in clinical practice using continuous variables. The co-occurrence of depression or anxiety symptoms in a psychotic patient might be measured using specific or cross-cutting rating scales. In this way, clinicians are also better able to describe hybrid models. In this chapter, we illustrate the usefulness of the Scale for the Rapid Assessment of Dimensional Psychopathology (SVARAD) [6] in the assessment of somatic symptom disorder, illness anxiety disorder, conversion disorder (functional neurological symptom disorder), and psychological factors affecting other medical conditions.

Categorical versus Dimensional Approach

Kraepelin has been a great advocate of the taxonomy of clear-cut clinical entities. Nevertheless, he stated the following: 'Wherever we try to mark out the frontier between mental health and disease, we find a neutral territory, in which the imperceptible change from the realm of normal life to that of obvious derangement takes place' [7]. The great variability in the clinical pictures of mental disorders and their 'continuums' can be explained in terms of the multifactorial, non-deterministic, stochastic models of their aetiologies and of the interactions between genetic-biological and environmental-psychosocial factors, disposition and resilience. It seems unlikely that the categorical model can accommodate and satisfactorily describe the continuous-quantitative rather than discrete-qualitative phenomenon of psychopathology and related symptoms, which are a function of a complex 'web of causation', implying a wide variety of risk factors ranging from genetic-neurochemical to interpersonal-motivational and from cognitive to cultural-psychosocial that interact with one another. In addition, modifiers and/or moderating variables play mediating roles, many of which are unknown but have been postulated, because for most mental disorders, currently known risk factors explain no more than 50% of the variance. As a consequence, one of the main goals of DSM-5 is to improve diagnoses on the basis of continuous measurements of psychopathology. Unfortunately, this model is not applicable for all mental disorders in terms of syndrome threshold and severity. However, it represents an attempt to overcome the prototypic structure of the DSM-IV TR, in which it was stated that 'There is no assumption that each category of mental disorder is a completely discrete entity with absolute boundaries dividing it from other mental disorders or from no disorder' [8]. The DSM-5, in fact, is also a categorical classification dividing mental disorders into types based on criterion sets with defining features. The prototypic, nomothetic nature of the categorical classification implies several disadvantages, such as extensive comorbidity. Most people who meet the criteria for a given mental disorder also meet criteria for one or more additional disorders.

'Concurrent diagnostic comorbidity is the norm rather than the exception, with the rate dramatically increasing if one considers lifetime comorbidity' [9]. Moreover, the categorical approach leads to extensive within-category heterogeneity. For example, individuals meeting the criteria for axis II personality disorders (5 out of 9) may share only one common feature.

Unresolvable boundary issues represent another problem. 'DSM-IV TR is replete with problematic boundary disputes, many of which could be the result of arbitrary categorical distinction being imposed along common, underlying domains of functioning' [10]. Despite the huge efforts of the authors who revised the DSM-5 and all contributors from several task forces, the afore-mentioned limitations of the DSM-IV have not been resolved in the DSM-5.

A dimensional model can effectively address the excessive comorbidity issue and boundary dispute present in the categorical model. Furthermore, in the categorical approach, the goal of validating categories and discovering common aetiologies has remained, to a large extent, elusive. In addition, epidemiologic studies have shown a high degree of short-term diagnostic instability for many disorders [10]. Finally, a lack of treatment specificity is the rule rather than the exception [11].

Treatment is one of the most important components of the very relevant issue of the clinical utility of a classification system, reliability and validity being other components affecting the appropriateness of clinical decisions. Categorical models of classification are easier to use and simpler to communicate, while dimensional models are definitely more complex but provide more specific, perhaps more valid, and certainly more precise information and a better individualised profile description of a patient's psychopathology that may, in turn, have more differentiated and specific treatment implications [10]. In line with the initial purposes of the fifth revision of the DSM, which were unfortunately not fulfilled at all, we suggest that in the assessment and treatment of psychosomatic patients with their complexity and multifaceted psychopathological suffering, the traditional categorical approach to psychiatric diagnosis would be better integrated with a dimensional approach. Our admittedly preliminary attempt to combine categorical and dimensional approaches could be of interest to psychiatrists working in different clinical settings and may better suit individual needs. The traditional categorical approach is based on standardised sets of criteria for mood or anxiety disorders. These categories guide protocols of psychotropic drug or combination treatments, such as counselling or psychotherapy for mild major depression, antidepressants for moderate-to-severe major depression, anxiolytics or psychotherapy for demoralisation or adjustment reactions, antipsychotics for delirium, and so on. This approach, according to our clinical experience, has some limitations.

Treatments might be improved by the addition of a dimensional approach, i.e., recognising prominent components of the presenting psychopathology of a given patient and addressing them with drugs according to their different underlying mechanisms, targeting circuits and neurotransmitters. Van Praag, a pioneer of psychopathology, proposed a shift from the nosological to the functional application of psychotropic drugs, in which functional psychopharmacology will be dysfunction-oriented and therefore inevitably geared towards utilising drug combinations [12].

Although we acknowledge that the application of such a dimensional model in psychiatry is at a very early phase, our preliminary experience with this new approach is promising and might improve patient care. In fact, the dimensional approach is regarded as interesting and intriguing by many clinicians, particularly in relation to difficulties and criticisms about categorical diagnoses in select clinical areas [13]. As formulated by Jaspers, the object of psychopathology denotes real, conscious psychic events that have consequences and relationships [14].

According to the categorical model, diagnostic criteria are summed only until a specified number is deemed to be present, after which the diagnosis is considered valid. The presence of more or fewer features than the threshold is not considered to have any significance.

The dimensional representation of psychopathology has a different structure; the model is cumulative, and the number of diagnostic features observed is an index of the degree to which the diagnostic entity is present [15]. The concept of psychopathological dimension is derived from psychometrics and is defined as an altered psychic function phenomenologically expressing itself through a set of symptoms or signs, indicating and specifying an altered function on a continuum ranging from extreme pathology to normality [13].

Giving its atheoretical assumption, this approach should be able to identify psychopathological dimensions that are not categorically expected. Studies conducted on primary unipolar depressed patients have revealed the presence of anger or an activation dimension [16–18] not included in the DSM-IV criteria for depressive disorder but previously described by ancient Greek physicians. We also detected an anger dimension in depressed cancer patients using a simple dimensional rating scale [19]. A dimensional diagnosis of depression implies that clinicians have to listen more accurately to the principal complaints of the patient. The categorical and dimensional approaches are complementary and represent two successive phases of a process aimed at therapy optimisation. To broadly frame a patient's clinical condition, we suggest that a categorical diagnosis should be first identified, which could be followed by a dimensional diagnosis, allowing for psychiatrists to tailor a treatment to an individual's needs. In fact, dimensional diagnosis entailing a reclassification of psychotropic drugs provides the opportunity to use drugs according to a pathophysiological rationale that has not been followed to date. Given their different drug actions and clinical effects, terms such as antidepressant or mood stabiliser are not very specific. Furthermore, both patients and non-psychiatrist doctors are generally puzzled by the conciseness of psychotropic drug terminology. Presently, in psychiatry, psychotropics are summarised in antidepressants, mood-stabilisers, antipsychotics and anxiolytics, while pharmacodynamics are referred to only in academic terminology. In contrast, hypertensive patients, for example, know well whether they are being treated with sartans or beta-blockers.

According to Pancheri, the pathophysiology of a given psychopathological dimension (sadness, fear, anger, activation, impulsivity, obsessiveness, apathy, reality distortion, and so on) could be better matched with a specific drug acting on a given neurotransmitter circuit rather than with a diagnostic DSM-IV category; that is, we can plan a more specific psychotropic drug treatment following a dimensional approach to psychopathology [13]. From this perspective, we do not consider anxiety or adjustment disorders as separate entities from depression. Anxiety could be a symptom of depression, particularly in patients prone to experience anxiety even when they are not depressed that may have personalities characterised by anxiety traits. With regard to adjustment disorders, the threshold between a normal response and a pathological response is arbitrary and not culture-oriented. In addition, the severity of the condition is less relevant than its duration. As a consequence, a subject diagnosed with an adjustment disorder might fulfil the criteria for a major depressive episode after a few weeks but not be prescribed a pharmacological intervention. Consequently, the treatment strategies discussed here not only refer to DSM-5 diagnoses but also integrate dimensional principles. Although evidence has been anecdotal until now and has been limited as far as clinical trials are concerned, we suggest the consideration of a dimensionally oriented drug treatment, which in our experience integrates well with the traditional DSM-5 categorical approach.

In our previous research, we have illustrated a clinical application of functional psychopharmacology using a combination of a selective serotonin reuptake inhibitor (SSRI) and an anticonvulsant in patients with unipolar depression with prominent anger, irritability, hostility, and aggressiveness [20]. Our findings suggest that adding an anticonvulsant affecting the GABAergic and glutamatergic systems is useful in depressed patients with dysphoric mood.

The Scale for the Rapid Assessment of Dimensional Psychopathology

Many clinical instruments allow for a dimensional approach to psychiatry and psychosomatic medicine, including the Symptom Check List-90 [21] or the Brief Psychiatric Rating Scale [22]. Because of the difficulties and time pressures experienced by psychiatrists in their real-life clinical practice, we have developed a specific psychopathological tool, the SVARAD (Appendix 1) [6]. The SVARAD was constructed to provide a rapid and efficient measurement of an individual's placement upon a continuum between pathology and normality. The SVARAD is a 10-item instrument specifically developed for the rapid assessment of some major psychopathological dimensions. A validation study has shown its satisfactory inter-rater reliability, content validity, and criterion validity [20]. It is thus a reliable and valid dimensional tool in both research and clinical settings. The items are rated on a 5-point scale ranging from 0 to 4, with higher scores indicating greater severity. Scores of 1 indicate the presence of a condition intermediate between normality and psychopathology, while scores of 2 or more indicate the presence of symptoms of definite clinical relevance.

The items explore the following dimensions: apprehension/fear, sadness/demoralisation, anger/aggressiveness, obsessiveness, apathy, impulsivity, reality distortion, thought disorganisation, somatisation, and activation.

Every dimension has been defined with both psychopathological and functioning criteria. The 10 items are described as follows:

Apprehension/fear: a condition of apprehension or fear, a sensation of imminent danger, a sensation of constraint, or feelings of nervousness or anxiety.

Sadness/demoralisation: self-dislike, pessimism, reduced creativity, or anhedonia.

Anger/aggressiveness: irritation, anger, resentment, irritability, quarrelsomeness, hostility, or verbal or physical violence.

Obsessiveness/iterativity: doubtfulness, inflexibility, preciseness, checking or preventing behaviours, or the presence of obsessions or compulsions.

Apathy: indifference, distance, flattened affectivity or drive or reduced planning.

Impulsivity: a sudden tendency to behave in an inadequate or potentially harmful way without sufficient reflection on the causes or consequences of one's own actions.

Reality distortion: effort distinguishing between reality and imagination, proneness to attributing unusual senses or relevance to neutral stimuli, or the presence of delusions or hallucinations.

Thought disorganisation: disorganised thinking as evidenced by disorganised speech.

Somatisation: an increased focus on body sensation, somatic symptoms without organic

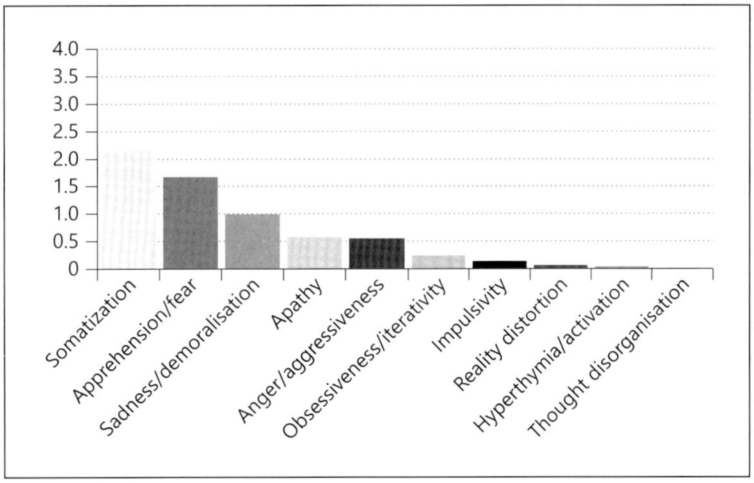

Fig. 1. Dimensional assessment of patients affected by somatoform disorder (n = 26) according to SVARAD.

evidence, excessive worrying about health, or a lack of justification for the fear of being sick.

Activation: increased motor activity, acceleration of ideas, disinhibition, increased energy and self-confidence, euphoria or irritability.

Dimensional Psychopharmacology Approach to Somatic Symptom Disorders

As mentioned in the introduction section, these disorders appear to be less discrete syndromes compared with other mental disorders. The boundaries between pathology and normalcy are difficult to determine due to their low degrees of severity, whereas a patient with a severe illness anxiety disorder may experience thought distortion or ruminative thoughts. Thus, using the SVARAD in the assessment of these disorders may highlight symptoms or dimensions that are unique to the patient and their culture. In a previous study, we evaluated 26 patients affected by somatoform disorder according to the DSM-IV, employing the SVARAD [23].

As shown in figure 1, in this sample, the main psychopathological dimensions are in line with the categorical criteria with the exception of the low level of anger/aggressiveness. The categorical diagnosis of a somatoform disorder as well as its distribution, explained in terms of mean values, are not very useful to clinicians in making treatment choices, whereas a dimensional profile (as illustrated below) of a single patient is more immediate and clear, illustrating the prominent dimension of suffering facilitating the decision-making process.

Interestingly, the results we obtained with the sample of somatoform disorder patients are similar to the findings obtained using the Symptom Check List-90-R to assess a sample of gastrointestinal patients [24]. Otherwise, two common clinical manifestations of somatisation are irritable bowel syndrome and fibromyalgia. The pathophysiologies of both of these conditions are not yet fully understood.

However, several psychotropic drugs are used to treat these conditions. In their review, Bundeff and Woodies have illustrated that fluoxetine, citalopram and paroxetine are useful for the treatment of irritable bowel syndrome, but the available data evaluating these agents are conflicting [25]. The same conclusion was drawn for atypical antipsychotics [26]. Regarding fibromyalgia, different antipsychotics have been employed with limited efficacy [27]. Several different medications, including serotonin and

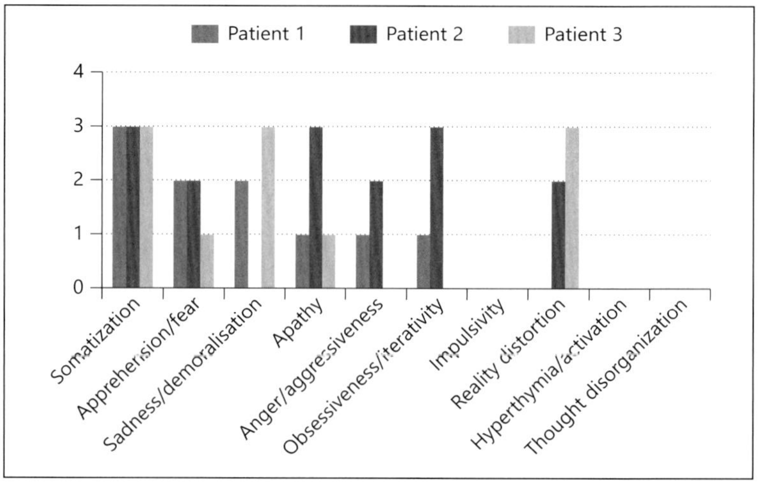

Fig. 2. Different dimensional profiles of three patients affected by illness anxiety disorder.

norepinephrine reuptake inhibitors, duloxetine and milnacipran and pregabalin have been approved by the Food and Drug Administration for the management of fibromyalgia based on their clinically meaningful and durable effects on pain in monotherapy trials. They also have been shown to beneficially affect patient global impressions of change and function and other key symptom domains, such as fatigue, sleep disturbance and cognition [28]. Researchers have established a core set of dimensions constituting the condition of fibromyalgia, including pain, fatigue, sleep and mood disturbance and cognitive dysfunction.

Pharmacological treatments are chosen on the basis of the prevailing dimensions for each individual. Therefore, the SVARAD would be useful when applied to a single patient affected by these two conditions. Similarly, subjects with the same stressors might receive the same categorical diagnosis of somatic symptom disorder but their dimensional profiles might strongly differ, leading to distinct treatments. Here, we illustrate the dimensional profiles of three patients affected by illness anxiety disorders (conversion disorder (functional neurological symptom disorder), according to the DSM-IV criteria), three patients affected by fibromyalgia, and three patients affected by inflammatory bowel syndrome (fig. 2–5). These clinical pictures may help psychiatrists with their prescription choices.

In fact, among the patients affected by an illness anxiety disorder, the first patient may be treated with an SSRI due to the predominance of sadness and apprehension, whereas the second patient may be treated with an SSRI for apprehension, apathy and obsessiveness plus a mood stabiliser or a D2 blocker for the moderate presence of anger and reality distortion. The third patient may be treated with the combination of an SSRI and a D2 blocker because sadness and reality distortion are the main clinical manifestations.

Among the patients affected by conversion disorder (functional neurological symptom disorder), the first patient may be treated with an SSRI or a tricyclic antidepressant with prominent serotonergic properties because of the moderate presence of apprehension, apathy, and obsessiveness. The second patient may be treated first with a mood stabiliser, such as valproate, plus a benzodiazepine because of the mild presence of anger, impulsivity and activation, while the third patient may be treated with an serotonin and noradrenaline reuptake inhibitor or SSRI plus a mood stabiliser, such as valproate or gabapentin, for the presence of sadness, apathy and anger.

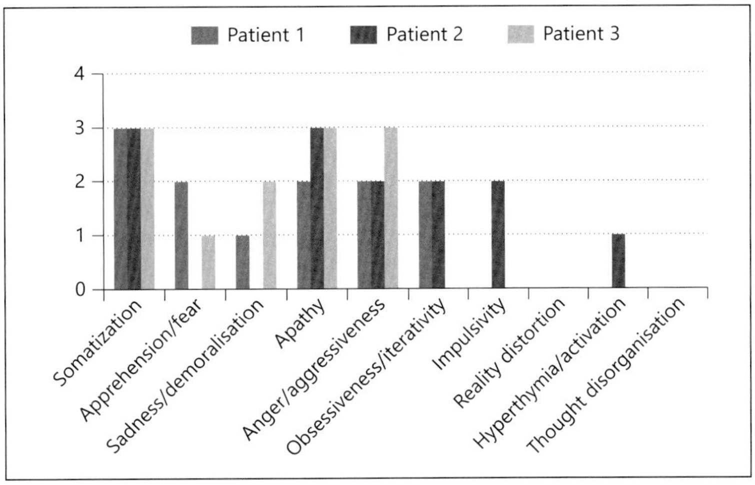

Fig. 3. Different dimensional profiles of three patients affected by conversion disorder.

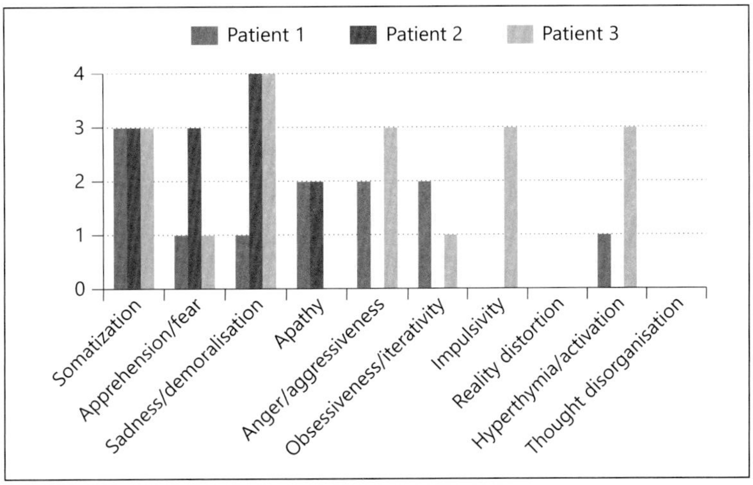

Fig. 4. Different dimensional profiles of three patients affected by fibromyalgia.

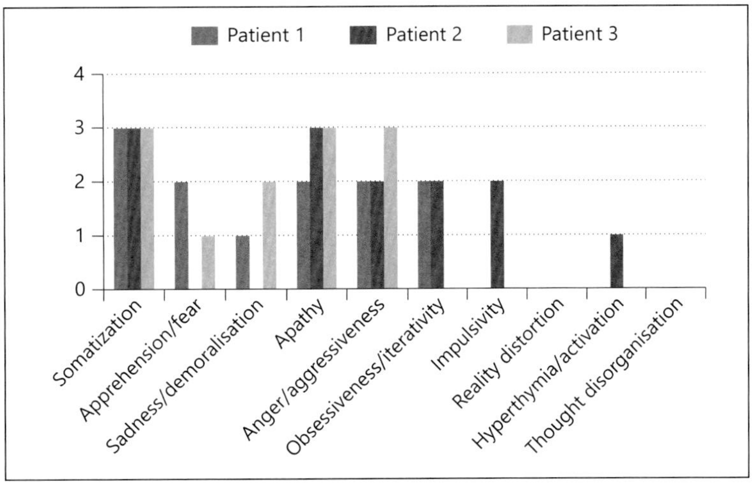

Fig. 5. Different dimensional profiles of three patients affected by inflammatory bowel syndrome.

Among the patients affected by fibromyalgia, the first patient may be treated with an SSRI for the presence of sadness, apprehension, apathy, and obsessiveness plus a mood stabiliser because of the mild presence of anger and activation. The second patient may be treated with an serotonin and noradrenaline reuptake inhibitor, SSRI or mirtazapine for the predominance of sadness and apprehension plus amisulpride for apathy, while the third patient may be treated with the combination of an SSRI plus a mood stabiliser for the presence of anger and activation in addition to sadness and low levels of apprehension and obsessiveness.

Among the patients affected by inflammatory bowel syndrome, the first patient may be treated initially with an SSRI or a tricyclic antidepressant with prominent serotonergic properties due to the presence of apprehension, apathy and obsessiveness and with a mood stabiliser, such as valproate, lamotrigine or gabapentin, for anger. Patient 2 may be treated the first time with a mood stabiliser because of the presence of anger, impulsivity and activation and a second time with an SSRI for obsessiveness and apathy. Patient 3 may be treated with the combination of an SSRI plus a mood stabiliser for the presence of anger in addition to sadness and apathy.

Antidepressants seem to be effective against somatisation and related disorders [29], although an extensive review of randomized controlled trials conducted on somatoform disorders as a group has summarised that there is not yet conclusive evidence for the use of antidepressants in their treatment [30]. There are differences in the efficacy of antidepressants for treating somatoform and conversion disorders that could explained by the different associated pathophysiological mechanisms. Several variables may be used to guide prescriptions under these conditions. According to a dimensional approach, different dimensions may prevail in the clinical presentation of a categorical diagnosis of depressive disorder. Clinicians should choose an antidepressant with a dopaminergic or noradrenergic profile if the apathy dimension prevails.

The presence of an activation dimension, insomnia, and anxiety might suggest the employment of an antagonist of postsynaptic serotonin receptors (5-HT2 and 5-HT3) and an H1 antagonist, such as mirtazapine or trazodone. When obsessiveness/iterativity prevail, a serotonergic agent, such as an SSRI or clomipramine, may be helpful. On the other hand, a combination of an SSRI and an anticonvulsant, typically valproate, may provide benefit when anger or irritability is the predominant dimension [20]. The presence of a slight degree of reality distortion may suggest treatment with a low dose of an atypical antipsychotic or a typical D2 blocker before prescription of an antidepressant. Finally, as suggested by Oulis et al. [31], adding a low dose of amisulpride may help in the treatment of conversion disorders.

Conclusions

In summary, a brief assessment of the prevailing dimensions of a categorical diagnosis could be suitable for the psychopharmacological targeting of individual profiles of suffering. The lack of evidence-based data is the main limitation of this approach; however, in everyday clinical practice, clinicians often choose a treatment using predominant symptomatic criteria and the personal or cultural characteristics of the patient. Dimensional psychopharmacology implies function-oriented prescriptions rather than categorically based ones. Thus, patients with the same diagnosis will receive a drug treatment tailored to their main psychopathology and specific dimensional profile (anxiety, apathy, anger/irritability, activation, sadness, etc.). The functional/dimensional perspective allows for the increased individualisation of psychotropic drug management compared with categorical models. Finally, the SVARAD can help make dimensional assessments and decision-making processes more efficient.

Appendix 1

The Scale for the Rapid Assessment of Dimensional Psychopathology, S.VA.RA.D. Paolo Pancheri, Massimo Biondi, Paola Gaetano, Angelo Picardi

Name	Surname	Age	Date of evaluation

Apprehension/fear: A condition of apprehension or fear, a sensation of imminent danger, a sensation of constraint, or feelings of nervousness or anxiety.

0 Absent
1 Mild: occasionally present or present following stressful events and not pervasive with good functioning in all areas.
2 Moderate: frequent, not pervasive, and induced by non-relevant stimuli with good functioning in all areas.
3 Severe: quite persistent and pervasive with moderate difficulties in social or work activities.
4 Very Severe: continuous and pervasive with serious impairments in social or work activities.

Sadness/demoralisation: Self-dislike, pessimism, reduced creativity, or anhedonia.

0 Absent
1 Mild: changeable by positive stimuli and experienced in few areas with good functioning in all areas.
2 Moderate: barely changeable and experienced in several areas with mild difficulties in social or work activities.
3 Severe: unchangeable and pervasive with moderate difficulties in social or work activities.
4 Very Severe: unchangeable and pervasive with extreme difficulties in social or work activities.

Anger/aggressiveness: Irritation, anger, resentment, irritability, quarrelsomeness, hostility, or verbal or physical violence.

0 Absent
1 Mild: occasionally present, but the patient has control over his/her anger.
2 Moderate: frequent but generally controlled.
3 Severe: pervasive and very frequently uncontrolled with social impairments.
4 Very Severe: pervasive, continuous, and uncontrolled with serious legal consequences.

Obsessiveness/iterativity: Doubtfulness, inflexibility, preciseness, checking or preventing behaviours, or the presence of obsessions or compulsions.

0 Absent
1 Mild: present without obsessions or compulsions.
2 Moderate: occasional presence of obsessions and compulsions that are not intrusive and are generally controlled with good functioning in all areas.
3 Severe: presence of obsessions and compulsions that are intrusive and uncontrolled with mild impairment in all areas.
4 Very Severe: intrusive obsessions and compulsions that are experienced all day and are uncontrolled with social impairment.

Apathy: Indifference, distance, flattened affectivity or drive or reduced planning ability.

0 Absent
1 Mild: mild and variable or changeable with a moderate planning ability and good functioning in all areas.
2 Moderate: evident but changeable by positive stimuli with a reduced planning ability and fair global functioning.
3 Severe: continuous and unchangeable with difficulty in social or work activities.
4 Very Severe: unchangeable and pervasive with an inability to plan daily routines and extreme difficulties in social or work activities.

Appendix 1 Continued

Name	Surname	Age	Date of evaluation

Impulsivity: The tendency to suddenly behave in an inadequate or potentially harmful way without sufficient reflection on the causes or consequences of one's own actions.

0 Absent
1 Mild: impulsive reactions that are generally controlled, sporadic, and induced by relevant stimuli.
2 Moderate: impulsive reactions that are partially controlled, infrequent, and induced by irrelevant stimuli with moderate functional impairment.
3 Severe: impulsive reactions that are poorly controlled and frequent with relevant social consequences.
4 Very Severe: lack of control over impulsivity with severe social or legal consequences.

Reality distortion: Effort to distinguish between reality and imagination, proneness to attributing unusual senses or relevance to neutral stimuli, or the presence of delusions or hallucinations.

0 Absent
1 Mild: tendency to attribute unusual or non-shareable meanings to events or uncommon perceptions.
2 Moderate: delusions without certainty or infrequent hallucinations that are perceived in particular conditions and are partially criticised.
3 Severe: non-pervasive structured delusions that are poorly criticised or frequent hallucinations that are not continuous and not criticised.
4 Very Severe: undeniable delusions that are pervasive with certainty or hallucinations that are unbearable and continuous and not criticised.

Thought disorganisation: Disorganised thinking as evidenced by disorganised speech.

0 Absent
1 Mild: occasionally present during free speech or induced by particular stimuli.
2 Moderate: frequent during free speech but less evident during conversation with efficient communication.
3 Severe: continuous during free speech and evident during conversation with altered communication.
4 Very Severe: continuous and pervasive with unintelligible communication.

Somatisation: Increased focus on body sensations, the presence of somatic symptoms without organic evidence, excessive worrying about health, or an unjustified fear of being sick.

0 Absent
1 Mild: infrequent, mild, and modifiable by reassurance.
2 Moderate: frequent and poorly modifiable by reassurance with mild global impairment.
3 Severe: quite continuous, stable, and temporarily modifiable with evident global impairment.
4 Very Severe: continuous, pervasive, not modifiable by reassurance, and invalidating.

Activation: increased motor activity, the acceleration of ideas, disinhibition, increased energy and self-confidence, euphoria or irritability.

0 Absent
1 Mild: mild expansiveness, irritability, disinhibition, restlessness, and good insight.
2 Moderate: increased energy and irritability, evident disinhibition, increased motor activity, potentially dangerous activities, and fluctuating insight.
3 Severe: euphoria or dysphoria, manifested disinhibition, and dangerous hyperactivity with poor insight.
4 Very Severe: acceleration of ideas and manic behaviours with no insight.

☐ Total Score

References

1 Abbey SE: Somatization and somatoform disorders; in Wise MG, Rundell JR (eds): The American Psychiatric Publishing Textbook of Consultation-Liaison Psychiatry: Psychiatry in the Medically Ill, ed 2. Washington DC, American Psychiatric Publishing, 2002, pp 361–392.
2 American Psychiatric Association: Diagnostic and Statistical Manual of Mental Disorders, ed 5. Arlington, VA, American Psychiatric Publishing, 2013.
3 Regier DA: Dimensional approaches to psychiatric classification; in Helzer JE, Kraemer HC, Frueger RF, Wittchen HU, Sirovatka PJ, Regier DA (eds): Dimensional Approaches in Diagnostic Classification. Refining the Research Agenda for DSM-V. Arlington, American Psychiatric Association, 2008, pp 17–23.
4 Hudziak JJ, Achenbach TM, Althoff RR, Pine DS: A dimensional approach to developmental psychopathology; in Helzer JE, Kraemer HC, Frueger RF, Wittchen HU, Sirovatka PJ, Regier DA (eds): Dimensional Approaches in Diagnostic Classification. Refining the Research Agenda for DSM-V. Arlington, American Psychiatric Association, 2008, pp 101–114.
5 Slade T, Andrews G: Latent structure of depression in a community sample: a taxonometric analysis. Psychol Med 2005;35:489–497.
6 Pancheri P, Picardi A, Gaetano P, Pasquini M, Puzella A, Di Fabio F, Biondi M: Validazione della scala per la valutazione rapida dimensionale 'SVARAD'. Riv Psichiatr 1999;34:84–93.
7 Kraepelin E: Lectures on clinical psychiatry, ed 3. New York, William Wood, 1917.
8 American Psychiatric Association: Diagnostic and Statistical Manual of Mental Disorders, DSM, ed 4, text revision. Washington DC, American Psychiatric Publishing, 2000.
9 Brown TA, Campbell LA, Lehman CL, Grisham JR, Mancill RB: Current and life-time comorbitity of DSM-IV anxiety and mood disorders in a large clinical sample. J Abnorm Psychol 2001;110: 585–599.
10 Widiger TA, Samuel DB: Diagnostic categories or dimensions? A question for DSM-IV- Fifth Edition. J Abnorm Psychol 2005;III:494–504.
11 Kupfer DJ, First MB, Regier DE: A research agenda for DSM-V. Washington, DC, American Psychiatric Association, 2002, pp 15–24.
12 Van Praag HM, Asnis GM, Kahn RS, Brown SL, Korn M, Harkavy-Friedman JM, Wetzler S: Nosological tunnel vision in biological psychiatry. A plea for a functional psychopathology. Ann NY Acad Sci 1990;600:501–510.
13 Pancheri P: Approccio dimensionale e approccio categoriale alla diagnosi psichiatrica. Giorn Ital Psicop 1995;1–3: 8–23.
14 Jaspers K: General Psychopathology – Volumes 1 & 2. Translated by Hoenig J and Hamilton MW. Baltimore and London, Johns Hopkins University Press, 1997.
15 Blashfield RK, Livesley WJ: Classification; in Millon T, Blaney PH, Davis RD (eds): Oxford Textbook of Psychopathology. New York, Oxford University Press, 1999, pp 3–28.
16 Fava M: Depression with anger attacks. J Clin Psychiatry 1998;59:18–22.
17 Pasquini M, Picardi A, Biondi M, Gaetano P, Morosini P: Relevance of anger and irritability in outpatients with major depressive disorder. Psychopathology 2004;37:155–160.
18 Biondi M, Picardi A, Pasquini M, Gaetano P, Pancheri P: Dimensional psychopathology of depression: detection of an 'activation' dimension in unipolar depressed outpatients. J Affect Disorders 2005;84:33–39.
19 Pasquini M, Biondi M, Costantini A, Cairoli F, Ferrarese G, Picardi A, Sternberg C: Detection and treatment of depressive and anxiety disorders among cancer patients: feasibility and preliminary findings from a liaison service in an oncology division. Depress Anxiety 2006;23:441–448.
20 Pasquini M, Picardi A, Speca A, Orlandi V, Tarsitani L, Morosini P, Cascavilla I, Biondi M: Combining an SSRI with an anticonvulsant in depressed patients with dysphoric mood: an open study. Clin Pract Epidemiol Ment Health 2007;3:3.
21 Derogatis LR, Lipman RS, Rickels K, Uhlenhuth EH, Covi L: The Hopkins Symptom Checklist (HSCL). A measure of primary symptom dimensions. Mod Probl Pharmacopsychiatry 1974;7:79–110.
22 Overall JE, Gorham DR: The brief psychiatric rating scale. Psychol Rep 1962; 10:799–812.
23 Picardi A, Morosini P, Gaetano P, Pasquini M, Biondi M: Higher levels of anger and aggressiveness in major depressive disorder than in anxiety and somatoform disorders. J Clin Psychiatry 2004;65:442–443.
24 Kovács Z, Seres G, Kerékgyártó O, Czobor P: Psychopathological symptom dimensions in patients with gastrointestinal disorders. J Clin Psychol Med Settings 2010;17:378–386.
25 Bundeff AW, Woodis CB: Selective serotonin reuptake inhibitors for the treatment of irritable bowel syndrome. Ann Pharmacother 2014;48:777–784.
26 Pae CU, Lee SJ, Han C, Patkar AA, Masand PS: Atypical antipsychotics as a possible treatment option for irritable bowel syndrome. Expert Opin Investig Drugs 2013;22:565–572.
27 Calandre EP, Rico-Villademoros F: The role of antipsychotics in the management of fibromyalgia. CNS Drugs 2012; 26:135–153.
28 Mease PJ, Dundon K, Sarzi-Puttini P: Pharmacotherapy of fibromyalgia. Best Pract Res Clin Rheumatol 2011;25:285–297.
29 Somashekar B, Jainer A, Wuntakal B: Psychopharmacotherapy of somatic symptoms disorders. Int Rev Psychiatry 2013;25:107–115.
30 Kroenke K: Efficacy of treatment for somatoform disorders: a review of randomized controlled trials. Psychosom Med 2007;69:881–888.
31 Oulis P, Kokras N, Papadimitriou GN, Masdrakis VG: Adjunctive low-dose amisulpride in motor conversion disorder. Clin Neuropharmacol 2009;32:342–343.

Massimo Pasquini
Department of Neurology and Psychiatry, SAPIENZA University of Rome
Viale dell'Universita 30
IT–00185 Rome (Italy)
E-Mail massimo.pasquini@uniroma1.it

Balon R, Wise TN (eds): Clinical Challenges in the Biopsychosocial Interface. Update on Psychosomatics for the 21st Century. Adv Psychosom Med. Basel, Karger, 2015, vol 34, pp 36–48 (DOI: 10.1159/000369083)

Forensic Issues in Medical Evaluation: Competency and End-of-Life Issues

Sherif Soliman[a] · Ryan C.W. Hall[b]

[a]Case Western Reserve University, School of Medicine, Northcoast Behavioral Healthcare, Northfield, Ohio, [b]Psychiatry, Department of Medical Education, University of Central Florida College of Medicine, and Department of Psychiatry, University of South Florida, and Barry University Dwayne O. Andreas School of Law, Orlando, Fla., USA

Abstract

Decision-making capacity is a common reason for psychiatric consultation that is likely to become more common as the population ages. Capacity assessments are frequently compromised by misconceptions, such as the belief that incapacity is permanent or that patients with dementia categorically lack capacity. This chapter will review the conceptual framework of decision-making capacity and discuss its application to medical decision-making. We will review selected developments in capacity assessment and recommend an approach to assessing decision-making capacity. We will discuss the unique challenges posed by end-of-life care, including determining capacity, identifying surrogate decision-makers, and working with surrogate decision-makers. We will discuss clinical and legal approaches to incapacity, including advance directives, surrogate decision-makers, and guardians. We will discuss the legal standards based on which surrogates make medical decisions and outline options for resolving disagreements between clinical staff and surrogate decision-makers. We will offer recommendations for approaching decision-making capacity assessments.

Introduction

In a recent survey of 288 members of the Academy of Psychosomatic Medicine, nearly two thirds of respondents rated capacity assessments as more challenging and more time consuming than other psychiatric consultations [1]. In this survey, one in six consultations was for decision-making capacity [1]. These consultations are likely to increase as the population ages since the elderly are at greater risk for dementia, delirium, and other conditions impairing cognition. Risk factors for incapacity in the elderly include acute or chronic medical illness, a lower educational level, and lower vocabulary [2]. The issue of the capacity to make treatment decisions at the end of life can be particularly challenging, both because terminally ill patients are at greater risk of having impaired capacity and because terminally ill patients who have capacity may rationally decide to forego treatment against the wishes of family members. It is therefore critical that the psychiatrists performing these consultations be familiar with the relevant ethical, clinical, and legal principles that underlie these assessments.

Capacity is a clinically determined ability to perform a specific task or tasks, such as consenting to medical treatment, living independently, or managing finances. Competence is a legally determined ability to perform a specific task. The criteria for specific competencies are sometimes defined in statutes or case law. However, the terms 'competence' and 'capacity' are often used interchangeably in both medical and legal settings [3].

Assessments of decision-making capacity involve the clinical task of describing an individual's abilities as they relate to the capacity in question as well as the ethical task of determining what degree of capacity is sufficient. These assessments require carefully weighing the ethical principles of autonomy and beneficence.

Over the past four decades, research has focused on formulating a conceptual framework for capacity assessments as well as on developing instruments to assist evaluators in assessing different capacities. Simultaneously, laws regarding competence, surrogate decision-making, and guardianship have been rapidly evolving in an attempt to protect incompetent patients while preserving their autonomy in areas where they retain competence. One example of this is the increased popularity of limited guardianships, which specifically limit the powers of a guardian, recognizing that people may be incompetent in some areas while competent in others.

In this chapter, we will discuss the ethical and legal principles that underlie capacity assessment and the conceptual framework of capacity assessments. We will review strategies for assessing capacity and will discuss the unique challenges posed by end-of-life care. We will offer recommendations for approaching these challenging consultations.

Ethical and Legal Principles

Determining precisely how much 'capacity' is sufficient to make a particular decision requires balancing the competing ethical principles of autonomy and beneficence. Respect for autonomy requires providing a competent patient with all relevant information and respecting the decision that he or she makes with regard to treatment. Beneficence requires the physician to act in the best interest of the patient. It sometimes requires seeking the legal authority to act against the stated wishes of an incompetent patient to provide necessary treatment. Although overriding the stated wishes of an incompetent patient may appear to violate the principle of autonomy, it often does not. In many cases, the patient, if competent, would have wanted the treatment, as evidenced by the patient's previously stated wishes, the opinion of relatives close to the patient, or the patient's opinion if he or she regains competence.

The analogous legal principles of *parens patriae* (the state's responsibility to provide for impaired individuals) and individual liberty are balanced by courts and policy makers. These competing concerns factor into a variety of decisions, such as determining when guardianship is appropriate, granting authority for involuntary treatment, and determining legal standards for civil commitment. Physicians strike this balance when they determine whether a particular patient lacks capacity and whether to seek authorization to treat the patient against the patient's wishes. Courts must balance similar factors in determining whether to override a patient's wishes through an involuntary treatment order or the appointment of a guardian. Legislative bodies and appellate courts consider these factors in determining statutory standards under which the courts consider individual cases.

Principles of Capacity Assessment

The most widely used conceptual framework for capacity assessment was developed by Appelbaum and Grisso and is discussed by Appelbaum and Guthiel [4, 5] (table 1). They list four abilities: the ability to communicate a choice, the ability to

Table 1. Components of Decisional Capacity [4, 5]

Component	Description	Example(s) of Deficits
Communication of choice	The patient should be able to state his or her decision in a reasonably stable manner. The communication need not be verbal.	A delirious patient repeatedly and without explanation states inconsistent choices.
Factual understanding of issues	The patient should understand key issues, including the risks and benefits of and alternatives to the proposed treatment.	Cognitive disorders may impair the ability to comprehend and retain key information. Psychosis may impair a patient's ability to accept information about his or her health.
Appreciation of situation and likely consequences	The patient should cognitively and affectively understand the likely consequences of selecting each of the viable options. He or she should also be able to apply the facts, in a rational manner, to his or her own situation.	Lack of insight may cause a patient to fail to apply his or her factual understanding of the issues to his or her own situation. Severe affective disorders may distorted the patient's assessment of likely consequences. A severely depressed patient may have such negative thinking that he or she only sees negative outcomes as plausible.
Rational manipulation of information	The reasoning process itself, rather than the decision, is the key issue. The process should be rational, and one thought should logically flow from the previous.	Psychosis can impair rational thought, either by causing the patient to make decisions based on delusional beliefs or by causing thought disorganization. Individuals with cognitive disorders may not have the ability to rationally weigh complex data.

factually understand the relevant information, the ability to appreciate the situation and its likely consequences, and the ability to rationally manipulate information. These standards are also often applied by courts, though courts (depending on the jurisdiction) may apply all of these or any combination of these factors.

The ability to communicate a choice need not be verbal [3]. It simply requires that the patient recognize that he or she has a choice and can, in a reasonably stable manner, indicate the choice that he or she has made. This does not mean that a patient cannot change his or her mind. However, substantial instability of a decision on a critical matter should raise concerns about capacity. Assessing this aspect requires asking the patient whether he or she is aware of the decision to be made and asking him or her to state his or her decision.

The patient's factual understanding of the issues involved is primarily a cognitive ability. When applied to the capacity to make a medical decision, this would entail an understanding of the condition and the treatment options, including the risks and benefits of the proposed treatment and of each of the treatment alternatives. An understanding of the risks and benefits of foregoing treatment is also included. In many cases, deficits in this area can flow from inadequate disclosure of information to the patient or from not spending enough time explaining the information to the patient. A consulting psychiatrist should first have a thorough understanding of the medical condition and treatment. The psychiatrist should then determine the patient's understanding and attempt to fill in any gaps by educating the patient. Finally, the psychiatrist should test the patient's understanding and ability to retain the information for a reasonable period.

Appreciation of the situation and its likely consequences requires a higher degree of 'knowing' than mere factual understanding. It requires the patient to apply the information to himself or herself. The patient should be able to acknowledge the likely consequences of accepting or rejecting treatment. Reasoning, insight, and affect can all impair appreciation. For example, patients with delusional disorder often have the ability to intellectually understand the generic risks and benefits of antipsychotic medication treatment. However, they do not have the ability to give informed consent because they lack insight into the benefits of treatment for them specifically by lacking insight into their illness. Affective states can also affect appreciation. Bursztajn et al. discussed this phenomenon and described a case of pathological grief impairing appreciation [6].

The ability to rationally manipulate information, or reasoning ability, refers to the patient's thought process, rather than to the actual decision reached. The decision cannot be substantially influenced by delusional thinking or gross impairments in reasoning ability. One pitfall is equating a decision that the physician endorses with competence. For example, a delusional patient may give assent for an appendectomy, a decision that seems rational. However, when asked why he wants the surgery, he may reveal that he believes that the surgeon will remove a chip that the government implanted. This is an example of a 'correct' decision that is nevertheless incompetent. The four factors provide a useful conceptual framework that can guide clinical assessments of capacity. Appelbaum and Guthiel additionally provide specific questions relevant to each of the components of capacity [5].

In determining whether impairment is sufficiently severe to render a patient incompetent, Appelbaum recommends utilizing a 'sliding scale' approach, requiring a greater degree of capacity to make decisions that are high risk and low benefit while requiring less capacity to make low-risk/high-benefit decisions [3]. Another important contextual factor is whether the patient's capacity impairment is temporary or permanent. If the decision can be deferred, the physician can treat the patient to restore his or her decision-making capacity. Treatable conditions that can impair capacity include infections causing delirium, exacerbation of schizophrenia in a patient who had attained remission, and medications' side effects.

While this section has focused on the medical decision-making capacity, it is important to keep in mind that there are several other capacities that a psychiatrist may be asked to assess. For example, guardianship evaluations require an assessment of the capacity to perform daily activities such as cooking, bill paying, performing basic hygiene, obtaining medical care, and responding to emergencies. Other capacities include testamentary capacity (the ability to make a will), contractual capacity (the ability to enter into contracts), and adjudicative capacity (the ability to stand trial as a criminal defendant).

Standardized Tests and Instruments

The use of standardized testing is sometimes helpful in difficult cases. Standardized tests in capacity evaluations can be broadly divided into measures of general cognitive ability and instruments specifically designed to assess the domains of capacity.

One of the most ubiquitous screening tests for general cognitive capacity is the Mini-Mental State Examination (MMSE) [7]. Because it is such a widely used measure, attempts have been made to correlate MMSE scores with measures of the capacity to consent to treatment. Kim et al. found that in patients with Alzheimer's disease, a score below 19 identified incompetent patients with a specificity of 84–94%. However, sensitivity at this cutoff was low, only detecting 39–54% of incompetent patients. A cutoff of 26 increased the sensitivity to 91–100% but decreased specificity to 29–36% [8]. Karlawish summarizes his data on the MMSE scores of Alzheimer's disease patients being assessed for the capacity to consent to treatment by noting that scores above 23 were associated with increased sensitivity (to detect incompetence), while scores of 19 and below were associated with increased specificity. He characterized scores of 20–22 as a 'gray zone' [9]. General measures of cognition, such as the MMSE, should never be used as proxies for a capacity assessment. Rather, a reasonable way to apply these data would be to recommend that primary care physicians consider a low MMSE score as one indication for assessing capacity. Scores below 19 should indicate a relatively high risk of impaired decision-making capacity.

The most widely used and studied instrument for assessing capacity is the MacArthur Competence Assessment Tool for Treatment, developed by Appelbaum and Grisso [10]. The authors estimate that it takes 15–20 minutes to administer. It is a semi-structured interview focusing on the patient's condition, treatment options, and decision regarding treatment. It is divided into the four areas of capacity previously described. Each question is scored on a 0–2 scale (0, inadequate; 1, partial; and 2, adequate). The authors did not establish cutoff scores for capacity, noting that specific impairments must be considered in the context of other clinical factors when determining whether a patient has the capacity to make a specific decision.

In a review of 23 instruments for assessing the decision-making capacity to consent to treatment and research, the MacArthur instruments (regarding consenting to treatment and research) were found to have the most empirical support [11]. Another review characterized the MacArthur instruments as the 'gold standards' [12]. Other instruments include the Hopkins Competency Assessment Test, the Informed Consent Survey, and the California Scale of Appreciation (regarding research consent) [11, 13].

There are some advantages to using standardized instruments. They help to guide assessments in close cases, to structure interviews around relevant issues, and to improve inter-rater reliability and can be useful in helping medical students and residents to learn to perform assessments. However, there are also several drawbacks, including the tendency to accord too much weight to the results of an instrument; the risk of viewing capacity as a categorical yes-no determination, rather than a continuum of abilities; insufficient flexibility in performing assessments; and failing to consider contextual factors in assessments.

Kapp and Mossman caution against the development of a 'capacimeter', or the 'Holy Grail' of capacity assessment [14]. They raise several concerns, including the inevitability of clinical judgment in determining which patients are assessed, the need to consider the specific decision to be made, differing legal competence standards, and the risk of physicians and courts assigning too much weight to the 'capacimeter' result.

In summary, specific instruments may be helpful in assessing decision-making capacity, especially in equivocal cases. General cognitive measures should never be used in place of a capacity assessment, though they may help to identify patients who are at risk for incapacity. Standardized instruments should be used in conjunction with, and not instead of, a complete clinical assessment and should be interpreted in light of contextual factors such as the decision to be made, the relevant legal standard, and the nature of the patient's impairment.

Overview of Options for Treating Incompetent Patients

Physicians have an obligation to treat patients in a medical emergency, with some exceptions. In some cases, patients will have stated their wishes in a living will or advance directive. These are legal documents in which a competent patient expresses his or her wishes in the event that he or she becomes incompetent. In addition, the patient may have a durable power of attorney, which authorizes another person to make medical decisions should the patient be deemed to lack decision-making capacity by his or her attending physician. The role of surrogates is discussed more fully below.

In cases where no surrogate decision-maker has been designated, most state statutes contain a hierarchy of default surrogate decision-makers. While there is some variance, the order is usually spouse, adult child, and parents [15]. In cases where there are no appointed or default surrogate decision-makers, courts may appoint guardians to make decisions for an incapacitated patient. Guardianship can be generally sought on an emergency basis, though states differ in their legal procedures. It is important for physicians to clearly communicate the prognosis to courts in order to assist the courts in tailoring a guardianship to the needs of a particular patient. Some U.S. states allow for limited guardianships, which specifically delineate the limits of the guardian's decision-making authority. Courts should also be advised of whether the impairment is expected to be temporary or permanent.

Misconceptions and Pitfalls

Consulting psychiatrists should be aware of prevalent misconceptions regarding capacity assessments when providing consultation to general medical physicians. Common misconceptions include failing to distinguish between legal competence and capacity, failing to understand that capacity is task specific, and failing to recognize that incapacity is not necessarily permanent.

In a survey of 395 members of the Academy for Psychosomatic Medicine, geriatricians, psychologist members of the Gerontological Society of America, and chairs of ethics committees, Ganzini et al. asked respondents to rate a list of 23 pitfalls on prevalence, importance to patient care, and importance to medical education. In total, 36% of respondents rated medical education as most important, believing that incapacity to make one medical decision meant incapacity to make all medical decisions [16]. Additionally, 79% of respondents rated failure to ensure that the patient has been given adequate information before making a treatment decision as very important to patient care.

Ganzini et al. subsequently utilized data from the same survey to identify the following ten 'common myths' about decision-making capacity [17]:

(1) Decision-making capacity and competence are the same.

(2) A lack of capacity can be presumed when patients go against medical advice.

(3) There is no need to assess decision-making capacity unless patients go against medical advice.

(4) Decision-making capacity is an 'all-or-nothing' phenomenon.

(5) Cognitive impairment equals a lack of decision-making capacity.

(6) A lack of decision-making capacity is a permanent condition.

(7) Patients who have not been given relevant and consistent information about their treatment lack decision-making capacity.

(8) All patients with certain psychiatric disorders lack decision-making capacity.

(9) Patients who have been involuntarily committed lack decision-making capacity.

(10) Only mental health experts can assess decision-making capacity.

Decision-Making Capacity at the End of Life

When evaluating capacity and end-of-life decisions, a physician has to balance the wishes of the patient, if known; the patient's condition; medical ethics; and professional discretion [18–20]. This can be particularly difficult in end-of-life decisions, when patients most likely do not have capacity due to the stage of their illness and/or medications that they are being prescribed [21–23]. Some studies have found that as few as 5% of critically ill patients have the capacity to make end-of-life decisions, with only 20% of surrogates actually knowing beforehand what a patient would want in a situation [19, 21]. However, Kova et al. recently reported a study of decision-making capacity in a series of 24 patients diagnosed with terminal illness [24]. The researchers administered the MacArthur Competence Assessment Tool for Treatment (see above) and found that only one third of participants were significantly impaired in one or more of the four domains of decision-making capacity. They note that this sample was likely skewed toward more cognitively intact patients because the sample consisted of patients identified by their physician as capable of completing the testing. Nevertheless, this study suggests that there is usually a window during which a significant proportion of terminally ill patients have capacity and can engage in planning for the future by executing advance directives and other documents.

The term 'end of life' has different research and policy definitions [25]. Some studies define it as the care received during a set time frame, such as during the last 6 months of life or the last treatment encounter (e.g. last hospital admission, period in palliative care), while others define end-of-life care as the time when certain decisions have to be made, such as withdrawal of or not initiating certain medical techniques, including ventilator support, peripheral feeding, and hydration [21, 25, 26]. Some 'end-of-life decisions', such as being identified as Do Not Resuscitate, may actually occur many years prior to one's death [23, 25]. Medical decision-making at the end of life can be challenging due to difficulty in defining the prognosis, the relative benefit of treatment, and quality of life.

Although laws vary, when an individual is not able to make an end-of-life decision, many U.S. states require that a surrogate or legal guardian use 'substituted judgment' in making treatment decisions [19, 21, 27–29]. Substituted judgment requires the surrogate to take the course of action that the patient would have wanted if he or she were able to make the decision; this course of action is based on the patient's beliefs, values, and past actions [27]. A key challenge of substituted judgment is determining what the person would have wanted if competent [30–32]. Several factors, including religious beliefs and previously expressed wishes, need to be weighed [32]. If substituted judgment cannot be determined, then the 'best-interest standard' is usually applied.

Advance Directives

Over the last 20 years, policy makers and health care professionals have focused on encouraging patients to prepare advance directives [27], which consist of living wills and health care or full powers of attorney [33]. Families have reported an easier experience with end-of-life treatment in part from having had discussions with loved ones regarding death when the document was drafted [30, 32, 34].

In some jurisdictions, care-related statements made to a physician can be memorialized by the physician as Physician Orders on Life-Sustaining Treatment [33]. Although the Patient Self-Determination Act of 1994 requires hospitals, long-term care facilities, and health plans to inquire about advance directives and to potentially assist in the creation of advance directives, it is estimated that only 20–66% of patients over age 60 actually do have valid instruments [22, 23, 25, 32, 33, 35]. Barriers to completing advance directives include access to the documents, social and cultural taboos related to contemplating death and sickness, confusion over what advance directives are, and the belief that people with advance directives will not receive 'aggressive treatment for normal situations' [35].

Though helpful, advance directives can still leave many questions unanswered. An advance directive has to be activated (usually based on two physicians' opinion that the individual has lost capacity) [33]. Once activated, the document may only give broad guidance [21, 33, 36]. In addition, the directive may use vague language [33]. There may be ambiguity about whether a particular treatment is 'heroic' when placed in the context of the patient's likelihood of recovery (e.g. in the case of pneumonia in an older but 'otherwise healthy' individual) compared with use of a ventilator with a low chance of 'long-term recovery'. Finally, an advance directive drafted many years prior may not reflect a patient's current views [19, 25, 32, 37].

How Surrogates Make Decisions

Surrogates can be identified through documents such as advance directives or medical powers of attorney or are appointed by a court. In cases where a surrogate has not previously been identified, many jurisdictions will use a hierarchical structure based on family relationships [20, 21, 26, 33]. At times, even with hierarchies and clear surrogates in place, there can be a legal conflict between interested parties, as was seen in the drawn-out Florida case of Terri Schiavo. In this case, her husband (the court-appointed guardian) and her parents disagreed about the removal of a feeding tube that had been placed due to her being in a persistent vegetative state [38].

Even for people who have prepared advance directives, the surrogate's job can still be challenging. For example, an advance directive may comment on use of a ventilator but may give no indications about use of dialysis. This may lead to a speculative conclusion about if the patient viewed ventilation and dialysis in the same way [27, 32]. In general, research involving hypothetical situations shows that surrogates and patients make the same decision about 60–70% of the time [25, 29, 39]. This rate is even lower for more speculative or ambiguous decisions, such as about participation in a research study [27, 29, 31]. There is also concern that for end-of-life questions where there is ambiguity, the surrogate will make decisions based on what the surrogate would have wanted or a reasonable person's standard, and not necessarily on subjective judgment [25, 27, 32].

Religious beliefs and how they are interpreted can also influence decision-making. Studies have found that approximately 50–60% of the public believes that miracles or divine intervention can occur for people in poor health or persistent vegetative states, compared with only 20% of health care providers [19, 25, 37]. There are also times when surrogates may conflate or misapply religious beliefs.

In a study done by Chidwick et al., looking at cases taken to a dispute resolution board (Consent and Capacity Board) in Ontario, Canada, it was noted that there were certain characteristics seen in the surrogates involved in the cases [37]. The surrogates believed that the patient would have wanted to suffer or 'accepted the pain' due to the high value that the patient placed on life. At times, general values or positions were interpreted as expressed wishes for end-of-life care (e.g. he did not like to miss meals, so he would want a feeding tube). The surrogates were found to have an 'unrealistic hope for recovery' for the patient, which was thought to negatively affect their ability to perform their function as surrogates. Some of the surrogates would not believe or accept the physician's diagnoses, prognosis, or medical opinion. In cases where the surrogate rejected the doctor's expertise, the surrogate often relied on intangible aspects of the patient's character to justify the opinion (e.g. the patient 'is a fighter', so the prognosis is not as grim or is wrong). Many surrogates also believed that the patient would improve if 'more time' was allowed for current treatments to work. In addition, the surrogates involved in the disputed cases frequently reported having an ability to communicate with the person that was greater than what the staff perceived, such as making meaningful eye contact; subtle body movements; and, in one case, being able to read the patient's mind to know what that person wanted for his or her care. In many of these cases, it was found that the surrogates 'needed education on their role and responsibilities', such as about substituted judgment being what the patient would have wanted, and not the surrogates' personal judgment. An additional feature of the cases was that most of them included treatment plans that involved 'palliative care' as well as withholding and/or withdrawal of life-sustaining treatment. The majority of the board's decisions were in favor of the physicians, but even with the third-party involvement of an ideally neutral board, 25% of the cases underwent further appeals. In some cases, the designated surrogate may not be competent to make end-of-life decisions or able to carry out the duties [30, 32]. This can occur due to advance directives and other end-of-life documents being established years prior to being needed. When these documents are finally activated, it may be discovered that the surrogate's own mental state or personal knowledge/relationship with the individual is no longer adequate [25, 30]. Surrogates may also lack capacity due to being emotionally overwhelmed with the responsibility of being a surrogate or due to a pre-existing cyclical mental disorder, such as bipolar disease [25, 30, 40]. If the surrogate lacks the capacity for informed consent, then the medical team has an ethical and legal obligation to switch to an already identified alternate surrogate or to have a new surrogate identified [27, 28, 31, 41].

Physicians' Involvement in End-of-Life Decisions

Doctors rarely ever occupy the surrogate role. There are two U.S. states that place doctors in the hierarchy as a decision-makers for patients, but only if the physician has knowledge of the patient's wishes prior to the time of incapacity and if no other surrogate is available [26, 42, 43]. In general, it is not recommended for physicians to serve as both the treater and the surrogate because it is difficult to effectively carry out both roles and because this situation raises concerns over whose interest the doctor is actually serving and could potentially have negative legal repercussions for the doctor, such as civil or criminal action [21, 22, 43]. Physicians may also be less accurate than patient-appointed or next-of-kin surrogates in making substituted-judgment decisions for patients [21, 42].

In exercising professional judgment, doctors can withhold or discontinue treatments that are futile since the ineffective treatment is not providing benefits and likely will harm the patient [21, 26, 41, 44]. There are two broad categories of futility of care: physiologic futility and medical futility. Physiologically futility (e.g. vasoconstrictors no being longer effective for maintaining blood pressure) is easier to document and less subjective than medical futility. Medical futility refers to the determination that even though treatment may be providing some benefit, it will ultimately not restore or 'reasonably' maintain the patient's health [25, 26, 41, 44].

Palliative or comfort care focuses on achieving comfort and ensuring respect for patients nearing death and often includes symptom management, social support, psychological treatment, and practical caregiver support [21, 37]. It is important for physicians to educate people about what palliative care is and that it is not 'giving up', is not euthanasia, and is not just 'killing the loved one'. The U.S. Supreme Court has heard cases discussing euthanasia and palliative care, such as *Washington v Glucksberg* and *Vacco v Quill* [45, 46]. In those cases, the Court ruled that the 'double effect' (the notion that a treatment may have two outcomes, such as relieving pain and hastening death) is permissible, as long as the treatment is being prescribed for the beneficial purpose (e.g. relieving suffering) [26].

Table 2. Documentation of End-of-Life Care

Key Elements of Documentation
1. Treatment plan
2. How arrived at determination of prognosis
3. Severity of illness (score if standardized scale is utilized)
4. Relevant literature underlying decisions (journal articles if novel or off-label treatment)
5. Alternatives considered
6. Second opinions or consults obtained
7. Knowledge of patient's expressed wishes (e.g., advance directive reviewed, re-reviewed)
8. Education provided to surrogate
9. Statements made by surrogate and team's responses (e.g., hospital chaplain consult)
10. Documented team meetings about concerns

Conflicts between Surrogates and Treatment Teams

If there is a conflict between a treatment team and a surrogate on the best course of action for a patient, it is generally necessary to reach some level of resolution prior to involving the courts [21]. Although the courts are unavoidable at times, getting court approval is often time consuming, costly, and inconvenient; distracts from treatment of the patient due to the adversarial nature of the court system; and is not guaranteed to result in a decision that better represents the patient's interests or wishes [21, 41, 42].

Improving communication between the treatment team and the surrogate can sometimes obviate the need for formal legal proceedings. Early stages of communication should include education for the surrogate on his or her role and what standard (e.g. substituted judgment, best interest) should be applied [23]. If a resolution is not obtained, the next level would be involvement of a second opinion, involvement of an ombudsman, or another level of treatment review (e.g. review by an ethics committee or multidisciplinary board, if available) [21, 40]. This allows for additional input, for potential grievances to be voiced, for resolution of personality conflicts, for people to have the opportunity to save face, and for additional information to be gathered and presented [19, 21, 40, 43]. The treatment team should document every action taken, which may be needed if a court decision is required [19, 21, 26, 40] (table 2).

Euthanasia

Due to its complexity and evolving position in American medical culture (e.g. two U.S. states allow some form, with the first being Oregon in 1994, when a euthanasia-friendly Hippocratic Oath was created), a thorough review of the topic of euthanasia is beyond the scope of this chapter [25, 35, 47]. In general, when a patient expresses the desire to end his or her life, whether the patient's mental state is abnormal or the patient's symptom management is suboptimal needs to be considered [35]. The withdrawal of life support is not considered as an act of euthanasia [28]. In jurisdictions and countries where physicians can prescribe medications with the intent to cause death (physician-assisted suicide), the patient has to have documented capacity in order for the physician to legally participate [25].

Suggested Approach to Capacity Consultation

While no approach will be appropriate for every evaluation, the following framework provides a systematic method for thinking about the issues of capacity and end-of-life decision-making. It is based in part on the approach to psycho-legal consultations for the elderly proposed by Soliman [48].

(1) Understand the context of the evaluation, including the specific decision(s) to be made, relevant legal standards for capacity, and the information that has been given to the patient.

(2) Conduct a focused psychiatric and cognitive evaluation.

(3) Interview the patient regarding the specific elements of decision-making capacity:

(a) Ability to communicate a choice.

(b) Factual understanding of the issues involved (current condition, risks, benefits, and alternatives).

(c) Appreciation of the likely consequences of accepting each of the possible treatments and of foregoing treatment.

(d) Ability to rationally manipulate information.

If the patient lacks capacity, consider the cause. If the cause is reversible and the decision can be deferred, initiate treatment to restore capacity.

If the cause is not reversible in a reasonable time period, explore whether the patient has a surrogate decision-maker or an advance directive. If not, attempt to identify a surrogate decision-maker if the law allows for default surrogate decision-makers, such as a spouse or adult children. Alternatively, a court may appoint an emergency guardian to make decisions.

Conclusion

Decision-making capacity is a dynamic construct. It can vary with time, the intellectual and emotional state, and the task involved. It is important for psychiatrists to be familiar with relevant legal standards in their jurisdiction before assessing capacity. Psychiatrists should utilize a systematic approach grounded in an understanding of the conceptual framework of capacity. The most commonly accepted framework consists of the ability to communicate a choice, factually understand the relevant issues, appreciate the situation and its likely consequences, and rationally manipulate information. Structured instruments for assessing capacity can be helpful but should never replace a thorough clinical evaluation. The instrument should also be appropriate to the clinical situation, patient population, and legal standard. The psychiatrist should be aware of the instrument's limitations. Patients with critical illnesses are at uniquely elevated risk for incapacity. Primary prevention of end-of-life conflicts surrounding treatment consists of careful planning. Patients can express their wishes in the event that they lose decision-making capacity by executing advance directives, powers of attorney, and living wills. In the event that there is no surrogate decision-maker, many state statutes define a succession of surrogate decision-makers. Conflicts sometimes arise between treatment teams and surrogate decision-makers based on values, interpretation of the patient's wishes, and medical opinion. These conflicts are best resolved through improved communication. If the conflict cannot be resolved between the parties, involving an ombudsman or review board can be helpful. As a last resort, courts can determine the appropriate course of action.

While any physician can and should be able to assess capacity, psychiatric consultation is appropriate in difficult or close cases. Psychiatrists are uniquely qualified to assess cognitive functioning, the impact of psychiatric illness on decision-making capacity, and rational thinking. Psychiatrists working in general medical settings have a unique opportunity to educate their colleagues about capacity assessment and to dispel some of the myths about decision-making capacity.

References

1 Seyfried L, Kerry A, Kim SYH: Assessment of decision-making capacity: views and experiences of consultation psychiatrists. Psychosomatics 2013;54:115–123.
2 Christensen K, Haroun A, Schneiderman LJ, Jeste DV: Decision-making capacity for informed consent in the older population. Bull Am Acad Psychiatry Law 1995;23:353–365.
3 Appelbaum PS: Assessment of patients' competence to consent to treatment. N Engl J Med 2007;357:1834–1840.
4 Appelbaum PS, Grisso T: Assessing patients' capacities to consent to treatment. N Engl J Med 1988;319:1635–1638.
5 Appelbaum PS, Gutheil TG: Clinical Handbook of Psychiatry and the Law. Philadelphia, Lippincott Williams & Wilkins, 2007.
6 Bursztajn HJ, Harding HP, Gutheil TG, Brodsky A: Beyond cognition: the role of disordered affective states in impairing competence to consent to treatment. Bull Am Acad Psychiatry Law 1991;19:383–388.
7 Folstein MF, Folstein SE, McHugh PR: Mini-Mental State Examination: a practical method for grading the cognitive states of patients for the clinician. J Psychiatr Res 1975;12:189–198.
8 Kim SYH, Caine ED: Utility and limits of the Mini Mental State Examination in evaluating consent capacity in Alzheimer's disease. Psychiatr Serv 2002;53:22–24.
9 Karlawish J: Measuring decision making capacity in cognitively impaired individuals. Neurosignals 2008;16:91–98.
10 Grisso T, Appelbaum PS, Hill-Fotouhi C: The MacCAT-T: a clinical tool to assess patients' capacities to make treatment decisions. Psychiatr Serv 1997;48:1415–1419.
11 Dunn LB, Nowrangi MA, Palmer BW, Jeste DV, Saks ER: Assessing decisional capacity for clinical research or treatment: a review of instruments. Am J Psychiatry 2006;163:1323–1334.
12 Sturman ED: The capacity to consent to treatment and research: a review of standardized assessment tools. Clin Psychol Rev 2005;25:954–974.
13 Janofsky JS, McCarthy RJ, Folstein MF: The Hopkins Competency Assessment Test: a brief method for evaluating patients' capacity to give informed consent. Hosp Community Psychiatry 1992;43:132–136.
14 Kapp MB, Mossman D: Measuring decisional capacity: cautions on the construction of a capacimeter. Psychol Public Policy Law 1996;2:73–95.
15 American Bar Association Commission on Law and Aging: Default Surrogate Consent Statutes as of November 2009. Washington, DC, American Bar Association, 2009. http://www.americanbar.org/content/dam/aba/migrated/aging/PublicDocuments/famcon_2009.authcheckdam.pdf (accessed July 23, 2014).
16 Ganzini L, Volicer L, Nelson W, Derse A: Pitfalls in assessment of decision-making capacity. Psychosomatics 2003;44:237–243.
17 Ganzini L, Volicer L, Nelson W, Fox E, Derse AR: Ten myths about decision making capacity. J Am Med Dir Assoc 2005;6:S100–S104.
18 Mendelson D: Roman concept of mental capacity to make end of life decisions. Int J Law Psychiatry 2007;30:201–212.
19 Sibbald RW, Chidwick P: Best interests at end of life: a review of decisions made by the Consent and Capacity Board of Ontario. J Crit Care 2010;25:171–177.
20 Derse AR: Making decisions about life sustaining medical treatment in patients with dementia: the problem of patient decision-making capacity. Theor Med Bioeth 1999;20:55–67.
21 Luce JM: End of life decision making in the intensive care unit. Respir Crit Care Med 2010;182:6–11.
22 Weiss BD, Berman EA, Howe CL, Fleming RB: Medical decision making for older adults without family. J Am Geriatr Soc 2012;60:2144–2150.
23 Torke AM, Sachs GA, Helft PR, Montz K, Hui SL, Slaven JE, Callahan CM: Scope and outcome of surrogate decision making among hospitalized older adults. JAMA Intern Med 2014;174:370–377.
24 Kolva E, Rosenfeld B, Brescia R, Comfort C: Assessing decision making capacity at end of life. Gen Hosp Psychiat 2014;36:392–397.
25 Guerts M, Macleod MR, Van Thiel GJ, Van Gijn, Kappelle LJ, Van der Worp HB: End of life decisions in patients with severe acute brain injury. Lancet 2014;13:515–524.
26 Luce JM, Alpers A: End of life care: what do the American courts say? Crit Care Med 2001;29(2 suppl):N40–N45.
27 Kapp MB: Medical decision making for incapacitated elders: a 'therapeutic interests' standard. Int J Law Psychiatry 2010;33:369–374.
28 Kirshner HS: Determination of mental competency: a neurological perspective. Curr Neurol Neurosci Rep 2013;13:356.
29 Bryant K, Skoaris LE, Smith B, Adelman EE, Meurer WJ: The accuracy of surrogate decision makers: informed consent in hypothetical acute stroke scenarios. BMC Emerg Med 2013;13:18.
30 Vig EK, Starks H, Taylor JS, Hopley EK, Fryer-Edwards K: Surviving surrogate decision making: what helps and hampers the experience of making medical decisions for others. J Gen Intern Med 2007;22:1274–1279.
31 Mayo AM, Wallhagen MI: Considerations of informed consent and decision making competence in older adults with cognitive impairment. Res Gerontol Nurs 2009;2:103–111.
32 Fritsch J, Petronio SM, Helft PR, Torke AM: Making decisions for hospitalized older adults: ethical factors considered by family surrogates. J Clin Ethics 2013;24:125–134.
33 Limehouse WE, Feeser VR, Bookman KJ, Derse A: A mode for emergency department end-of-life communications after acute devastating events – part I: decision making capacity, surrogates, and advance directives. Acad Emerg Med 2012;19:E1068–E1072.
34 Ferris FD, Von Gunten CF, Emanuel LL: Competency in end-of-life care: last hours of life. J Palliat Med 2003;6:605–613.
35 Valente SM: End of life challenges: honoring autonomy. Cancer Nurs 2004;27:314–319.
36 Olga R: Here we (neurologists) go again – brain death news invites some old, some new questions. Neurology Today 2014;14:5–6.

37 Chidwick P, Sibbald R, Hawryluck L: Best interests at the end of life: an updated review of decisions made by the Consent and Capacity Board of Ontario. J Crit Care 2013;28:22–27.

38 Kollas CD, Boyer-Kollas B: Evolving medico-legal issues in palliative medicie. J Palliat Med 2007;10:1395–1401.

39 Shalowitz D, Garrett-Mayer E, Wendler D: The accuracy of surrogate decision makers: a systematic review. Arch Intern Med 2006;166:493–497.

40 Bramstedt KA: Questioning the decision-making capacity of surrogates. Intern Med J 2003;33:257–259.

41 Kasman D: When is medical treatment futile? A guide for students, residents, and physicians. J Gen Intern Med 2004; 19:1053–1056.

42 Varma S, Wendler D: Medical decision making for patients without surrogates. Arch Intern Med 2007;167:1711–1715.

43 White DB, Curtis JR, Lo B, Luce JM: Decisions to limit life-sustaining treatment for critically ill patients who lack both decision-making capacity and surrogate decision-makers. Crit Care Med 2006; 34:2053–2059.

44 Fullbrook S: End-of-life challenges: honoring autonomy. Cancer Nurs 2004;16: 816–818.

45 Washington v. Glucksberg. 521 U.S. 702. U.S. Supreme Court, 1997.

46 Vacco v. Quill. 521 U.S. 793. U.S. Supreme Court, 1997.

47 Hall RCW, Hall RCW, Chapman M: Identifying geriatric patients at risk for suicide and depression. Clin Geriatr 2003;11:36–44.

48 Soliman S: Psychiatric consultation: legal issues in older psychiatric patients. Curr Psychiatr 2012;11:39–54.

Sherif Soliman, MD
Case Western Reserve University, School of Medicine, Northcoast Behavioral Healthcare
1756 Sagamore Rd.
Northfield, OH 44067 (USA)
E-Mail docsoli@gmail.com

Balon R, Wise TN (eds): Clinical Challenges in the Biopsychosocial Interface. Update on Psychosomatics for the 21st Century. Adv Psychosom Med. Basel, Karger, 2015, vol 34, pp 49–60 (DOI: 10.1159/000369839)

Then and Now ... HIV Consultation Psychiatry Update

Harold W. Goforth[a] • Matthew Bader[b] • Francisco Fernandez[c]

[a]Cleveland Clinic Foundation, Neurological Institute, Neurological Center for Pain, Department of Psychiatry & Psychology, Cleveland, Ohio, [b]Cognitive Psychiatry of Chapel Hill, Chapel Hill, N.C., and [c]School of Medicine, Medical Affairs, University of Texas Rio Grande Valley, Harlington, Tex., USA

Abstract

Over the last 2 decades, human immunodeficiency virus (HIV) illness has transformed to a chronic disease model. However, challenges, including the effects of co-morbid illnesses and the challenge of preventing future spread of the disease, continue to confront those infected with HIV. Addictions remain an important problem and a serious contributor to overall morbidity and mortality in this population. This book chapter seeks to illustrate the new developments in the treatment of these addictions as well as provide an overview of the medical updates regarding HIV and hepatitis C virus exposure prophylaxis and how they relate to the consultant psychiatrist.

Introduction

In the last 15 years, human immunodeficiency virus (HIV) infection has transformed from an often-seen, acute illness with shortened life expectancy and dismal prognosis to a disease that is most often addressed with a chronic-care model of disease, such as that for diabetes or chronic hypertension [1]. This chapter seeks to update the practitioner on the current medical concerns regarding HIV infection that may present to the consultant psychiatrist. This chapter will also focus on the medical updates concerning the ongoing management of HIV disease as well as on the updates regarding the overlying psychiatric issues commonly seen in HIV-infected patients, including substance abuse.

Substance Abuse Issues During Human Immunodeficiency Virus Infection

One of the more novel developments in substance abuse and HIV infection has been the emergence of HIV antiretroviral (ARV) drugs as a category of prescription drug misuse and abuse. A recent, excellent review looking at media reports over the last 5 years suggests that ARV drug diversion is a growing issue among drug-abusing individuals in large urban centers. Portions of this drug diversion appear to be due to the recreational value of ARV drugs; however, the drug diversion also appears to be due to enhancement of the intoxicating properties of other more commonly abused drugs by ARV medications. Reports from Durban, South Africa, note that mixtures of efavirenz and other drugs such as cannabis, cocaine or heroin, also known as whoonga, are mixed to enhance their intoxicating effects. Efavirenz appears to be the agent most often used in this manner due to its hallucinogenic potential and typical side effect of vivid dreams. Smoking efavirenz has been noted to produce multiple effects, including euphoria, dizziness, and a sense of depersonalization. This is not without controversy, as other small studies suggest that whoonga does not contain ARV substances but rather may be a mixture of other agents unrelated to HIV medications [2].

Another study of prescription drug diversion in Miami, FL, demonstrated that there was a significant market for ARV medications, although the motivation that supported this underground market was unclear. A survey of 25 HIV-seropositive men and women found that the majority had been approached on multiple occasions to sell their HIV medications, with many acknowledging that they had sold medications for cash or traded them for illicit drugs. Focus group participants also noted that medications such as ritonavir heightened the psychoactive effects of methamphetamine and ecstasy, that efavirenz was sought for its intoxicating properties, and that methamphetamine users were among the major purchasers of diverted HIV medications [2, 3].

Zidovudine, stavudine, lamivudine, nevirapine, efavirenz, and indinavir show high penetrance into the cerebrospinal fluid (CSF). Zidovudine in high doses has been linked to delusions, mania, and hallucinations. Abacavir has been associated via case reports with mood changes and hallucinations, and nevirapine and efavirenz have been linked to mania and hallucinations. Efavirenz remains the most widely abused ARV, and it is highly penetrant into the CSF, which is the same property that allows it to be such an effective ARV in the treatment of HIV [2].

Multiple case reports and series have described the potential neuropsychiatric effects of efavirenz, especially among naïve users. When initiating this agent for treatment of HIV, up to 90% of users have vivid dreams or nightmares, and this appears to correlate with the effective CSF concentration of the agent. Over a period of 3 months, the incidence of these side effects is markedly reduced, and after 3 months, only approximately 5% of individuals continue to have these dreams. Isolated case reports indicate that this agent may trigger mania, suicidality, hallucinations, and psychosis in susceptible individuals. These side effects, however, are relatively rare and do not appear to be systematically present in studied populations [4].

Cannabis Abuse and Human Immunodeficiency Virus

There are reports of combining cannabis and HIV medications – efavirenz – to produce heightened euphoria via CYP3A4 inhibition and of the resultant, slowed elimination of cannabis toxins from the body. While efavirenz has been most commonly noted to induce the CYP3A4 enzyme, this process occurs over days to weeks following an immediate period of CYP3A4 inhibition. This initial inhibition followed by induction is another potential reason for the production of the early neuropsychiatric side effects of efavirenz, which diminish over time. For sporadic abusers of cannabis/efavirenz combinations, however, CYP3A4 inhibition by efavirenz is likely to produce heightened levels of delta-9-THC and immediate increased drug effects for the occasional user [2].

Opioid and Human Immunodeficiency Virus Epidemiology

Treatment of opioid dependence in acute inpatient medical units is becoming more common with the proliferation of opioid abuse in the United States and with the growing availability of illicit opioids such as heroin [5, 6]. Substance abuse issues are coming to the forefront of consultation liaison psychiatry and now represent one of the most common reasons for psychiatric consultation in inpatient medical-surgical units. Acute opioid withdrawal is generally characterized by two phases: (a) acute withdrawal and (b) prolonged abstinence. The acute withdrawal syndrome tends to last from 5 to 14 days, depending upon the half-life of the opioid, and consists of gastrointestinal distress, insomnia, myalgias & arthralgias, anxiety, dysphoria, and thermal dysregulation. This acute syndrome is not life-threatening in the absence of other co-occurring medical issues, although it is severely uncomfortable, which can provoke continued opioid use [7].

Opioid-based, medically supervised withdrawal can be accomplished in an inpatient medical-surgical unit, with the substituted opioid being slowly weaned to avoid precipitating acute withdrawal. Methadone is the most commonly used opioid for medical withdrawal because of its long half-life and once-daily administration. However, methadone has significant properties, including QTc prolongation, which can make it difficult to use, if not outright contraindicated, with co-occurring illnesses such as cardiovascular disease in the medical setting. Care must also be taken to avoid methadone accumulation over the initial few days, which would result in iatrogenic overdose. Outpatient withdrawal using methadone must be performed in a federally licensed opioid treatment program, which complicates its use in most medical-surgical settings. For individuals already participating in a methadone-treatment program, their home dose of methadone can be continued while they are admitted to a medical-surgical hospital but cannot be tapered or altered, except in cases of medical necessity [7].

Other options for the treatment of opioid withdrawal and dependence include buprenorphine, which also has a long half-life. Buprenorphine has been approved for office-based, medically supervised withdrawal, so it can be used in the general medical-surgical hospital setting without the same restrictions as methadone. For individuals demonstrating iatrogenic opioid dependence in the setting of chronic pain (prescription opioids), one can substitute any long-acting agent, such as morphine extended-release capsules (Kadian), and gradually taper their use each day [7, 8].

It is the practice of some consultation programs to utilize only nonopioid-based management of withdrawal while in medical-surgical units. This can be done but has generally been associated with a higher degree of patient discomfort than opioid-based protocols. Clonidine is an alpha-2-agonist that has been shown to diminish opioid withdrawal symptoms and is most effective for suppressing autonomic signs and symptoms of opioid withdrawal. Regimens of 0.1–0.2 mg orally every 4 h have been suggested in clinical trials based on tolerability and blood pressure monitoring. Other adjuvants, including antimotility agents for diarrhea and antinausea agents for nausea & vomiting, may be required if using a clonidine-based opioid withdrawal protocol. Lofexidine, which is a centrally acting alpha-2-agonist, has been extensively studied for use in opioid withdrawal and appears to be more sparing of blood pressure effects than clonidine [7].

In addition to the setting of acute withdrawal, which is likely to be encountered by consultant psychiatrists, one is more likely to encounter patients in the maintenance phase of treatment, given the increasing prevalence of opioid-use disorders. Medications used in this phase may include chronic opioid replacement therapy with buprenorphine or methadone, intramuscular depot formulations of naltrexone, oral naltrexone, or the combination of these in the setting of pregnancy and acute pain crises. Naltrexone is an opioid antagonist that provides essentially complete blockade of opioid receptors and can be administered orally or with an intramuscular depot formulation. It essentially blocks the reinforcing properties of opioids and is nonaddicting, so it is becoming a preferred alternative for ongoing opioid maintenance treatment. However, clinical retention rates are low for this agent and average 20–30% at 6 months. Additionally, craving for opioids may continue during naltrexone treatment, and at least one meta-analysis has shown no support for this treatment modality. In unusual circumstances, naltrexone has been shown to be associated with liver injury that resolves with discontinuation of the offending agent. Therefore, monitoring of hepatic function tests is required when using this form of therapy. Additionally, naltrexone cannot be used in individuals currently receiving opioids, as it will provoke immediate opioid withdrawal. Ultimately, naltrexone therapy appears to be similar to the use of disulfiram in alcohol-dependent patients, in that it is useful for a small but highly motivated cohort of individuals who wish to avoid opioid replacement therapy for their opioid dependence [7, 9, 10].

Methadone-based opioid replacement therapy has long been the standard of care for heroin addiction treatment in HIV-seropositive individuals, and it is devoid of significant long-term side effects, with the exception of hypogonadism and QTc prolongation with risk of progression to torsades de pointes. This therapy has been associated with good treatment retention, improved psychosocial adjustment, and reduction in criminal activity. It has also been shown to reduce injection-associated risk factors that contribute to HIV seroconversion as well as improve combination antiretroviral therapy (cART) adherence and HIV-based outcomes, even in HIV/hepatitis C virus (HCV) coinfection models [7, 11].

Daily methadone doses of greater than 60 mg are the norm, and it appears that patients maintained on higher doses perform better than those on lower doses. Factors that influence the breakdown of methadone include the presence of chronic disease, such as hepatic dysfunction and chronic renal disease, and medication interactions. This is especially true for HIV- and tuberculosis-based therapies, such as rifampin and efavirenz, and antiepileptics, such as phenytoin and carbamazepine. Finally, alterations in physiology, such as pregnancy, can also result in increased methadone needs. Individuals receiving methadone replacement therapy also have high rates of other drug abuse, including cocaine and alcohol (30–40%), which may increase the risk of complicated withdrawal syndromes when admitted to general medical-surgical units [7].

When faced with an acute pain syndrome in a methadone-maintained patient, it is important to realize that one is dealing with an already highly opioid-tolerant individual. The patient's standard daily dose of methadone should be maintained throughout hospitalization, if medically safe, and this can be done effectively in the medical-surgical setting. Failure to maintain the person on their home regimen will precipitate opioid withdrawal. Any opioid-based medication used to treat acute pain should be administered in addition to the patient's regularly scheduled methadone, and an increase in total morphine oral equivalents of 20% should be considered a reasonable starting point for these patients to treat acute pain syndromes [7].

Buprenorphine has been shown to be an effective alternative to methadone for opioid replacement therapy in HIV populations. Buprenorphine treatment produces significant and substantial improvements in psychosocial functioning over time and can aid the pursuit of sobriety by stabilizing cravings in early abstinence. It is significantly safer in overdose, and its partial agonism may limit abuse and diversion liability. It is safer in the setting of medical disease in that it has fewer effects on respiratory depression than full agonists as well as a more favorable QTc effect on electrocardiogram. Buprenorphine appears effective for the concurrent treatment of either acute or chronic pain, with a reduction in opioid sensitization that appears to occur with full agonists via agonism of the opioid-like receptor [12].

There have been reports of opioids being combined with HIV medications, but from a pharmacological perspective, there is little interaction between these two classes of drugs. The most commonly abused illicit opioid is heroin, which is metabolized through plasma esterases to morphine and then glucuronidated and excreted. Therefore, there would not be any expected increase in the potency or half-life of these agents with enzyme inhibitors. Among the iatrogenically provided and abused agents, oxycodone is primarily metabolized by CYP2D6, and hydrocodone utilizes both CYP2D6 and CYP3A4 for its metabolism to hydromorphone. A CYP2D6 inhibitor such as ritonavir could theoretically increase oxycodone levels but would also theoretically decrease hydromorphone levels in the setting of hydrocodone abuse by preventing the conversion of hydrocodone to a more potent opioid. While CYP3A4 inhibitors could potentially increase methadone levels, methadone is commonly recognized as one of the least euphorigenic opioids. Additionally, consistent blending of efavirenz or nevirapine with methadone has been demonstrated to markedly reduce the effective blood concentrations of methadone to the point of provoking opioid withdrawal by inducing CYP3A4. Little clinically significant interaction has been seen with buprenorphine and ARV agents [2].

3,4-Methylenedioxymethamphetamine and Club Drugs and Human Immunodeficiency Virus

3,4-Methylenedioxymethamphetamine (Ecstasy; MDMA) remains one of the most popular club drugs and has been associated with heightened rates of HIV among regular users [13]. MDMA is primarily metabolized via CYP2D6, and concomitant administration with a CYP2D6 inhibitor such as ritonavir can lead to potentially toxic increases in amphetamine exposure. Cases linking ritonavir to cases of fatal MDMA use have been reported and are supportive of this potential drug-drug interaction. All protease inhibitors can inhibit CYP3A4, so this potentially fatal combination needs to be noted when evaluating these individuals during a consultation psychiatry service. Similar patterns of toxicity have been identified in case studies of 4-hydroxybutanoic acid poisoning [2].

New Guidelines for Human Immunodeficiency Virus Exposure

In October 2014, the New York State Department of Health AIDS Institute published an update on HIV prophylaxis following occupational and other exposures. Post-exposure prophylaxis (PEP) is supported by several clinical studies that demonstrated significantly reduced transmission rates following administration of retroviral agents. Vertical transmission rates between mother and child were dramatically decreased in studies in which single-dose nevirapine was administered at the time of delivery compared to zidovudine treatment. A Centers for Disease Control (CDC) retrospective, case-control study of zidovudine use demonstrated an 81% risk reduction following occupational HIV exposure in healthcare workers. Currently, the CDC and other expert bodies recommend a three-drug regimen for all significant risk exposure to ensure the suppression of viral replication and to shift the biologic advantage to the host cellular immune system [14, 15].

Following inoculation with the virus, experimental models suggest a stepwise progression of local HIV replication in tissue macrophages or dendritic cells at the site of viral entry. In 2–3 days, the viral replication pattern spreads to the lymph nodes, and viremia occurs within 3–5 days following inoculation. This process has major implications for PEP and illustrates that regimens with the most rapid onset of activity, multiple sites of antiviral action, and the greatest strength are potentially most effective [14, 16].

Viral transmission rates following inoculation vary depending upon the source of entry and the viral load of the contributing source. The estimated probability of contracting HIV following a blood transfusion is 90+%, but percutaneous needle stick injuries appear to result in only a 0.3% risk. Mucosal exposures to infected sources are orders of magnitude lower and have been estimated to be 0.09%. Other exposures, including biting, spitting, and exchange of bodily fluids, have a negligible risk of transmission [14].

The Medical Care Criteria committee now recommends tenofovir + emtricitabine plus either raltegravir or dolutegravir as the preferred initial PEP regimen. Zidovudine is no longer recommended as the preferred PEP regimen because of its significantly higher rates of side effects and it having no clear advantage over more tolerable regimens. All of these agents block HIV replication prior to viral integration with the cellular DNA, which provides a theoretical advantage for preventing the establishment of HIV infection [14].

Of the ARV drugs, efavirenz should be avoided as a component of PEP because its central nervous system (CNS) side effects complicate the need to be able to provide an initial dose at any point during the day. These CNS effects may impair one's ability to return to work following the initial and subsequent doses. Efavirenz use also needs to be avoided in pregnant women or women of childbearing potential who are not using effective birth control. Substantial efavirenz resistance is found in community samples of HIV isolates. Nevirapine is contraindicated in PEP due to risk of hepatotoxicity, and abacavir should not be used due to the risk of hypersensitivity reactions. Furthermore, elfinavir, indinavir, stavudine, and didanosine should not be used in PEP due to poor tolerability and risk of toxicities, and CCR5 co-receptor antagonists should not be used due to lack of activity against CXCR4 tropic virus. Rilpivirine and etravirine have not been commonly used in PEP, so data are lacking regarding these agents [14].

In addition to the new PEP medication recommendations, plasma HIV RNA testing of the source patient is recommended with HIV serological screening in settings where the source patient's HIV screening test is negative. However, if the risk for HIV exposure in the previous 6 weeks or if the HIV screening is positive but the confirmatory assay is nonreactive or indeterminate, PEP should be continued until the results of the plasma HIV RNA assay are available [14].

Studies have demonstrated improved tolerability and increased rates of adherence when tenofovir + emtricitabine/lamivudine have been used as components of the ARV regimen. This combination has been highly successful in recent studies of pre-exposure prophylaxis [14].

Occupational exposure requires urgent medical evaluation, and one should strive to initiate PEP as soon as possible, ideally within 2 h of exposure. The first dose of PEP should be offered immediately while the evaluation is underway and should never be delayed while awaiting information about the source patient or results of the baseline HIV test. Baseline HIV testing should always be obtained following an occupational exposure, even in the setting of an exposed patient declining PEP. Repeat HIV serological testing should be repeated at 4 and 12 weeks, and routine testing at 6 months is no longer recommended. If the source patient is known to be infected with HIV or refuses HIV testing, the exposed patients should complete a 28-day regimen, unless they are showing signs of HIV viral conversion, in which case, the treatment may be extended for a longer duration. If the source patient is known to be HIV positive and his/her present ART experience, current level of viral suppression, or resistance profile is known, then the treating clinician may be able to individualize the PEP regimen in consultation with an experienced provider who is knowledgeable about HIV and PEP [14].

Individuals who are on PEP should use condoms during this time to prevent potential sexual transmission, avoid pregnancy and breastfeeding, avoid needle sharing, and refrain from donating blood, plasma, organs, tissue, or semen. Acute

HIV infection typically occurs within 2–4 weeks following exposure and will present with symptoms largely consistent with influenza, including fever; however, rash, mucocutaneous ulcers, thrush, and meningismus are more specific for the HIV seroconversion reaction. The CDC currently recommends fourth-generation antibody/antigen combination immunoassays for initial HIV screening, which can simultaneously detect HIV1 and HIV2 antibodies and HIV1 p-24 antigens and will generally be positive within 2 weeks of infection. Western blotting is no longer recommended as the confirmatory test. Instead, an HIV1/HIV2 antibody-differentiation assay is now the recommended test for confirmatory analysis [14].

When occupational exposure occurs, the source patient should be evaluated for both Hepatitis B and C. The risk of transmission of hepatitis B virus (HBV) following a needle stick is upwards of 30%, and the risk of HCV following a needle stick is approximately 1.8%. The hepatitis B vaccine series should be initiated in non-HBV immune-exposed workers who are exposed to blood or bodily fluids from a source patient with acute or active HBV infection; afterwards, hepatitis B immunoglobulin (HBIG) should be administered. Both should ideally be administered within 24 h of exposure, but HBIG should be administered no later than 14 days following exposure. Administration of the HBV vaccine series within 12–24 h of exposure has been demonstrated to be between 70 and 90% effective in preventing HBV infection, and HBIG treatment provides a similar level of efficacy. Neither immunoglobulin nor antivirals are recommended for HCV PEP. Early detection of infection and treatment of acute HCV with an interferon-based regimen is highly effective – upwards of 98%, but no randomized controlled trials exist to guide this acute treatment of HCV infection [14].

Nonoccupational exposure to HIV is managed in a similar manner to occupational exposure, but it is worthwhile for consultant psychiatrists to be familiar with this, as they may encounter these situations more readily than occupational exposures in their practice. The most effective way to prevent HIV transmission is to protect against exposure by limiting unsafe practices, but nonoccupational PEP (nPEP) can be a way to prevent HIV transmission when HIV exposure does occur. nPEP is based upon data for occupational exposure, but there is a lack of definitive evidence concerning its efficacy to support this practice [14].

nPEP should incorporate a systematic assessment of HIV risk following exposure, HIV and sexually transmitted disease testing and treatment, prevention and risk-reduction counseling, clinicians with expertise in the administration of ART, and timely access to the initiation of nPEP. It is recommended that, when deciding whether to administer nPEP, the clinician should assess the patient's risk of HIV acquisition based on exposure type, and nPEP should not be prescribed when there is a negligible or very low risk of transmission. Additionally, nPEP should not be dismissed solely on the basis of repeated high-risk behavior. Rather, those individuals who have high rates of high-risk behavior should have more intensive counseling, education, and preventive services. If the high-risk behaviors continue, then the patient can be assessed for pre-exposure prophylaxis [14].

High-risk exposures include receptive and insertive vaginal or anal intercourse, needle sharing, and injuries with exposure to blood or other potentially infected fluids. A case-by-case analysis of oral-vaginal contact, oral-anal contact, and all types of oral-penile contact should be undertaken. Factors that may increase this risk include high viral loads of the source person, nonintact oral mucosa, blood exposure, or the presence of a genital ulcer or other sexually transmitted disease. If any of these mitigating factors are present, then nPEP should be offered. No-risk exposures include kissing, oral-oral contact without mucosal damage, human bites not involving blood, exposure to solid-bore needles or sharps not in recent contact with blood, and mutual masturbation in the absence of skin breakdown or blood exposure [14].

If nPEP is recommended, then it should be initiated as soon as possible, with a goal of 2 h, but within 36 h of exposure, and it should involve the same recommended regimen of tenofovir + emtricitabine plus raltegravir or dolutegravir, as used in PEP. Baseline testing of the exposed person should include HIV, pregnancy testing, *Neisseria gonorrhoeae/Chlamydia trachomatis* tests, and rapid plasma regain tests. Baseline and follow-up testing for HIV, HBV, and HCV remain the same as with occupational exposure [14].

Hepatitis C and Human Immunodeficiency Virus Co-Infection: Updates

With the initiation of ARV in 1996 and the transformation of HIV into a model of sustained control and chronic disease, patients have had markedly decreased HIV-associated morbidity and mortality. However, liver disease as a result of chronic HCV co-infection has emerged as an important cause of morbidity and mortality that is not associated with acquired immune deficiency syndrome (AIDS) in HIV-infected patients. It is estimated that approximately one-quarter of all HIV patients have concurrent HCV infection [17].

In the absence of treatment, HIV/HCV co-infection leads to faster progression to hepatic fibrosis, and this is especially true in those with an AIDS-defining condition. This faster progression has been hypothesized to be secondary to the direct fibrotic effect of HCV on the liver and a consequence of HIV on the innate and adaptive immune systems leading to inflammation, apoptosis, and fibrosis. Successful control of HIV can lead to a slowing of the pro-fibrotic effect of HIV; therefore, it is important to keep dually infected individuals well treated and in a state of clinical control. However, in spite of successful HIV treatment, patients do progress, with a portion developing frank cirrhosis and hepatocellular carcinoma. Treatment of HCV remains a high priority in the comorbidly infected [17, 18].

Treatment of HCV was revolutionized with the use of pegylated interferon and ribavirin combination therapy (PegIFN/RBV). However, among patients with HCV genotype 1 or 4, the sustained virological response rates were disappointingly low and averaged 25–35%. Direct-acting antivirals (DAAs) against HCV have again marked a sea change for the treatment of HCV and have increased treatment responses to 60–80%. However, treatment of HCV in HIV-infected individuals remains complex, given that there appears to be higher rates of adverse events and difficult drug-drug interactions between DAAs and highly active antiretroviral therapy [17, 19].

A phase IIa double-blind study of 98 HCV-genotype 1/HIV patients investigated the safety and efficacy of boceprevir in combination with PegIFN/RBV. More than 90% of the patients were taking protease inhibitor-based therapies and had largely undetectable viral loads. At the end of week 24, 63% had a sustained virological response compared to 29% of the control group. However, the boceprevir group had more adverse events, including anemia, pyrexia, anorexia, dysgeusia, vomiting, and neutropenia [17, 20].

A similar phase IIa study looking at the role of telaprevir in HIV/HCV-infected patients found that the patients responded at a rate of 74 vs. 45%. Two patients experienced HCV breakthrough due to telaprevir-resistant variants, but no patient receiving ARV therapy experienced HIV breakthrough. ARV exposure was not significantly modified by telaprevir, and serious adverse events occurred in 5% of the group receiving telaprevir vs. 0% of the control group. Both pilot trials demonstrated superior outcomes in dually infected patients receiving DAA-based HCV therapy [17, 21].

Other studies have addressed the role of DAAs in patients with HIV/HCV coinfection who had been previously exposed to PegIFN/RBV therapy and who failed to demonstrate or sustain a complete response. The patients started with a 4-week lead-in of PegIFN/RBV, and then telaprevir was added for 12 weeks. Baseline CD4 counts and viral loads were within the normal range and undetectable, respectively, in these patients. Eighty-eight percent of the patients achieved undetectable HCV RNA levels at the end of week 16; and grade 3–4 anemia, erythropoietin use, transfusion, or RBV dose reduction was recorded in 61% of individuals, but treatment effect and size based on ART or previous response type to PegIFN/RBV did not appear to matter. A second trial looking at the use of boceprevir in triple ARV therapy in this population found that 63% achieved undetectable HCV levels at week 15. Anemia occurred in 42% of the patients, but only 5% developed Grade 3–4 anemia. Forty-two percent of the patients received concomitant erythropoietin. Both studies demonstrated early treatment response rates independent of baseline fibrosis stage, although it remains to be seen whether relapse following discontinuation of therapy is higher for HIV/HCV comorbid patients than other patient groups or whether the sustained virological response can be maintained for a long-term cure [17, 22].

The cure rates for HCV therapy during HIV co-infection have been demonstrated to increase with improving baseline CD4 counts. HIV RNA also appears to be independently associated with improved sustained virological response rates to anti-HCV therapies. In patients with CD4 counts less than 500 cells/mm^3, early ART initiation is recommended to optimize HCV outcome. In patients who are not currently receiving ART, only those with CD4 counts greater than 500 should be considered for HCV therapy. Telaprevir can only be safely combined with boosted atazanavir, raltegravir, maraviroc, rilpivirine, etravirine, or efavirenz used in combination with tenofovir, abacavir, or emtricitabine vs. with lamivudine, while boceprevir can only be safely combined with raltegravir, rilpivirine, or etravirine in combination with tenofovir, abacavir, or emtricitabine vs. with lamivudine. Other DAAs are currently in the approval process and are anticipated to be brought to market in the coming months. Given these complexities of care, it is important that these patients be managed in major centers that have experience in managing co-infected HIV/HCV patients [17, 23].

Drug-Drug Interactions in the Setting of Hepatitis C Virus Treatment

Cytochrome P450 is the main enzyme for the metabolism and oxidation of medications, and this, combined with conjugation, allows most medications to be excreted with the bile or urine. It has been noted that antidepressants, sedatives, and antipsychotics are frequently used by individuals at risk for HCV. The majority of these agents are metabolized by cytochrome P450 2D6, 3A4, and 2C19. The area under the curve (AUC) for escitalopram was reduced by approximately 35%, but the telaprevir concentration was not significantly affected. No relevant interactions between escitalopram and boceprevir have been observed. Hence, it is thought that escitalopram can be safely used with both DAA agents. However, agents relying upon CYP3A4 metabolism show significant increases in AUC concentrations, with the AUC concentrations of triazolam being increased by almost 800% and 430% with telaprevir and boceprevir, respectively. Alprazolam showed a 35% increase in the presence of telaprevir. Other agents having a substantial drug-drug interaction with DAAs include fluoxetine, paroxetine, sertraline and, to some extent, mirtazapine. Olanzapine is metabolized by 1A2, so it is considered safe when used in combination with DAAs [24].

Methadone has high protein binding and is metabolized primarily by CYP3A4. Telaprevir and boceprevir were noted to increase the AUC by 29 and 22%, respectively, by displacing protein-bound methadone, but dose adjustment is not recommended, except in individual cases. Similarly, buprenorphine appears to be safe in these combinations, with its AUC being increased by 4% with telaprevir and by 19% with boceprevir, and there were no significant changes in the concentrations of the DAAs. No pharmacological data are available with respect to their impact upon heroin concentrations, but given that it is metabolized by CYP3A4, an increase in drug levels is possible and of concern for potentially increasing the risk of heroin overdose [24, 25].

Marijuana compounds are unlikely to be significantly affected by the presence of a DAA, in that they are metabolized via multiple routes. Amphetamine, cocaine, and ecstasy, however, are, in part, substrates of CYP3A4 and CYP2D6 and have a low toxicity threshold, so concomitant use should be avoided. Barbiturates are generally metabolized by CYP3A4 and can be strong inducers of CYP3A4, likely resulting in significant increases in barbiturate levels and decreases in DAA levels [24, 26].

Updates in Human Immunodeficiency Virus-Associated Cognitive Disorders

In 2007, the National Institute of Mental Health and National Institute of Neurological Disorders and Stroke updated the HIV-associated neurocognitive disorder (HAND) criteria to define three stages of increasing severity of cognitive impairment that are associated with HIV infection: HIV-associated asymptomatic neurocognitive impairment (ANI), HIV-associated mild neurocognitive disorder and HIV-associated dementia (HAD). The incidence of HAD has decreased markedly with the advent of cART, but the incidences of ANI and mild neurocognitive disorders have increased. Similarly, prior to cART therapy, the progression to HAD was a predictor of deaths within months, but now, individuals with HAND remain stable for many years. Other studies note that individuals with HAND may suffer a fluctuating course from abnormal to normal over the course of their illness [27].

Aging remains an important contributor to the overall clinical impact of HIV on cognition, and by 2015, it is estimated that half of all HIV-seropositive individuals will be older than 50 years of age. More than 75% of seropositive individuals die from non-HIV related disease, and this has enormous implications for the care of aging HIV-seropositive individuals in that cognitive dysfunction will begin to have multiple contributors, such as non-HIV-related cerebrovascular disease and primary dementing illness. Already, data demonstrate an increase in amnestic neurocognitive disorders among older individuals with HIV compared to their seronegative counterparts. Motor symptoms of HIV infection have been noted to decrease in individuals on cART, but with aging, there may be an increase in motor signs with a concurrent increase in subcortical diseases of aging, such as Parkinson's disease [27, 28].

Asymptomatic neurocognitive impairment is an increasingly important diagnostic category, although not without controversy. Some believe that the incidence of neurocognitive disorders in HIV patients are overestimated by this category. However, evidence supports the presence of neuronal injury occurring early in the course of HIV disease, even when individuals remain asymptomatic. Those with ANI are 2–5 times more likely than others to progress to symptomatic neurocognitive impairment, which illustrates the need to identify these individuals and screen for other potential causes of impairment and treatment early in the course of disease [27, 29].

Treatment of HAND is largely via the initiation or optimization of cART with agents that have superior penetration into the CNS. However, this approach is controversial, and randomized data comparing highly penetrant CNS regimens with those that are less penetrant do not appear to demonstrate superior outcomes with HAND, even though the data do demonstrate improved CNS HIV viral suppression. Other controversial data show that individuals who were followed for approximately 3 years and who began highly

CNS-penetrant cART had actual increases in the risk of HAD, suggesting a potential deleterious effect from CNS exposure to these agents. Additional trials and observational data are required prior to being able to issue definitive recommendations regarding the use of these agents [27].

Numerous small trials have examined the utility of non-cART agents in modifying the course of HAND, including memantine, minocycline, selegiline, and nimodipine, but all failed to demonstrate sustained benefit. Both valproate and lithium, which affect glycogen synthase kinase-3 beta and the selective serotonin reuptake inhibitors paroxetine and citalopram, have been hypothesized to down-regulate HIV replication and neuroinflammation, but they have also failed to demonstrate clinical benefit. Trials on rivastigmine failed to show benefit in terms of cognitive performance, but there were some secondary improvements in processing speed and executive function. To date, the therapeutic options for HAND appear limited to none [27, 30–32].

Conclusion

HIV-AIDS psychiatry and medicine, as it relates to consultation-liaison psychiatry, has been transformed in recent years. Highly active antiretroviral therapy has transformed the management of HIV into that of a chronic disease. However, the burdens of hepatitis C and its associated infections remain problematic and life-limiting for a significant proportion of patients. Now, with the advent of new therapies directed towards HCV, this serious disease is also slowly coming under control. Addictions in the HIV, HCV, and HIV/HCV populations perhaps remain the most challenging problems of all, and this group is the most likely to experience life-limiting infections and succumb to death as a direct result of ongoing substance abuse. Future treatment will require additional data-based addiction practices for the optimal care of this group of individuals.

References

1 Maartens G, Celum C, Lewin SR: HIV infection: epidemiology, pathogenesis, treatment, and prevention. Lancet 2014; 384:258–271.

2 Davis GP, Surratt HL, Levin FR, Blanco C: Antiretroviral medication: an emerging category of prescription drug misuse. Am J Addict 2014;23:519–525.

3 Inciardi JA, Surratt HL, Kurtz SP, Cicero TJ: Mechanisms of prescription drug diversion among drug-involved club- and street-based populations. Pain Med 2007;8:171–183.

4 Kenedi CA, Goforth HW: A systematic review of the psychiatric side-effects of efavirenz. AIDS Behav 2011;15:1803–1818.

5 Jones CM, Paulozzi LJ, Mack KA: Alcohol involvement in opioid pain reliever and benzodiazepine drug abuse-related emergency department visits and drug-related deaths – United States, 2010. MMWR Morb Mortal Wkly Rep 2014; 63:881–885.

6 Chen LH, Hedegaard H, Warner M: Drug-Poisoning Deaths Involving Opioid Analgesics: United States, 1999–2011. NCHS Data Brief, No. 166. Hyattsville, MD, National Center for Health Statistics, 2014.

7 Stine SM, Kosten TR: Pharmacologic interventions for opioid dependence; in Ries RK, Fiellin DA, Miller SC, Saitz R (eds): The ASAM Principles of Addiction Medicine, ed 5. Philadelphia, Wolters Kluwer Publishers, 2014, pp 735–758.

8 Fingerhood MI, King VL, Brooner RK, Rastegar DA: A comparison of characteristics and outcomes of opioid-dependent patients initiating office-based buprenorphine or methadone maintenance treatment. Subst Abus 2014;35:122–126.

9 Di Paola A, Lincoln T, Skiest DJ, Desabrais M, Altice FL, Springer SA: Design and methods of a double blind randomized placebo-controlled trial of extended-release naltrexone for HIV-infected, opioid dependent prisoners and jail detainees who are transitioning to the community. Contemp Clin Trials 2014; 39:256–268.

10 Dennis BB, Naji L, Bawor M, Bonner A, Varenbut M, Daiter J, Plater C, Pare G, Marsh DC, Worster A, Desai D, Samaan Z, Thabane L: The effectiveness of opioid substitution treatments for patients with opioid dependence: a systematic review and multiple treatment comparison protocol. Syst Rev 2014 DOI: 10.1186/2046-4053-3-105.

11 Wang M, Mao W, Zhang L, Jiang B, Xiao Y, Jia Y, Wu P, Cassell H, Vermund S: Methadone maintenance therapy and hiv counseling and testing are associated with lower frequency of risky behaviors among injection drug users in China. Subst Use Misuse 2015;50:15–23.

12 Fiellin DA, Weiss L, Botsko M, Egan JE, Altice FL, Bazerman LB, Chaudhry A, Cunningham CO, Gourevitch MN, Lum PJ, Sullivan LE, Schottenfeld RS, O'Connor PG; BHIVES Collaborative: Drug treatment outcomes among HIV-infected opioid-dependent patients receiving buprenorphine/naloxone. J Acquir Immune Defic Syndr 2011; 56(suppl 1):S33–S38.
13 Palamar JJ, Kiang MV, Storholm ED, Halkitis PN: A qualitative descriptive study of perceived sexual effects of club drug use in gay and bisexual men. Psychol Sex 2014;5:143–160.
14 New York State Department of Health. HIV prophylaxis following occupational exposure. http://www.hivguidelines.org/clinical-guidelines/post-exposure-prophylaxis/hiv-prophylaxis-following-occupational-exposure/ (accessed November 4, 2014).
15 Kuhar DT, Henderson DK, Struble KA, Heneine W, Thomas V, Cheever LW, Gomaa A, Panlilio AL; for the US Public Health Service Working Group: Updated US Public Health Service guidelines for the management of occupational exposures to human immunodeficiency virus and recommendations for postexposure prophylaxis. Infect Control Hosp Epidemiol 2013;34:875–892.
16 Clerici M, Levin JM, Kessler HA, Harris A, Berzofsky JA, Landay AL, Shearer GM: HIV-specific T-helper activity in seronegative healthcare workers exposed to contaminated blood. JAMA 1994;271:42–46.
17 Rockstroh JK, Bhagani S: Managing HIV/hepatitis C co-infection in the era of direct acting antivirals. BMC Med 2013;11:234.
18 Lacombe K, Rockstroh J: HIV and viral hepatitis coinfections: advances and challenges. Gut 2012;61(suppl 1):i47–i58.
19 Rodriguez-Torres M, Slim J, Bhatti L, Sterling R, Sulkowski M, Hassanein T, Serrão R, Sola R, Bertasso A, Passe S, Stancic S: Peginterferon alfa-2a plus ribavirin for HIV-HCV genotype 1 coinfected patients: a randomized international trial. HIV Clin Trials 2012;13: 142–152.
20 Sulkowski MS, Sherman KE, Dieterich DT, Bsharat M, Mahnke L, Rockstroh JK, Gharakhanian S, McCallister S, Henshaw J, Girard PM, Adiwijaya B, Garg V, Rubin RA, Adda N, Soriano V: Combination therapy with telaprevir for chronic hepatitis C virus genotype 1 infection in patients with HIV: a randomized trial. Ann Intern Med 2013; 159:86–96.
21 Cotte L, Braun J, Lascoux-Combe C, Vincent C, Valantin MA, Sogni P, Lacombe K, Neau D, Aumaitre H, Batisse D, de Truchis P, Gervais A, Michelet C, Morlat P, Vittecoq D, Rosa I, Bertucci I, Chevaliez S, Aboulker JP, Molina JM; for the French National Agency for Research on AIDS and Viral Hepatitis (ANRS) HC26 Study Group: Telaprevir for HIV/hepatitis C virus-coinfected patients failing treatment with pegylated interferon/ribavirin (ANRS HC26 TelapreVIH): an open-label, single-arm, phase 2 trial. Clin Infect Dis 2014;59: 1768–1776.
22 Poizot-Martin I Bellissant E, Piroth L, Renault A, Quertainmont Y, Rosenthal E, Alric L, Guyader D, Bourliere M, Molina J, ANRS-HC27 BOCEPREVIH Study Group: ANRS-HC27 BOCEPREVIH interim analysis: high early virologic response with boceprevir + pegylated interferon + ribavirin in hepatitis c Virus/HIV co-infected patients with previous failure to pegylated interferon + ribavirin. 20th Conference on Retroviruses and Opportunistic Infections, Atlanta. 2013. Abstract 37.
23 Martel-Laferrière V, Bichoupan K, Dieterich DT: Hepatitis C direct-acting antiviral agents: changing the paradigm of hepatitis C treatment in HIV-infected patients. J Clin Gastroenterol 2014;48: 106–112.
24 Mauss S, Klinker H: Drug-drug interactions in the treatment of HCV among people who inject drugs. Clin Infect Dis 2013;57(suppl 2):S125–S128.
25 Burger D, Back D, Buggisch P, Buti M, Craxí A, Foster G, Klinker H, Larrey D, Nikitin I, Pol S, Puoti M, Romero-Gómez M, Wedemeyer H, Zeuzem S: Clinical management of drug-drug interactions in HCV therapy: challenges and solutions. J Hepatol 2013;58:792–800.
26 Hariparsad N, Nallani SC, Sane RS, Buckley DJ, Buckley AR, Desai PB: Induction of CYP3A4 by efavirenz in primary human hepatocytes: comparison with rifampin and phenobarbital. J Clin Pharmacol 2004;44:1273–1281.
27 Sacktor N, Robertson K: Evolving clinical phenotypes in HIV-associated neurocognitive disorders. Curr Opin HIV AIDS 2014;9:517–520.
28 Brew BJ, Chan P: Update on HIV dementia and HIV-associated neurocognitive disorders. Curr Neurol Neurosci Rep 2014;14:468.
29 Grant I, Franklin DR Jr, Deutsch R, Woods SP, Vaida F, Ellis RJ, Letendre SL, Marcotte TD, Atkinson JH, Collier AC, Marra CM, Clifford DB, Gelman BB, McArthur JC, Morgello S, Simpson DM, McCutchan JA, Abramson I, Gamst A, Fennema-Notestine C, Smith DM, Heaton RK; CHARTER Group: Asymptomatic HIV-associated neurocognitive impairment increases risk for symptomatic decline. Neurology 2014;82:2055–2062.
30 Simioni S, Cavassini M, Annoni JM, Métral M, Iglesias K, Rimbault Abraham A, Jilek S, Calmy A, Müller H, Fayet-Mello A, Giacobini E, Hirschel B, Du Pasquier RA: Rivastigmine for HIV-associated neurocognitive disorders: a randomized crossover pilot study. Neurology 2013; 80:553–560.
31 Schifitto G, Zhong J, Gill D, Peterson DR, Gaugh MD, Zhu T, Tivarus M, Cruttenden K, Maggirwar SB, Gendelman HE, Dewhurst S, Gelbard HA: Lithium therapy for human immunodeficiency virus type 1-associated neurocognitive impairment. J Neurovirol 2009;15:176–186.
32 Ances BM, Letendre SL, Alexander T, Ellis RJ: Role of psychiatric medications as adjunct therapy in the treatment of HIV associated neurocognitive disorders. Int Rev Psychiatry 2008;20:89–93.

Harold W. Goforth, MD
Cleveland Clinic Foundation, Neurological Institute, Center for Functional Restoration
9500 Euclid Ave, C-21
Cleveland, OH 44195 (USA)
E-Mail goforth@ccf.org

Balon R, Wise TN (eds): Clinical Challenges in the Biopsychosocial Interface. Update on Psychosomatics for the 21st Century. Adv Psychosom Med. Basel, Karger, 2015, vol 34, pp 61–77 (DOI: 10.1159/000369085)

Fibromyalgia and Chronic Fatigue: The Underlying Biology and Related Theoretical Issues

Graziella F. Romano[a] · Simona Tomassi[b] · Alice Russell[a] · Valeria Mondelli[a] · Carmine M. Pariante[a]

[a]Stress, Psychiatry and Immunology Laboratory, Department of Psychological Medicine, Institute of Psychiatry, King's College London, London, UK; [b]Section of Psychiatry, Department of Public Health and Community Medicine, University of Verona, Verona, Italy

Abstract

There is an increasing interest in understanding the biological mechanism underpinning fibromyalgia (FM) and chronic fatigue syndrome (CFS). Despite the presence of mixed findings in this area, a few biological systems have been consistently involved, and the increasing number of studies in the field is encouraging. This chapter will focus on inflammatory and oxidative stress pathways and on the neuroendocrine system, which have been more commonly examined. Chronic inflammation, together with raised levels of oxidative stress and mitochondrial dysfunction, has been increasingly associated with the manifestation of symptoms such as pain, fatigue, impaired memory, and depression, which largely characterise at least some patients suffering from CFS and FM. Furthermore, the presence of blunted hypothalamic-pituitary-adrenal axis activity, with reduced cortisol secretion both at baseline and in response to stimulation tests, suggests a role for the hypothalamic-pituitary-adrenal axis and cortisol in the pathogenesis of these syndromes. However, to what extent these systems' abnormalities could be considered as primary or secondary factors causing FM and CFS has yet to be clarified.

Introduction

In recent years, an increasing amount of attention has been given to further understanding the biology underlying fibromyalgia (FM) and chronic fatigue syndrome (CFS). CFS is a complex, debilitating disorder that is characterised by persistent fatigue lasting for at least 6 months and is neither related to overexertion nor alleviated by rest. Associated symptoms, such as cognitive impairment, flu-like symptoms, muscle and joint pain in the absence of swelling, and unrefreshing sleep, must also be present to a degree [1–3]. FM is also complex, causing significant disability in those individuals who suffer from the condition. In contrast to CFS, FM is predominantly characterised by widespread pain; however, overlapping symptoms with CFS include cognitive impairment, sleep disturbances, and a persistent lack of energy [4, 5]. Indeed, it has been proposed that such similar disorders be considered on a continuum, as opposed to distinct diagnoses: that is, to be viewed according to a dimensional approach, as opposed to a categorical approach [6].

Biological, psychological, and social factors have been implicated in the pathogenesis and the maintenance of these disorders, although the degree to which each of these factors contributes to these processes has been a source of debate, with more debate arising in recent years as further biological evidence has mounted [7, 8]. Indeed, research in the field has increasingly focussed on the biological processes putatively underlying these disorders, in an attempt to make further progress in understanding the mechanisms that may lead to advances in treatment and improvement of outcomes. The current paucity of treatment options has contributed to the increased level of disability, and without a medical explanation for their symptoms, patients feel increasingly stigmatised. To date, the results of biological studies are mixed, largely due to unclear diagnoses at recruitment, the heterogeneity of the diagnostic criteria applied, small sample sizes, and a small number of studies examining each biological mechanism proposed. Despite this, some replicated findings are emerging, and the increasing number of studies in the field is encouraging. As such, this chapter will focus on the inflammatory and oxidative stress pathways and the neuroendocrine system, as these biological systems are more commonly examined and have somewhat clearer results.

The Role of the Immune System and Its Implication in Chronic Fatigue Syndrome/Fibromyalgia

The main recognised role of the immune system is the defence of the human body against pathogens and infections. It is divided into two subsystems: innate and adaptive/acquired immunity. The innate immune system reacts to pathogen-associated molecular patterns by activating the production and secretion of inflammatory mediators, such as histamines, prostaglandins, bradykinin, serotonin, and leukotrienes. These factors attract macrophages that release cytokines, namely, tumour necrosis factor (TNF)-α, interleukin (IL)-1, and IL-6, in order to prolong the systemic inflammatory response and stimulate the adaptive/acquired immune system. The latter system principally functions to create and maintain the immune system's memory and is mainly mediated by T and B cells, or lymphocytes playing a central role in cell-mediated immunity [9]. Furthermore, IL-6 stimulates the release of acute-phase proteins such as C-reactive protein (CRP), which originates in the liver. Under normal circumstances, inflammation is accompanied by an anti-inflammatory response. IL-4 and IL-10 are among the factors contributing to decreased production of TNF-α, IL-1, IL-6, and IL-8 and are defined as anti-inflammatory cytokines. However, comorbidities and other factors can influence a patient's ability to respond appropriately [10].

Interestingly, the increased production of pro-inflammatory cytokines can contribute to the development of a range of symptoms and behavioural changes that both humans and animals experience when affected by physical illnesses and that resemble those in CFS/FM. These changes and symptoms are often referred to as 'sickness behaviour' and include symptoms such as fatigue, pain, low mood, and cognitive impairment. While this is an evolutionary adaptive response during infection because it facilitates the body's fight against virus or bacteria, more recently, it has been suggested that when such changes occur in the absence of infection, they may contribute to pathology [11]. Administration of TNF-α and IL-1β in rats and mice induces dose- and time-dependent behavioural changes typical of sickness behaviour: the animals tend to stay in a corner of their cage and lose interest in the physical and social environment, and decreased motor activity and reduced food and water intake are also observed. Furthermore, they show increased pain sensitivity and decreased resistance to forced exercise, induced mostly by IL-1 administration [12, 13]. Similarly, cytokine-based immunotherapy with interferon-α in patients affected by hepatitis C virus induces similar symptoms, such as depression; severe fatigue; and somatic symptoms, including pain. In patients undergoing interferon-α treatment, both depression and fatigue show a correlation with high levels of pro-inflammatory cytokines [14, 15] and are influenced by genetic variants in immune genes [16, 17]. Of interest, blocking pro-inflammatory status with medications has been found to alleviate fatigue and pain in patients with rheumatoid arthritis and psoriasis [18, 19]. Such evidence for the role of inflammation in these symptoms forms part of a growing body of research, with several studies reporting activation of the immuno-inflammatory pathway in a considerable number of psychiatric disorders [20, 21] and chronic illnesses characterised by chronic, unexplained fatigue [22–24]. Evidence for increased inflammation in CFS/FM will now be discussed.

Elevated Inflammatory Markers in Chronic Fatigue Syndrome/Fibromyalgia

Increased levels of pro-inflammatory cytokines, such as IL-1β, TNF-α, and IL-6, have been reported in people affected by CFS; in these subjects, IL-1 and TNF-α levels were significantly positively correlated with fatigue, sleep, appetite disturbances, and flu-like symptoms [25, 26]. Raised levels of anti-inflammatory and immunosuppressive cytokines, such as IL-10 and transforming growth factor-β1, have also been shown in CFS patients [27, 28], although another study observed lowered transforming growth factor-β1 production [29]; these conflicting data may have resulted from different methodological approaches, with the last study measuring levels of cytokines in vitro rather than in vivo. Other molecules triggered by cytokines that have been observed to be elevated in CFS patients include lysozyme and polymorphonuclear neutrophil elastase (enzymes secreted by leukocytes) and cyclooxygenase (COX)-2 and neopterin (synthesised by macrophages) [30]. Furthermore, elevated levels of cytokines, such as IL-1, TNF-α, IL-6, IL-8, and IL-10, have been found in FM patients, suggesting that activation of the pro-inflammatory pathway contributes to the pathogenesis of both CFS and FM [31, 32]. A study reported high levels of IL-10 at night time, showing a correlation with sleep disturbances and unrefreshing sleep [33]. Interestingly, a second study then reported that levels of IL-10 were inversely correlated with the duration of sleep and that this correlation was stronger in patients with comorbid CFS/FM [34]. Finally, a strong correlation between higher levels of IL-8 and pain intensity has been reported in FM patients [35, 36].

Higher levels of CRP have also been detected in the blood of CFS patients compared with healthy controls [37–39]. Interestingly, patients suffering from CFS have a similar CRP profile as subjects experiencing fatigue who do not meet the criteria for CFS, suggesting a possible association with the symptom of fatigue, rather than with the syndrome specifically. Serum CRP levels have also been found to be higher in FM patients compared with healthy controls, showing a significant correlation with body mass index, the erythrocyte sedimentation rate, and IL-8 and IL-6 levels. Again, these findings suggest that inflammation plays a role in causing symptoms in both CFS and FM patients, especially when comorbid with obesity [31, 40].

Evidence of T cell subset alterations have also been reported in CFS patients [41, 42]. Elevated expression of CD38 and CD8 on T cells has been described [43], although a recent study showed higher expression of CD4 and reduced CD8/CD38 activity [44]. Reduced numbers and activity of natural killer (NK) cells have also been described [45, 46]. NK cells can be considered as the primary defence against pathogen invasion and may act as a regulator of autoimmunity by controlling T cell proliferation, activation, and differentiation. Furthermore, a recent review suggested that NK cells play a role in the pathogenesis of autoimmune diseases such as systemic lupus erythaematosus and multiple sclerosis [47]. Notably, raised levels of autoimmune markers have also been detected in CFS patients, such as higher numbers of mature CD19-, CD20- and CD21-expressing B cells, accompanied by increased production of antibodies against 5-hydroxytryptamine receptor 1A, dopamine receptor D2, cholinergic receptor muscarinic 1, and opioid receptor mu 1 [48, 49]. Hypogammaglobulinaemia, i.e., a deficiency of immunoglobulin G (IgG) 1 and IgG3, has also been observed in CFS patients. This condition may predispose an individual to chronic inflammation and recurrent infections due to dysfunction of the humoral response in adaptive immunity [50]. As in CFS, the presence of antibodies against serotonin and thromboplastin has also been reported in FM patients [51].

Another feature that may predispose an individual to chronic inflammation is a decreased ratio of omega 3 to omega 6 (ω3/ω6), which are types of polyunsaturated fatty acids (PUFAs). A PUFA is a type of fatty acid implicated in the pathogenesis of inflammation through the production of chemical mediators such as prostaglandin, thromboxane, and leukotriene as a consequence of its degradation. Notably, anti-inflammatory properties characterise ω3, whereas ω6 is pro-inflammatory. Indeed, a decreased ratio of ω3/ω6 has been shown in CFS patients [52]. Additionally, higher levels of free fatty acids, with low content of PUFAs, have been reported in FM patients [53].

Further support for the role of inflammation in CFS and FM comes from studies examining gene expression as well as genetic polymorphisms. Immune-related genes are differentially modulated in the blood of CFS patients [54–56]. Moreover, a TNF-α gene allele associated with increased inflammation has been shown to be more prevalent among patients who suffer from CFS [57].

A recent review highlighted the possibility of a role for the tryptophan pathway in the pathogenesis of CFS and FM, in view of the inflammation-induced shift in tryptophan catabolism towards the production of neurotoxic catabolites [58]. There have been two studies on tryptophan catabolism in CFS and FM patients, reporting conflicting data: one reporting no difference between CFS patients and healthy controls [59] and the other reporting low levels of tryptophan in the CFS group [60]. However, increased tryptophan degradation seems to be positively correlated with the severity of fatigue symptoms and with the prevalence of somatic symptoms in depressed and non-depressed patients [61]. Tryptophan catabolism is induced by two enzymes, indoleamine 2,3-dioxygenase and tryptophan 2,3-dioxygenase, which are activated by increased inflammation. Indoleamine 2,3-dioxygenase is mainly expressed in microglia and other immune cells, while tryptophan 2,3-dioxygenase is mainly expressed in hepatic cells, astrocytes, and neurons. Enhanced tryptophan catabolism results in its decreased availability for serotonin and in increased production of tryptophan catabolites such as kynurenic acid and quinolinic acid. Quinolinic acid has an excitotoxic effect on the glutamate N-methyl-D-aspartate receptor, the stimulation of which may result in hyperalgesia and central sensitisation, defined as an increased sensitivity to pain. Drugs blocking the glutamate N-methyl-D-aspartate receptor have been shown to be beneficial for pain in patients affected by FM and CFS [62].

The main findings about the immune system in CFS/FM are summarised in table 1.

Oxidative Stress and Mitochondrial Dysfunction in Chronic Fatigue Syndrome and Fibromyalgia

According to the literature, the putative chronic pro-inflammatory status in patients affected by CFS and FM is accompanied by an increased level of oxidative and nitrosative stress. This occurs as a result of the increased production of nitrates,

Table 1. Immune markers

	CFS	FM
Pro-Inflammatory cytokines	↑ IL-1β, TNF-α, IL-6	↑ TNF-α, IL-1, IL-6, IL-8
Anti-inflammatory/ immunosuppressive cytokines	↑ IL-10, TGF-β1	↑ IL-10 at night time
Acute-phase proteins	↑ CRP	↑ CRP
T and B cells	↑ $CD8^+$, $CD38^+$, $CD4^+$, $CD19^+$, $CD20^+$, $CD21^+$	
Antibodies	Anti: 5-HTR1A, DRD2, CHRM1, OPRM1, 5HT ↓ IgG1, IgG3	Anti: 5HT and thromboplastin
NK cells	↓ Number and activity of NK cells	
Pro-inflammatory Cytokines induced Tryptophan Metabolism	↑ Quinolinic acid ↓ Serotonin	↓ Serotonin
Fatty acids	↓ ω3/ω6 (ratio)	↑ Free fatty acids ↓ PUFAs

TGF-β1 = transforming growth factor-β1; 5-HTR1A = 5-hydroxytryptamine receptor 1A; DRD2 = dopamine receptor D2; CHRM1 = cholinergic receptor muscarinic 1; OPRM1 = opioid receptor mu 1, 5HT = 5-hydroxytryptamine.

such as nitrogen monoxide (NO) and peroxynitrite (ONOO), and reactive oxygen species (ROS), such as hydrogen peroxide (H_2O_2) and the superoxide radical (O^{2-}), in neutrophils and macrophages. This increased presence of nitrates and ROS can cause DNA fragmentation and membrane lipid oxidation [42]. The most important source of ROS in mammalian cells is the mitochondrion. It is in the mitochondrion that the principal production of adenosine triphosphate (ATP), the energy source of the human body, takes place through a system called the 'respiratory chain', which consists of a number of reductive and oxidative reactions combined with electron carriers that proceed to form molecular oxygen (O_2) [63] (see fig. 1). Under normal circumstances, ROS in mitochondria are generated through the progression of reductive and oxidative reactions but are neutralised by the scavenger activity of antioxidants. However, if the equilibrium between antioxidants and the oxidative status is compromised, the accumulation of ROS may damage the structure of the mitochondria, leading to dysfunction in the production of O_2 and ATP, which leads to cell death (apoptosis). Muscle and nerve cells are especially sensitive to mitochondrial defects because they need so much ATP and O_2 to function normally [64, 65].

In recent years, there has been an increasing interest in studying oxidative and nitrosative stress, together with mitochondrial dysfunction, as contributing factors to the pathogenesis of CFS and FM [66]. A recent review hypothesised that enhanced production of ROS, together with a chronic pro-inflammatory status, may cause impairment in mitochondrial function and the production of ATP in patients affected by CFS and FM. Indeed, a broad range of symptoms present in mitochondrial disorders, like intense malaise, fatigue, muscle weakness, cramps, pain, migraine, memory impairment, depression, and

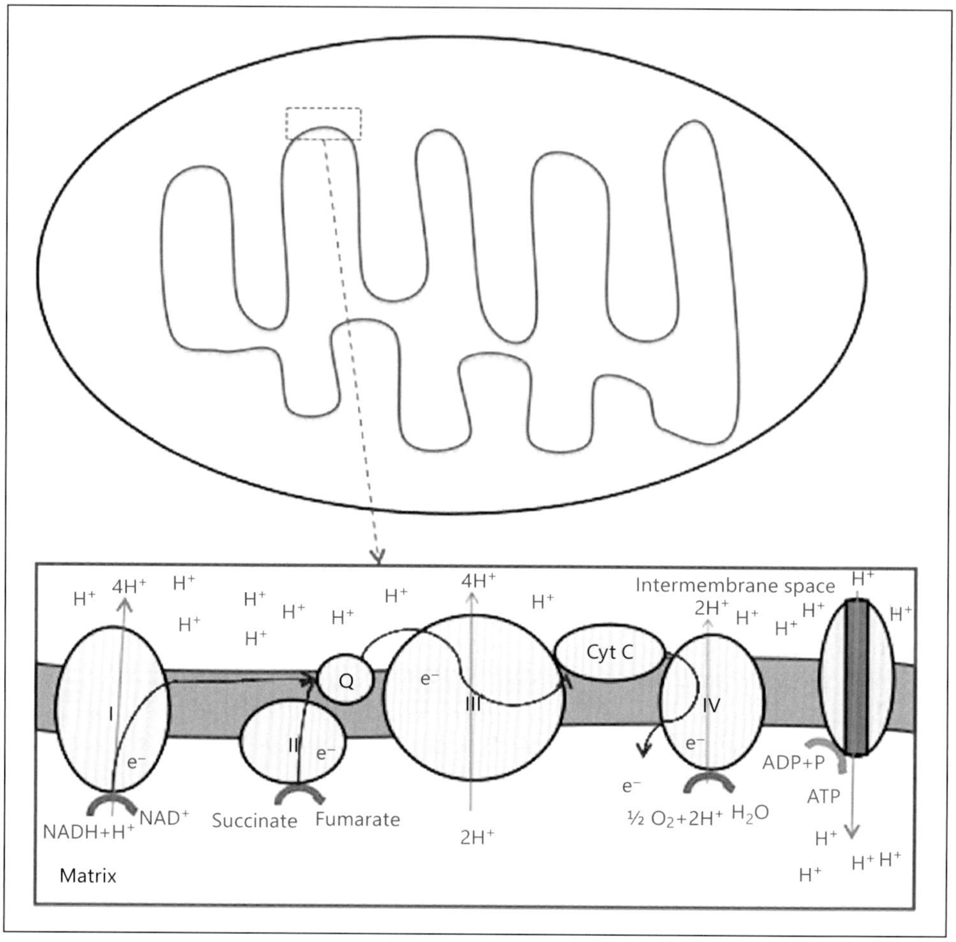

Fig. 1. Mitochondrial respiratory chain: A mitochondrion is bounded by two membranes, namely, the outer and inner membranes, which create two compartments: an internal one, called the 'matrix', and an external one, called the 'intermembrane space'. The latter is characterised by a composition similar to that of the cytosol because the outer membrane is rich in porins, which allow the passage of ions through it. Conversely, the inner membrane, organized into cristae, is impermeable to ions and contains a series of catalysts that form the respiratory chain, a system responsible for the generation of ATP. The respiratory chain consists of four complexes, named I, II, III, and IV in the figure, in which reductive and oxidative reactions take place. Electrons from NADPH and the other oxidisable substrates pass through the chain of complexes and carriers such as cytochrome C (Cyt C) and coenzyme Q (Q) in the inner membrane. The electron flow is accompanied by proton transfer across the membrane, producing both a chemical gradient and an electrical gradient. Due to the impermeability of the inner mitochondrial membrane to protons, protons can re-enter the matrix only through proton-specific channels that are coupled with ATP synthase (Murray, Granner, Mayes and Rodwell, 1999; Nelson and Cox, 2004).

exercise intolerance, are also detectable in CFS and FM patients. This similarity has led to the hypothesis that mitochondrial dysfunction is a possible factor in the onset of CFS and FM [67]. Evidence for mitochondrial dysfunction and for the presence of oxidative stress in CFS/FM will be discussed.

Pro-Oxidative Stress Status Mediators in Chronic Fatigue Syndrome/Fibromyalgia

In CFS patients, higher levels of COX-2 and inducible NO synthase (iNOS), an enzyme responsible for the intracellular production of NO, have been found to be positively related to aches and pains, a subjective feeling of infection, fatigue, muscular tension, failing memory, difficulties in concentration, and sadness [68]. Furthermore, significant positive correlations have been detected between levels of COX-2, iNOS, and nuclear factor-kB and the severity of the illness [68]. Both COX-2 and nuclear factor-kB have been previously reported to play a role in the production of nitrates and ROS [69, 70]. Moreover, increased levels of iNOS in the muscle cells of FM patients have been found to be negatively correlated with exercise [71]. In support of findings linking markers of oxidative stress with cognitive impairment, overexpression of COX-2 has also been found to be positively related to cognitive deficits in ageing-related disease [72, 73]. This suggests a role for COX-2 hyper-activity in the pathogenesis of both pain and cognitive symptoms in CFS/FM patients.

Several studies have shown a decreased antioxidant status in CFS/FM patients, as indicated by lower zinc, coenzyme Q_{10} (CoQ_{10}), glutathione, and dehydroepiandrosterone sulphate plasma levels (see Lorusso [41]). Perhaps the most frequently observed of these markers, CoQ_{10} is a strong antioxidant that confers resistance to mitochondrial damage induced by oxidative and nitrosative stress. Moreover, CoQ_{10} has neuroprotective properties, protecting neural cells against central neurotoxic damage. Lower plasma levels of CoQ_{10} have been found in depressed patients with comorbid CFS in comparison with depressed patients without CFS [74]. Low levels of CoQ_{10} in FM patients are also correlated with more severe headache and with higher levels of lipid peroxidation, a marker of ROS. Notably, in another study, supplementation with CoQ_{10} led to a significant recovery of oxidative stress levels and marked improvement in headache [75, 76].

Glutathione is another antioxidant that is upregulated by the transcription factor p53 following oxidative stress. A recent review reported low levels of glutathione as being positively correlated with the increased presence of oxidative stress in patients affected by CFS and depression [77]. Moreover, loss of p53 activity and transcription, as detected in CFS and FM patients, can impair mitochondrial function by reducing the activity of the respiratory chain and reducing the expression of genes encoding enzymes with antioxidant functions. This may result in a significant increase in intracellular ROS, which in turn may cause oxidative and nitrosative stress-mediated damage to mitochondria and mitochondrial DNA. Furthermore, loss of p53 can decrease exercise capacity and increase fatigability because skeletal muscle and brain cells have high metabolic rates and are very sensitive to ATP deprivation [78]. Low levels of CoQ_{10} have been detected in the peripheral blood mononuclear cells, skeletal muscle cells, and skin cells of CFS and FM patients [79–81].

The levels of products of oxidation, such as oxidised low-density lipoprotein, 8-isoprostaglandin, and F2α-isoprostane, have been reported to be significantly increased in those CFS patients who reported the most severe postexertional malaise and severe joint pain [82]. Furthermore, urinary F2-isoprostane has been found in FM patients who experience higher levels of fatigue [83]. While not products of oxidation themselves, peroxides are one type of ROS that can be found in peripheral blood and that indicate the presence of oxidative stress. Significant increments in peroxide levels, indicative of increased oxidative stress, have been detected in CFS patients, showing a positive correlation to symptoms such as headache. The levels of peroxides in CFS patients also correlate positively with levels of anti-oxidised low-density lipoprotein IgG, indicating that oxidation of LDL may depend on lipid peroxidation [84]. Significant correlations between oxygen consumption during exercise and increasing levels of oxidation products of polyunsaturated fatty acids, such as thiobarbituric acid-reactive substances, have also been detected in CFS patients [85]. Additionally, high levels of methaemoglobin, an oxidised form of haemoglobin, have been found in CFS patients [86]. Finally, nitration causes chemical modifications to proteins, creating NO derivatives such as nitro-tyrosine, nitrophenylalanine, nitro-arginine, nitro-tryptophan, and nitro-cysteine, which can elicit an autoimmune reaction. High levels of immunoglobulin M (IgM) against these compounds have been detected in CFS patients, potentially leading to a chronic, systemic inflammatory state [50, 87]. In CFS patients, raised levels of both IgM directed against oxidised fatty acids and toxic compounds resulting from the peroxidation of membrane lipids, such as malondialdehyde, have been found to be positively correlated with the severity of aches and pain, muscular tension, and fatigue [88].

Mitochondrial dysfunction and abnormal production of ATP have also been described in CFS/FM patients. The available data have been obtained mainly from white blood cells and muscle cells [89]. A limited number of studies addressing mitochondrial dysfunction in the muscle in CFS are available, and the data are conflicting; only some of these studies have shown abnormal mitochondrial degeneration and severe oxidative stress damage in mitochondrial DNA, resulting in decreased production of ATP and increased lactate concentrations. In FM, several studies have reported mitochondrial dysfunction in white blood cells and muscle cells using electron microscopy (see Klein and Berg [87]). During exercise, the production of lactate is greater in CFS patients, which may indicate a pathological response to demand for ATP [90–92]. Assessments of cardiac and peripheral muscle energetic and metabolic function have also been conducted in CFS patients by measuring the levels of phosphocreatine and ATP; positive correlations between PCr/ATP ratios and skeletal and cardiac muscle function in CFS patients demonstrate impaired bio-energetic function of both the skeletal and cardiac muscles, suggesting a shared underlying dysfunction in energy production. Another method for measuring the efficiency of ATP production is the ATP profile; using this technique, mitochondrial dysfunction has been observed in the neutrophils of CFS patients, accompanied by a lack of substrates or essential co-factors [93] and correlating with the severity of the illness [90].

The main findings about oxidative stress and mitochondrial dysfunction in CFS/FM are shown in table 2.

Hypothalamic-Pituitary-Adrenal Axis Abnormalities and Chronic Fatigue Syndrome/Fibromyalgia

Another biological system extensively studied in CFS/FM is the neuroendocrine system [94], and the hypothalamic-pituitary-adrenal (HPA) axis in particular. Broadly, the endocrine system coordinates functions among different organs through hormones (peptides, steroids, or amino acid derivatives) released into the bloodstream from the endocrine glands. Hormones determine the maintenance of homeostasis and affect target tissues' functions by binding selectively to receptors located inside or on the surface of cells. The HPA axis is one of the main neuroendocrine axes and is directly relevant to the biological responses to stress. Hypothalamic corticotropin-releasing hormone (CRH), one of the neurohormones produced in the paraventricular nucleus of the hypothalamus, reaches the anterior pituitary (called

Table 2. Oxidative and nitrosative stress and mitochondrial dysfunction markers

	CFS	FM
Oxidative stress products	↑ Ox-LDL, 8-isoprostaglandin, F2α-isoprostane, peroxides, Met-Hb, TBARS	↑ F2α-isoprostane
Anti-oxidants	↓ CoQ_{10}, glutathione	↓ CoQ_{10}
Antibodies vs. oxidative and nitrosative stress products	Anti: Oxidised fatty acids, MDA, nitro-tyrosine, nitro-phenylalanine, nitro-arginine, nitro-tryptophan, nitro-cysteine	Anti: Oxidised fatty acids and MDA
Enzymes	↑ COX-2, iNOS	
Transcription factors	↑ NF-kB ↓ p53	↓ p53
Mitochondrial dysfunction	↑ Lactic acid ↓ ATP, mtDNA	↓ ATP, mtDNA

Ox-LDL = oxidised low-density lipoprotein; Met-Hb = methaemoglobin; TBARS = thiobarbituric acid-reactive substances; MDA = malondialdehyde; NF-kB = nuclear factor-kB; mtDNA = mitochondrial DNA.

adenohypophysis) through a specialised portal vascular system and stimulates the synthesis and release of adrenocorticotropic hormone (ACTH) in the bloodstream. ACTH then acts on the fasciculate zone of the adrenal glands, inducing the release of glucocorticoids, such as 11-deoxycorticosterone, corticosterone, and cortisol. The glucocorticoids in turn act on the hypothalamus and pituitary levels through a negative feedback mechanism to suppress CRH and ACTH production [95]. The circadian secretion of cortisol starts with increasing cortisol secretion in the second part of the night and a peak in cortisol levels in the early morning hours, followed by a subsequent decline throughout the day, with the lowest levels during the first half of the night [96].

Hypothalamic-Pituitary-Adrenal Axis Activity in Chronic Fatigue Syndrome/Fibromyalgia

As mentioned above, the HPA axis is involved in controlling responses to stress; inducing behavioural changes [96]; and affecting many fundamental bodily functions, including immune system activity, mood and energy storage, and energy/fatigue [21, 97, 98]. The relevance of cortisol levels to CFS/FM was first considered based on the observation that conditions characterised by altered levels of glucocorticoids, such as Addison's and Cushing's diseases, have similar core symptoms, including fatigue, arthralgia, myalgia, sleep problems, and mood disturbances [99]. Furthermore, short-term fatigue seems to be alleviated by low doses of glucocorticoids [100]. The first study in which the presence of a mild adrenocortical insufficiency (low plasma cortisol levels) was described in patients with chronic fatigue was published in 1981 [101]. A decade later, Demitrack and colleagues [102] described a significant reduction of urinary free cortisol excretion over 24 hours and reduced basal glucocorticoid plasma levels in the evening. Moreover, they reported a lower ratio of ACTH/cortisol during stimulation with CRH, adrenocortical hyper-responsiveness to low-dose ACTH, and an attenuated response to higher doses of ACTH. More recently, several reviews on this topic have confirmed the evidence that HPA axis alterations might play a fundamental role in the development of CFS/FM [97, 103, 104]. Whether these abnormalities are a cause, a consequence, or a maintaining factor is, however, still under debate. We will now summarise this evidence.

While cortisol levels can be assessed in plasma, urine, and saliva, the third measurement has the advantage of being a more naturalistic test since it can be conducted at home, without the stress of venepuncture. The cortisol awakening response (CAR) and the cortisol circadian profile are the two measures most frequently used in conjunction with assessment of salivary cortisol levels. The CAR is a discreet and distinct component of the cortisol circadian cycle, independent of the circadian profile; it is a physiological response to the arousal of awakening, and it is considered to be a marker of the ability of the body to respond to stress [105]. This response is defined as a rapid increase in cortisol levels within 20–30 minutes after awakening in the morning [95].

In 2004, Roberts and colleagues [106], followed by Nater and colleagues in 2008 [107], found a reduced CAR; however, in the latter study, this was found to be present only in women, and not in men. Two recent studies found a reduced CAR in a large group of adolescents with CFS and in subjects with CFS and a history of childhood traumatic experience, with CFS patients without such a history showing normal cortisol levels [108, 109]. This seems to suggest a significant role for childhood trauma in influencing and shaping the individual stress response in the context of CFS [110]. With regard to the circadian levels, Strickland and colleagues [111] found significantly lower evening cortisol levels and a trend of lower morning cortisol levels in 1998. Furthermore, in 2005, Jerjes et al. [112] found that the amplitude (defined as half of the difference between nadir and peak) and the midline estimate statistic of rhythm (defined as the rhythm-adjusted mean salivary cortisol) were both significantly lower in CFS compared with controls. However, in 2009, Papadopoulus et al. [113] demonstrated significantly raised basal cortisol output in CFS compared with controls, independent of the presence or absence of depression. In contrast, previous studies found no differences in either the CAR or the circadian levels of salivary cortisol between CFS and controls [114–116]. More recently, Papadopoulus and Cleare reviewed results from studies measuring cortisol in blood samples and again found heterogenic results [103].

HPA axis stimulation and suppression tests aim to elucidate the mechanisms underlying putative HPA axis abnormalities. Commonly used stimulation tests are the insulin tolerance test, the Trier Social Stress Test, and the single-dose metyrapone test, measuring the HPA axis responses to hypoglycaemia, to an experimental psychological stress, and to a pharmacologically induced decrease in cortisol levels, respectively. In 2004, Gaab and colleagues [117] investigated insulin tolerance test results in CFS patients and found no differences in plasma or saliva cortisol levels but did find lower ACTH levels, correlating with increased duration and severity of CFS symptoms. A year later, using the Trier Social Stress Test, the same group also found significantly reduced ACTH levels in CFS patients [118]. At the same time, another study reported a reduced cortisol peak in response to ACTH testing and in 11-deoxycortisol response to metyrapone [119]. These results are consistent with those described in the literature, showing a reduced salivary cortisol response after dexamethasone suppression/CRH testing in CFS patients [120]. In contrast, only one study found no changes in plasma ACTH or cortisol in response to any challenge test performed [121].

The dexamethasone suppression test and the prednisolone suppression test can assess HPA feedback regulation and the related function of the glucocorticoid and mineralocorticoid receptors (the receptors for cortisol). Available data show significantly reduced salivary cortisol after both tests in CFS patients, indeed providing evidence for an enhanced negative feedback mecha-

Table 3. HPA axis abnormalities

	CFS	FM
Basal cortisol levels	↓ CAR ↓ Cortisol profile	↓ CAR ↓ Cortisol profile
Stimulation tests	↓ Cortisol after ITT and TSST ↓ Cortisol after ACTH and CRH test (hypo-responsiveness)	↓ Cortisol after ACTH test and ITT ↑ ACTH after CRH test Delayed ACTH release after IL-6 test (hypo-responsiveness)
Suppression test	↓ Cortisol after DST and PST (hyper-responsiveness)	↓ Cortisol after DST (hyper-responsiveness)

ITT = Insulin tolerance test; TSST = Trier Social Stress Test; DST = dexamethasone suppression test; PST = prednisolone suppression test.

nism as a result of hyper-responsiveness of both the glucocorticoid [116] and mineralocorticoid [122] receptors. Further support for these findings comes from in vitro studies [123, 124]. A history of early-life stress [125] and the presence of comorbid depression [113] appear to influence the results.

Studies on FM are again characterised by inconsistent findings. Several studies, reviewed recently by Tak and colleagues [104], have been conducted to analyse plasma and urine basal cortisol levels, with no clear or consistent results; for example, one study has shown increased basal saliva cortisol levels, while two other studies have shown a decreased CAR [104, 126–128], and yet others have shown no HPA axis abnormalities [129, 130]. Studies using stimulation tests have shown enhanced ACTH release after CRH release [131–133] and a lower peak cortisol level after ACTH release [134, 135] and exercise [136, 137]. Finally, the only study exploring the HPA axis response to a suppression test with dexamethasone again has shown decreased cortisol plasma levels in FM patients [138]. Taken together, the data indicate that it is clear that there is a degree of overlap in HPA abnormalities between CFS and FM.

The main findings about HPA axis abnormalities in CFS/FM are shown in table 3.

Summary of Findings and Concluding Remarks

We summarise all potential mechanisms in the model illustrated in figure 2. Overall, the large number of studies examining putative biological mechanisms in CFS/FM has identified some common themes underlying a plethora of less consistent findings. The existing data about an association between CFS and activation of the immune system are inconsistent, and a previous meta-analysis reported no clear abnormalities [139]. However, the largest study to date has identified increased CRP levels both in CFS patients and in subjects with chronic fatigue not meeting the CFS criteria [38]. Whether or not the inflammatory profile might be different in different forms of fatigue (i.e., in milder or shorter syndromes) has yet to be studied [140]. Abnormal oxidative and mitochondrial processes have been more consistently described, but studies have used a variety of approaches and biochemical indicators, making comparison between studies difficult. Moreover, it remains unclear whether mitochondrial abnormalities are primary or are the secondary effects of cellular hypoxia or increased oxidative stress [90]. The HPA axis also appears to be implicated in CFS (with much less evidence in FM), with blunted

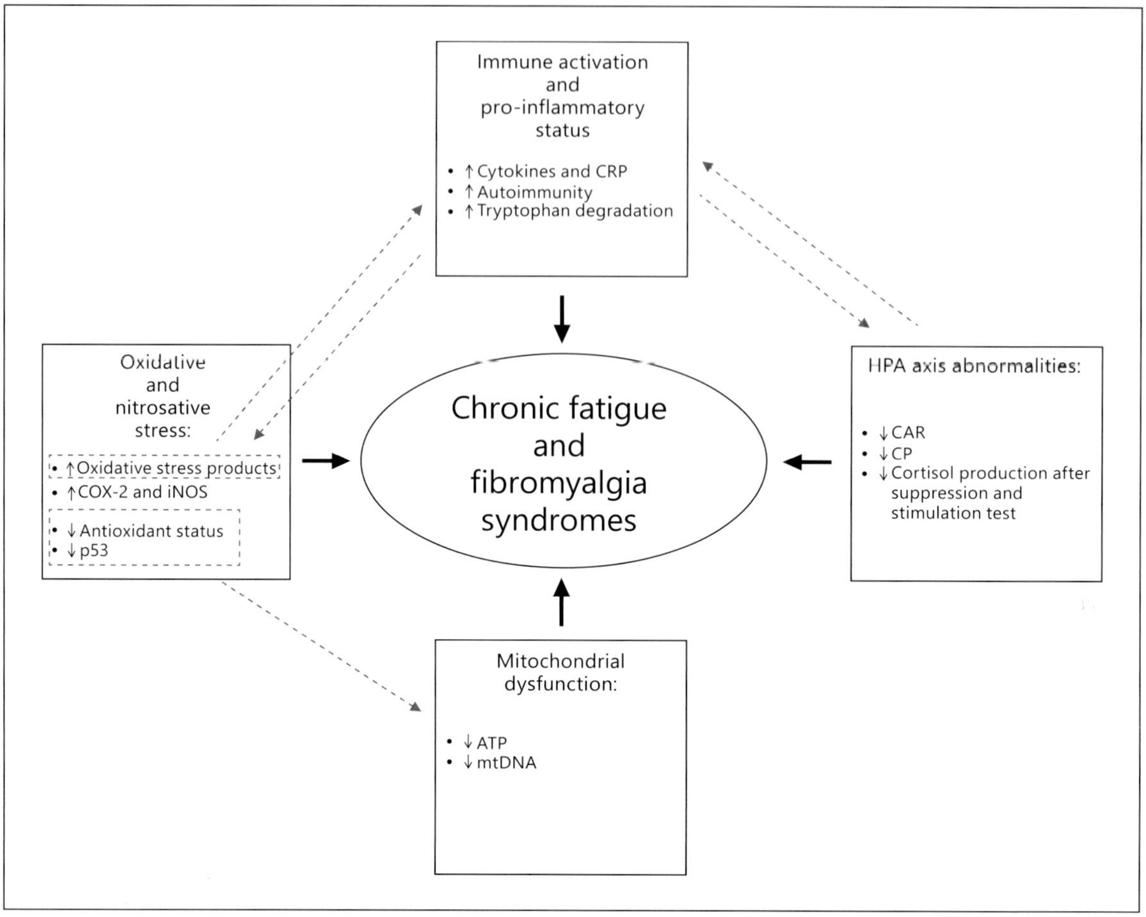

Fig. 2. Proposed systems involved in CFS/FM pathogenesis.

HPA axis activity both at baseline and in response to stimulation being the most (but not always) consistent findings, possible due to a hyper-sensitivity of cortisol receptors. However, again it is unclear whether the HPA axis is involved as a primary causal factor or as a secondary, maintaining factor, prolonging fatigue or worsening the outcome. Indeed, some authors suggest that HPA axis abnormalities develop later in the natural history of CFS due to sleep disturbances or inactivity [141]. Perhaps more in CFS/FM than in any other area, more biological research is truly needed in order to identify new targetable mechanisms that could be used a biomarkers for outcome prediction and for the discovery of new therapeutic interventions.

Acknowledgements and Conflicts of Interest

This work was supported by the Medical Research Council (UK) MR/J002739/1 and the NIHR Mental Health Biomedical Research Centre at the South London and Maudsley NHS Foundation Trust and King's College London. Professor Pariante has received research funding from pharmaceutical companies interested in the role of inflammation in mental health, but the work leading to this review was independent of this funding.

References

1 Centers for Disease Control and Prevention: Chronic Fatigue Syndrome (CFS) Case Definition. Atlanta, GA, Centers for Disease Control and Prevention, 2012.

2 Fukuda K, Straus SE, Hickie I, Sharpe MC, Dobbins JG, Komaroff A: The chronic fatigue syndrome: a comprehensive approach to its definition and study. International Chronic Fatigue Syndrome Study Group. Ann Intern Med 1994;121:953–959.

3 Reeves WC, Lloyd A, Vernon SD, et al: Identification of ambiguities in the 1994 chronic fatigue syndrome research case definition and recommendations for resolution. BMC Health Serv Res 1994;3: 1–9.

4 Centers for Disease Control and Prevention: Fibromyalgia. Atlanta, GA, Centers for Disease Control and Prevention, 2012.

5 Wolfe F, Clauw DJ, Fitzcharles MA, et al: The American College of Rheumatology preliminary diagnostic criteria for fibromyalgia and measurement of symptom severity. Arthritis Care Res 2010;62: 600–610.

6 Wessely S, Nimnuan C, Sharpe M: Functional somatic syndromes: one or many? Lancet 1999 Sep;354:936–939.

7 Maes M, Twisk FNM: Chronic fatigue syndrome: Harvey and Wessely's (bio) psychosocial model versus a bio(psychosocial) model based on inflammatory and oxidative and nitrosative stress pathways. BMC Med 2010;8: 35.

8 Harvey S, Wessely S: Chronic fatigue syndrome: identifying zebras amongst the horses. BMC Med 2009;7:58.

9 Abbas AK, Lichtman AHH, Pillai S: Cellular and Molecular Immunology: with STUDENT CONSULT Online Access, ed 7. Philadelphia, Elsevier Health Sciences, 2011.

10 Burdette SD, Parilo MA, Kaplan LJ, Bailey H: Systemic inflammatory response syndrome. 2014. http://emedicine.medscape.com/article/168943-overview (accessed June 19, 2014).

11 Dantzer R, Kelley KW: Twenty years of research on cytokine-induced sickness behavior. Brain Behav Immun 2007;21: 153–160.

12 Carmichael MD, Davis JM, Murphy EA, et al: Role of brain IL-1beta on fatigue after exercise-induced muscle damage. Am J Physiol Regul Integr Comp Physiol 2006;291:R1344–R1348.

13 Kelley KW, Bluthe RM, Dantzer R, et al: Cytokine-induced sickness behavior. Brain Behav Immun 2003;17:S112–S118.

14 Capuron L, Miller AH: Immune system to brain signaling: neuropsychopharmacological implications. Pharmacol Ther 2011;130:226–238.

15 Bonaccorso S, Marino V, Biondi M, Grimaldi F, Ippoliti F, Maes M: Depression induced by treatment with interferon-alpha in patients affected by hepatitis C virus. J Affect Disord 2002;72:237–241.

16 Bull SJ, Huezo-Diaz P, Binder EB, et al: Functional polymorphisms in the interleukin-6 and serotonin transporter genes, and depression and fatigue induced by interferon-alpha and ribavirin treatment. Mol Psychiatry 2009;14: 1095–1104.

17 Su K-P, Huang S-Y, Peng C-Y, et al: Phospholipase A2 and cyclooxygenase 2 genes influence the risk of interferon-alpha-induced depression by regulating polyunsaturated fatty acids levels. Biol Psychiatry 2010;67:550–557.

18 Strand V, Singh JA: Improved health-related quality of life with effective disease-modifying antirheumatic drugs: evidence from randomized controlled trials. Am J Manag Care 2007;13:S237–S251.

19 Tyring S, Gottlieb A, Papp K, et al: Etanercept and clinical outcomes, fatigue, and depression in psoriasis: double-blind placebo-controlled randomised phase III trial. Lancet 2006;367:29–35.

20 Baumeister D, Russell A, Pariante C, Mondelli V: Inflammatory biomarker profiles of mental disorders and their relation to clinical, social and lifestyle factors. Soc Psychiatry Psychiatr Epidemiol 2014;49:841–849.

21 Rosenblat JD, Cha DS, Mansur RB, McIntyre RS: Inflamed moods: a review of the interactions between inflammation and mood disorders. Prog Neuropsychopharmacol Biol Psychiatry 2014; 53C:23–34.

22 Lasselin J, Capuron L: Chronic low-grade inflammation in metabolic disorders: relevance for behavioral symptoms. Neuroimmunomodulation 2014; 21:95–101.

23 Silverman MN, Heim CM, Nater UM, Marques AH, Sternberg EM: Neuroendocrine and immune contributors to fatigue. PM R 2010;2:338–346.

24 Anderson G, Berk M, Maes M: Biological phenotypes underpin the physio-somatic symptoms of somatization, depression, and chronic fatigue syndrome. Acta Psychiatr Scand 2014;129:83–97.

25 Brenu EW, Huth TK, Hardcastle SL, et al: Role of adaptive and innate immune cells in chronic fatigue syndrome/myalgic encephalomyelitis. Int Immunol 2014;26:233–242.

26 Fletcher MA, Zeng XR, Barnes Z, Levis S, Klimas NG: Plasma cytokines in women with chronic fatigue syndrome. J Transl Med 2009;7:96.

27 Skowera A, Cleare A, Blair D, Bevis L, Wessely SC, Peakman M: High levels of type 2 cytokine-producing cells in chronic fatigue syndrome. Clin Exp Immunol 2004;135:294–302.

28 Zhang H-Y, Liu Z-D, Hu C-J, Wang D-X, Zhang Y-B, Li Y-Z: Up-regulation of TGF-β1 mRNA expression in peripheral blood mononuclear cells of patients with chronic fatigue syndrome. J Formos Med Assoc 2011;110:701–704.

29 Tomoda A, Joudoi T, Rabab E-M, Matsumoto T, Park TH, Miike T: Cytokine production and modulation: comparison of patients with chronic fatigue syndrome and normal controls. Psychiatry Res 2005;134:101–104.

30 Maes M, Twisk FNM, Kubera M, Ringel K: Evidence for inflammation and activation of cell-mediated immunity in Myalgic Encephalomyelitis/Chronic Fatigue Syndrome (ME/CFS): increased interleukin-1, tumor necrosis factor-alpha, PMN-elastase, lysozyme and neopterin. J Affect Disord 2012;136:933–939.

31 Bote ME, Garca JJ, Hinchado MD, Ortega E: Inflammatory/stress feedback dysregulation in women with fibromyalgia. Neuroimmunomodulation 2012;19: 343–351.

32 Wallace DJ, Linker-Israeli M, Hallegua D, Silverman S, Silver D, Weisman MH: Cytokines play an aetiopathogenetic role in fibromyalgia: a hypothesis and pilot study. Rheumatology (Oxford) 2001;40: 743–749.
33 Togo F, Natelson BH, Adler GK, et al: Plasma cytokine fluctuations over time in healthy controls and patients with fibromyalgia. Exp Biol Med (Maywood) 2009;234:232–240.
34 Nakamura T, Schwander SK, Donnelly R, et al: Cytokines across the night in chronic fatigue syndrome with and without fibromyalgia. Clin Vaccine Immunol 2010;17:582–587.
35 Gür A, Karakoç M, Nas K, et al: Cytokines and depression in cases with fibromyalgia. J Rheumatol 2002;29:358–361.
36 Wang H, Buchner M, Moser MT, Daniel V, Schiltenwolf M: The role of IL-8 in patients with fibromyalgia: a prospective longitudinal study of 6 months. Clin J Pain 2009;25:1–4.
37 Buchwald D, Wener MH, Pearlman T, Kith P: Markers of inflammation and immune activation in chronic fatigue and chronic fatigue syndrome. J Rheumatol 1997;24:372–376.
38 Raison CL, Lin JMS, Reeves WC: Association of peripheral inflammatory markers with chronic fatigue in a population-based sample. Brain Behav Immun 2009;23:327–337.
39 Spence VA, Kennedy G, Belch JJF, Hill A, Khan F: Low-grade inflammation and arterial wave reflection in patients with chronic fatigue syndrome. Clin Sci (Lond) 2008;114:561–566.
40 Xiao Y, Haynes WL, Michalek JE, Russell IJ: Elevated serum high-sensitivity C-reactive protein levels in fibromyalgia syndrome patients correlate with body mass index, interleukin-6, interleukin-8, erythrocyte sedimentation rate. Rheumatol Int 2013;33:1259–1264.
41 Lorusso L, Mikhaylova SV, Capelli E, Ferrari D, Ngonga GK, Ricevuti G: Immunological aspects of chronic fatigue syndrome. Autoimmun Rev 2009;8: 287–291.
42 Morris G, Maes M: A neuro-immune model of Myalgic Encephalomyelitis/Chronic fatigue syndrome. Metab Brain Dis 2013;28:523–540.
43 Robertson MJ, Schacterle RS, Mackin GA, et al: Lymphocyte subset differences in patients with chronic fatigue syndrome, multiple sclerosis and major depression. Clin Exp Immunol 2005; 141:326–332.
44 Curriu M, Carrillo J, Massanella M, et al: Screening NK-, B- and T-cell phenotype and function in patients suffering from Chronic Fatigue Syndrome. J Transl Med 2013;11:68.
45 Mihaylova I, DeRuyter M, Rummens J, Bosmans E, Maes M: Decreased expression of CD69 in chronic fatigue syndrome in relation to inflammatory markers: evidence for a severe disorder in the early activation of T lymphocytes and natural killer cells. Neuro Endocrinol Lett 2007;28:477–483.
46 Aoki T, Miyakoshi H, Usuda Y, Herberman R: Low NK syndrome and its relationship to chronic fatigue syndrome. Clin Immunol Immunopathol 1993;69: 253–265.
47 Poggi A, Zocchi MR: NK Cell autoreactivity and autoimmune diseases. Front Immunol 2014;5:27.
48 Bradley AS, Ford B, Bansal AS: Altered functional B cell subset populations in patients with chronic fatigue syndrome compared to healthy controls. Clin Exp Immunol 2013;172:73–80.
49 Tanaka S, Kuratsune H, Hidaka Y, et al: Autoantibodies against muscarinic cholinergic receptor in chronic fatigue syndrome. Int J Mol Med 2003;12:225–230.
50 Bassi N, Amital D, Amital H, Doria A, Shoenfeld Y: Chronic fatigue syndrome: characteristics and possible causes for its pathogenesis. Isr Med Assoc J 2008; 10:79–82.
51 Werle E, Fischer HP, Müller A, Fiehn W, Eich W: Antibodies against serotonin have no diagnostic relevance in patients with fibromyalgia syndrome. J Rheumatol 2001;28:595–600.
52 Maes M, Mihaylova I, Leunis JC: In chronic fatigue syndrome, the decreased levels of omega-3 poly-unsaturated fatty acids are related to lowered serum zinc and defects in T cell activation. Neuro Endocrinol Lett 2005;26:745–751.
53 Miyamae T, Seki M, Naga T, et al: Increased oxidative stress and coenzyme Q10 deficiency in juvenile fibromyalgia: amelioration of hypercholesterolemia and fatigue by ubiquinol-10 supplementation. Redox Rep 2013;18:12–19.
54 Steinau M, Unger ER, Vernon SD, Jones JF, Rajeevan MS: Differential-display PCR of peripheral blood for biomarker discovery in chronic fatigue syndrome. J Mol Med (Berl) 2004;82:750–755.
55 Fang H, Xie Q, Boneva R, Fostel J, Perkins R, Tong W: Gene expression profile exploration of a large dataset on chronic fatigue syndrome. Pharmacogenomics 2006;7:429–440.
56 Kerr JR, Petty R, Burke B, et al: Gene expression subtypes in patients with chronic fatigue syndrome/myalgic encephalomyelitis. J Infect Dis 2008;197: 1171–1184.
57 Carlo-Stella N, Badulli C, De Silvestri A, et al: A first study of cytokine genomic polymorphisms in CFS: positive association of TNF-857 and IFNgamma 874 rare alleles. Clin Exp Rheumatol 2006; 24:179–182.
58 Blankfield A: Kynurenine pathway pathologies: do nicotinamide and other pathway co-factors have a therapeutic role in reduction of symptom severity, including chronic fatigue syndrome (CFS) and fibromyalgia (FM). Int J Tryptophan Res 2013;6:39–45.
59 Badawy AA-B, Morgan CJ, Llewelyn MB, Albuquerque SRJ, Farmer A: Heterogeneity of serum tryptophan concentration and availability to the brain in patients with the chronic fatigue syndrome. J Psychopharmacol 2005;19: 385–391.
60 Vassallo CM, Feldman E, Peto T, Castell L, Sharpley AL, Cowen PJ: Decreased tryptophan availability but normal post-synaptic 5-HT2c receptor sensitivity in chronic fatigue syndrome. Psychol Med 2001;31:585–591.
61 Maes M, Galecki P, Verkerk R, Rief W: Somatization, but not depression, is characterized by disorders in the tryptophan catabolite (TRYCAT) pathway, indicating increased indoleamine 2,3-dioxygenase and lowered kynurenine aminotransferase activity. Neuro Endocrinol Lett 2011;32:264–273.
62 Nijs J, Meeus M, Van Oosterwijck J, et al: Treatment of central sensitization in patients with 'unexplained' chronic pain: what options do we have? Expert Opin Pharmacother 2011;12:1087–1098.
63 Nelson DDL, Lehninger AL, Cox MM: Lehninger Principles of Biochemistry, ed 6. New York, W.H. Freeman, 2013.
64 Alberts B, Bray D, Hopkin K, et al: Essential Cell Biology, ed 4. New York, Garland Science, 2013.

65 Murphy MP: How mitochondria produce reactive oxygen species. Biochem J 2009;417:1–13.
66 Maes M: Inflammatory and oxidative and nitrosative stress pathways underpinning chronic fatigue, somatization and psychosomatic symptoms. Curr Opin Psychiatry 2009;22:75–83.
67 Morris G, Maes M: Mitochondrial dysfunctions in myalgic encephalomyelitis/chronic fatigue syndrome explained by activated immuno-inflammatory, oxidative and nitrosative stress pathways. Metab Brain Dis 2014;29:19–36.
68 Maes M, Mihaylova I, Kubera M, Bosmans E: Not in the mind but in the cell: increased production of cyclo-oxygenase-2 and inducible NO synthase in chronic fatigue syndrome. Neuro Endocrinol Lett 2007;28:463–469.
69 Bazan NG: Metabolism of arachidonic acid in the retina and retinal pigment epithelium: biological effects of oxygenated metabolites of arachidonic acid. Prog Clin Biol Res 1989;312:15–37.
70 Closa D, Folch-Puy E: Oxygen free radicals and the systemic inflammatory response. IUBMB Life 2004;56:185–191.
71 McIver KL, Evans C, Kraus RM, Ispas L, Sciotti VM, Hickner RC: NO-mediated alterations in skeletal muscle nutritive blood flow and lactate metabolism in fibromyalgia. Pain 2006;120:161–169.
72 Chung HY, Lee EK, Choi YJ, et al: Molecular inflammation as an underlying mechanism of the aging process and age-related diseases. J Dent Res 2011;90: 830–840.
73 Melnikova T, Savonenko A, Wang Q, et al: Cycloxygenase-2 activity promotes cognitive deficits but not increased amyloid burden in a model of Alzheimer's disease in a sex-dimorphic pattern. Neuroscience 2006;141:1149–1162.
74 Maes M, Mihaylova I, Kubera M, Uytterhoeven M, Vrydags N, Bosmans E: Lower plasma Coenzyme Q10 in depression: a marker for treatment resistance and chronic fatigue in depression and a risk factor to cardiovascular disorder in that illness. Neuro Endocrinol Lett 2009; 30:462–469.
75 Cordero MD, Cano-Garcìa FJ, Alcocer-Gòmez E, de Miguel M, Sànchez-Alcàzar JA: Oxidative stress correlates with headache symptoms in fibromyalgia: coenzyme Q 10 effect on clinical improvement. PLoS One 2012;7:e35677.
76 Cordero MD, Cotàn D, Del-Pozo-Martìn Y, et al: Oral coenzyme Q10 supplementation improves clinical symptoms and recovers pathologic alterations in blood mononuclear cells in a fibromyalgia patient. Nutrition 2012;28:1200–1203.
77 Morris G, Anderson G, Dean O, et al: The glutathione system: a new drug target in neuroimmune disorders. Mol Neurobiol 2014;50:1059–1084.
78 Morris G, Maes M: Increased nuclear factor κβ and loss of p53 are key mechanisms in Myalgic Encephalomyelitis/chronic fatigue syndrome (ME/CFS). Med Hypotheses 2012;79:607–613.
79 Cordero MD, de Miguel M, Carmona-López I, Bonal P, Campa F, Moreno-Fernández AM: Oxidative stress and mitochondrial dysfunction in fibromyalgia. Neuro Endocrinol Lett 2010;31: 169–173.
80 Cordero MD, Moreno-Fernàndez AM, Carmona-Lòpez MI, et al: Mitochondrial dysfunction in skin biopsies and blood mononuclear cells from two cases of fibromyalgia patients. Clin Biochem 2010;43:1174–1176.
81 Castro-Marrero J, Cordero MD, Sáez-Francas N, et al: Could mitochondrial dysfunction be a differentiating marker between chronic fatigue syndrome and fibromyalgia? Antioxid Redox Signal 2013;19:1855–1860.
82 Kennedy G, Spence VA, McLaren M, Hill A, Underwood C, Belch JJF: Oxidative stress levels are raised in chronic fatigue syndrome and are associated with clinical symptoms. Free Radic Biol Med 2005;39:584–589.
83 Chung CP, Titova D, Oeser A, et al: Oxidative stress in fibromyalgia and its relationship to symptoms. Clin Rheumatol 2009;28:435–438.
84 Maes M, Kubera M, Uytterhoeven M, Vrydags N, Bosmans E: Increased plasma peroxides as a marker of oxidative stress in myalgic encephalomyelitis/chronic fatigue syndrome (ME/CFS). Med Sci Monit 2011;17:SC11–SC15.
85 Jammes Y, Steinberg JG, Mambrini O, Brégeon F, Delliaux S: Chronic fatigue syndrome: Assessment of increased oxidative stress and altered muscle excitability in response to incremental exercise. J Intern Med 2005;257:299–310.
86 Richards RS, Wang L, Jelinek H: Erythrocyte oxidative damage in chronic fatigue syndrome. Arch Med Res 2007;38: 94–98.
87 Klein R, Berg PA: High incidence of antibodies to 5-hydroxytryptamine, gangliosides and phospholipids in patients with chronic fatigue and fibromyalgia syndrome and their relatives: evidence for a clinical entity of both disorders. Eur J Med Res 1995;1:21–26.
88 Maes M, Mihaylova I, Leunis J-C: Chronic fatigue syndrome is accompanied by an IgM-related immune response directed against neopitopes formed by oxidative or nitrosative damage to lipids and proteins. Neuro Endocrinol Lett 2006;27:615–621.
89 Meeus M, Nijs J, Hermans L, Goubert D, Calders P: The role of mitochondrial dysfunctions due to oxidative and nitrosative stress in the chronic pain or chronic fatigue syndromes and fibromyalgia patients: peripheral and central mechanisms as therapeutic targets? Expert Opin Ther Targets 2013;17:1081–1089.
90 Myhill S, Booth NE, McLaren-Howard J: Chronic fatigue syndrome and mitochondrial dysfunction. Int J Clin Exp Med 2009;2:1–16.
91 VanNess JM, Stevens SR, Bateman L, Stiles TL, Snell CR: Postexertional malaise in women with chronic fatigue syndrome. J Womens Health (Larchmt) 2010;19:239–244.
92 Vermeulen RCW, Kurk RM, Visser FC, Sluiter W, Scholte HR: Patients with chronic fatigue syndrome performed worse than controls in a controlled repeated exercise study despite a normal oxidative phosphorylation capacity. J Transl Med 2010;8:93.
93 Booth NE, Myhill S, McLaren-Howard J: Mitochondrial dysfunction and the pathophysiology of Myalgic Encephalomyelitis/Chronic Fatigue Syndrome (ME/CFS). Int J Clin Exp Med 2012;5: 208–220.
94 Cleare AJ: The HPA axis and the genesis of chronic fatigue syndrome. Trends Endocrinol Metab 2004;15:55–59.
95 Baumeister D, Lightman S, Pariante C: The interface of stress and the HPA axis in behavioural phenotypes of mental illness. Curr Top Behav Neurosci 2014; 18:13–24.
96 Tsigos C, Chrousos GP: Hypothalamic-pituitary-adrenal axis, neuroendocrine factors and stress. J Psychosom Res 2002;53:865–871.

97 Powell DJH, Liossi C, Moss-Morris R, Schlotz W: Unstimulated cortisol secretory activity in everyday life and its relationship with fatigue and chronic fatigue syndrome: a systematic review and subset meta-analysis. Psychoneuroendocrinology 2013;38:2405–2422.
98 Silverman MN, Sternberg EM: Glucocorticoid regulation of inflammation and its functional correlates: from HPA axis to glucocorticoid receptor dysfunction. Ann N Y Acad Sci 2012; 1261:55–63.
99 Khani S, Tayek JA: Cortisol increases gluconeogenesis in humans: its role in the metabolic syndrome. Clin Sci (Lond) 2001;101:739–747.
100 Cleare AJ, Heap E, Malhi GS, Wessely S, O'Keane V, Miell J: Low-dose hydrocortisone in chronic fatigue syndrome: a randomised crossover trial. Lancet 1999:353:455–458.
101 Poteliakhoff A: Adrenocortical activity and some clinical findings in acute and chronic fatigue. J Psychosom Res 1981; 25:91–95.
102 Demitrack MA, Dale JK, Straus SE, et al: Evidence for impaired activation of the hypothalamic-pituitary-adrenal axis in patients with chronic fatigue syndrome. J Clin Endocrinol Metab 1991;73:1224–1234.
103 Papadopoulos AS, Cleare AJ: Hypothalamic-pituitary-adrenal axis dysfunction in chronic fatigue syndrome. Nat Rev Endocrinol 2012;8:22–32.
104 Tak LM, Cleare AJ, Ormel J, et al: Meta-analysis and meta-regression of hypothalamic-pituitary-adrenal axis activity in functional somatic disorders. Biol Psychol 2011;87:183–194.
105 Wilhelm I, Born J, Kudielka BM, Schlotz W, Wűst S: Is the cortisol awakening rise a response to awakening? Psychoneuroendocrinology 2007; 32:358–366.
106 Roberts AD, Wessely S, Chalder T, Papadopoulos A, Cleare AJ: Salivary cortisol response to awakening in chronic fatigue syndrome. Br J Psychiatry 2004;184:136–141.
107 Nater UM, Maloney E, Boneva RS, et al: Attenuated morning salivary cortisol concentrations in a population-based study of persons with chronic fatigue syndrome and well controls. J Clin Endocrinol Metab 2008;93:703–709.
108 Nijhof SL, Rutten JMTM, Uiterwaal CSPM, Bleijenberg G, Kimpen JLL, Putte EM: The role of hypocortisolism in chronic fatigue syndrome. Psychoneuroendocrinology 2014;42:199–206.
109 Heim C, Nater UM, Maloney E, Boneva R, Jones JF, Reeves WC: Childhood trauma and risk for chronic fatigue syndrome: association with neuroendocrine dysfunction. Arch Gen Psychiatry 2009;66:72–80.
110 Borsini a, Hepgul N, Mondelli V, Chalder T, Pariante CM: Childhood stressors in the development of fatigue syndromes: a review of the past 20 years of research. Psychol Med 2013;1–15.
111 Strickland P, Morriss R, Wearden A, Deakin B: A comparison of salivary cortisol in chronic fatigue syndrome, community depression and healthy controls. J Affect Disord 1998;47:191–194.
112 Jerjes WK, Cleare a J, Wessely S, Wood PJ, Taylor NF: Diurnal patterns of salivary cortisol and cortisone output in chronic fatigue syndrome. J Affect Disord 2005;87:299–304.
113 Papadopoulos A, Ebrecht M, Roberts ADL, Poon L, Rohleder N, Cleare AJ: Glucocorticoid receptor mediated negative feedback in chronic fatigue syndrome using the low dose (0.5 mg) dexamethasone suppression test. J Affect Disord 2009;112:289–294.
114 Young AH, Sharpe M, Clements A, Dowling B, Hawton KE, Cowen PJ: Basal activity of the hypothalamic-pituitary-adrenal axis in patients with the chronic fatigue syndrome (neurasthenia). Biol Psychiatry 1998;43:236–237.
115 Wood B, Wessely S, Papadopoulos A, Poon L, Checkley S: Salivary cortisol profiles in chronic fatigue syndrome. Neuropsychobiology 1998;37:1–4.
116 Gaab J, Hüster D, Peisen R, et al: Low-dose dexamethasone suppression test in chronic fatigue syndrome and health. Psychosom Med 2002;64:311–318.
117 Gaab J, Engert V, Heitz V, Schad T, Schürmeyer TH, Ehlert U: Associations between neuroendocrine responses to the Insulin Tolerance Test and patient characteristics in chronic fatigue syndrome. J Psychosom Res 2004;56:419–424.
118 Gaab J, Rohleder N, Heitz V, et al: Stress-induced changes in LPS-induced pro-inflammatory cytokine production in chronic fatigue syndrome. Psychoneuroendocrinology 2005;30: 188–198.
119 İzgi H, Gökçe C, Çals M, et al: Investigation of the hypothalamopituitary – adrenal axis by low-dose (1 g) adrenocorticotrophic hormone test and metyrapone test in patients with chronic fatigue syndrome. Endocrinologist 2005;15:89–92.
120 Van Den Eede F, Moorkens G, Van Houdenhove B, Cosyns P, Claes SJ: Hypothalamic-pituitary-adrenal axis function in chronic fatigue syndrome. Neuropsychobiology 2007;55:112–120.
121 Inder WJ, Prickett TCR, Mulder RT: Normal opioid tone and hypothalamic-pituitary-adrenal axis function in chronic fatigue syndrome despite marked functional impairment. Clin Endocrinol (Oxf) 2005;62:343–348.
122 Jerjes WK, Taylor NF, Wood PJ, Cleare AJ: Enhanced feedback sensitivity to prednisolone in chronic fatigue syndrome. Psychoneuroendocrinology 2007;32:192–198.
123 Visser J, Blauw B, Hinloopen B, et al: CD4 T lymphocytes from patients with chronic fatigue syndrome have decreased interferon-gamma production and increased sensitivity to dexamethasone. J Infect Dis 1998;177:451–454.
124 Visser J, Lentjes E, Haspels I, et al: Increased sensitivity to glucocorticoids in peripheral blood mononuclear cells of chronic fatigue syndrome patients, without evidence for altered density or affinity of glucocorticoid receptors. J Investig Med 2001;49:195–204.
125 Van Den Eede F, Moorkens G, Hulstijn W, et al: Combined dexamethasone/corticotropin-releasing factor test in chronic fatigue syndrome. Psychol Med 2008;38:963–973.
126 Catley D, Kaell a T, Kirschbaum C, Stone AA: A naturalistic evaluation of cortisol secretion in persons with fibromyalgia and rheumatoid arthritis. Arthritis Care Res 2000;13:51–61.
127 Klingmann PO, Kugler I, Steffke TS, Bellingrath S, Kudielka BM, Hellhammer DH: Sex-specific prenatal programming: a risk for fibromyalgia? Ann N Y Acad Sci 2008;1148:446–55.

128 Riva R, Mork PJ, Westgaard RH, Rø M, Lundberg U: Fibromyalgia syndrome is associated with hypocortisolism. Int J Behav Med 2010;17:223–233.
129 Macedo J a, Hesse J, Turner JD, Meyer J, Hellhammer DH, Muller CP: Glucocorticoid sensitivity in fibromyalgia patients: decreased expression of corticosteroid receptors and glucocorticoid-induced leucine zipper. Psychoneuroendocrinology 2008;33:799–809.
130 McLean S a, Williams D a, Harris RE, et al: Momentary relationship between cortisol secretion and symptoms in patients with fibromyalgia. Arthritis Rheum 2005;52:3660–3669.
131 Griep EN, Boersma JW, de Kloet ER: Altered reactivity of the hypothalamic-pituitary-adrenal axis in the primary fibromyalgia syndrome. J Rheumatol 1993;20:469–474.
132 Griep EN, Boersma JW, Lentjes EG, Prins AP, van der Korst JK, de Kloet ER: Function of the hypothalamic-pituitary-adrenal axis in patients with fibromyalgia and low back pain. J Rheumatol 1998;25:1374–1381.
133 Riedel W, Layka H, Neeck G: Secretory pattern of GH, TSH, thyroid hormones, ACTH, cortisol, FSH, and LH in patients with fibromyalgia syndrome following systemic injection of the relevant hypothalamic-releasing hormones. Z Rheumatol 1998; 57(suppl 2):81–87.
134 Calis M, Gökçe C, Ates F, et al: Investigation of the hypothalamo-pituitary-adrenal axis (HPA) by 1 microg ACTH test and metyrapone test in patients with primary fibromyalgia syndrome. J Endocrinol Invest 2004;27:42–46.
135 Kirnap M, Colak R, Eser C, Ozsoy O, Tutus A, Kelestimur F: A comparison between low-dose (1 microg), standard-dose (250 microg) ACTH stimulation tests and insulin tolerance test in the evaluation of hypothalamo-pituitary-adrenal axis in primary fibromyalgia syndrome. Clin Endocrinol (Oxf) 2001;55:455–459.
136 Van Denderen JC, Boersma JW, Zeinstra P, Hollander AP, van Neerbos BR: Physiological effects of exhaustive physical exercise in primary fibromyalgia syndrome (PFS): is PFS a disorder of neuroendocrine reactivity? Scand J Rheumatol 1992;21:35–37.
137 Gursel Y, Ergin S, Ulus Y, Erdogan MF, Yalcin P, Evcik D: Hormonal responses to exercise stress test in patients with fibromyalgia syndrome. Clin Rheumatol 2001;20:401–405.
138 Wingenfeld K, Wagner D, Schmidt I, Meinlschmidt G, Hellhammer DH, Heim C: The low-dose dexamethasone suppression test in fibromyalgia. J Psychosom Res 2007;62:85–91.
139 Lyall M, Peakman M, Wessely S: A systematic review and critical evaluation of the immunology of chronic fatigue syndrome. J Psychosom Res 2003;55:79–90.
140 Pariante C: Chronic fatigue syndrome and the immune system: 'findings in search of meanings'. Brain Behav Immun 2009;23:325–326.
141 Cleare AJ, O'Keane V, Miell JP: Levels of DHEA and DHEAS and responses to CRH stimulation and hydrocortisone treatment in chronic fatigue syndrome. Psychoneuroendocrinology 2004;29:724–732.

Prof. Carmine M. Pariante, MD, FRCPsych, PhD
Institute of Psychiatry, King's College London, Room 2–055, The James Black Centre
125 Coldharbour Lane
London SE5 9NU (UK)
E-Mail carmine.pariante@kcl.ac.uk

Balon R, Wise TN (eds): Clinical Challenges in the Biopsychosocial Interface. Update on Psychosomatics for the 21st Century. Adv Psychosom Med. Basel, Karger, 2015, vol 34, pp 78–91 (DOI: 10.1159/000369087)

Fibromyalgia and Chronic Fatigue Syndrome: Management Issues

Julius Bourke

Centre for Psychiatry at The Wolfson Institute for Preventive Medicine, Barts and The London School of Medicine and Dentistry, Queen Mary University of London, UK

Abstract

Fibromyalgia and chronic fatigue syndrome represent two of the most commonly encountered functional somatic syndromes in clinical practice. Both have been contentious diagnoses in the past, and this diagnostic dispute has resulted in a therapeutic nihilism that has been of great detriment to their management and to alleviation of the intense suffering and disability that they have caused their innumerable sufferers. A new age has dawned in terms of a better understanding of these syndromes' physiology and improved approaches to their management. Here, the diagnosis and management of these closely related disorders are discussed, with particular reference to the recent empirical evidence that has come to light as a consequence of neurophysiological insights and robustly designed randomised clinical trials. Much work remains to be done in this vein, but we are better placed to facilitate recovery from these disorders than we have been previously. Whilst remission should always be a goal, complete symptom resolution is not the norm, but 'moderate' improvements are certainly attainable with appropriate management.

Fibromyalgia

Once a diagnosis of contention, fibromyalgia is now an accepted medical diagnosis. Although its nomenclature was changed from 'fibrositis' when no consistent evidence could be found to support an inflammatory process in its pathophysiology, the diagnostic validity of fibromyalgia is now supported by a host of research that has identified augmented pain and sensory processing, highlighting a distinct clinical phenotype involving sensitisation of the central nervous system.

Fibromyalgia affects between 2 and 7% of the population [1, 2]. Most individuals diagnosed in clinics are young or middle aged, but population surveys suggest that it is a diagnosis that increases with age, with a maximum prevalence in the 60s [1, 3].

Diagnosis

Although a number of different diagnostic criteria have been proposed over the years, the most universally applied are those of the American

College of Rheumatology (ACR). These criteria used to rely upon the demonstration of 11 out of 18 possible 'tender points', in combination with careful medical screening, inclusive of history taking and examination followed by blood tests. These included a full blood count and tests for urea and electrolytes, thyroid function, C-reactive protein, erythrocyte sedimentation rate, and antinuclear antibodies.

Recently, these criteria were contested because 25% of patients with fibromyalgia do not necessarily have sufficient tender points; because patients often report additional or other areas of pain and tenderness, along with other symptoms and comorbid diagnoses; and because the use of tender points creates a bias towards the diagnosis being made in women, who are more tender than men [4].

As a consequence, the ACR criteria were updated in 2010 [4] and no longer require an examination of tender points. Instead, these new criteria combine the concept of chronic widespread pain (as a widespread pain index (WPI) covering 19 regions) with the presence of an additional measure for fatigue, sleep, cognitive symptoms, mood symptoms, and further sources of pain (as the symptom severity score). The combination of the WPI and the symptom severity (SS) score provides a maximum score of 31. For the diagnosis to be made, patients must score a minimum of 3 or more on the WPI, with a score totalling 12 when combined with the SS score. Additionally, symptoms must have been present for at least 3 months, in the absence of an alternative diagnosis that explains the pain [4].

The advantage of these new criteria is considered to be that they allow the syndrome to be conceptualised as a continuum of sensitivity and symptomology, rather than as a more purely binary diagnosis, as in its previous incarnation [1, 5]. Fibromyalgia is not considered as a diagnosis of exclusion and may co-exist with other sources of muscle and joint pain. However, caution should be exercised, as 37% of systemic lupus erythaematosus patients, 21% of rheumatoid arthritis patients, and 17% of osteoarthritis patients will fulfil the criteria for fibromyalgia using the ACR 2010 criteria.

Additional Symptoms and Comorbidities

The most common symptoms reported in addition to chronic pain are fatigue, disturbed sleep, problems concentrating, depression, and anxiety.

Fatigue. Chronic fatigue is common in fibromyalgia, to such an extent that, along with other symptoms, it has significant overlap with chronic fatigue syndrome (CFS) – so much so that some have argued that they are the same disorder [6].

Sleep. Fibromyalgia patients spend more time awake at night, and 90% of patients describe nonrestorative sleep. Research has isolated deficient stage IV (deep) sleep as the primary sleep architecture abnormality [7].

Cognitive Dysfunction. Forgetfulness, sensory overload, and difficulty processing thoughts and following conversations are frequent problems. Patients often report this as their 'thinking feels slowed'. It has been estimated that cognitive deficits in fibromyalgia are equal to those found in healthy controls who are 20 years older [8].

Depression and Anxiety. A clinical overlap exists between fibromyalgia and major depressive disorder (MDD) [9]. There is a high lifetime prevalence of MDD in fibromyalgia patients [10], with 62% of fibromyalgia patients experiencing MDD. The same is true of anxiety disorders, which affect nearly two-thirds of fibromyalgia sufferers. Given the high prevalence of these disorders, it has been suggested that the presence of anxiety and depression splits fibromyalgia patients into three patient subgroups [11, 12]:

Group 1: Not very tender, low levels of depression/anxiety, low levels of catastrophising, and moderate control over pain. In this group, psychological factors, such as catastrophising, are thought to play little role in the stability or fluctuation of symptoms.

Group 2: Tender, high levels of depression/anxiety, very high catastrophising, and no control over pain. In this group, psychological factors are thought to play an important role in the worsening of symptoms.

Group 3: Extremely tender, low levels of depression/anxiety, very low catastrophising, and high control over pain. In this group, psychological factors are thought to play an important role in the improvement of symptoms.

Management

The most important domains for patients tend to include pain, fatigue, quality of life, and physical function. It often helps to make a note of these in order to assess clinical progress that is also meaningful to the patient.

The management of fibromyalgia should involve a biopsychosocial approach and will invariably require the involvement of a multidisciplinary team that includes psychiatrists, pain specialists (usually rheumatologists and anaesthetists), psychologists, physiotherapists, and occupational therapists. The make-up of teams will vary between services; effective multidisciplinary work and communication are the keys to effective management.

Pharmacological Approaches

The current pharmacological options available for the treatment of fibromyalgia have a similar degree of efficacy as those available for other chronic pain states [13], but effect sizes for pain and quality of life remain small to moderate in most drug studies [14]. The choice of drug should target the symptoms that are most problematic for the patient, and it is important to be aware that multiple drugs are often required [15]. It is often of use to explain this to patients early in the course of management. The mainstays of drug treatment are currently antidepressants and α2δ ligands.

Antidepressants

Tricyclic antidepressants (TCAs). The effects of TCAs are independent of their antidepressant actions [16], which is unsurprising, given the small doses that are normally used (e.g. amitriptyline 25–100 mg). Their primary benefit in the management of pain may be their ability to restore aberrant sleep patterns, which consistently demonstrate the greatest response [17]. Amitriptyline is the most commonly used antidepressant in the treatment of fibromyalgia [17] and may be more effective when combined with the selective serotonin reuptake inhibitor (SSRI) fluoxetine [18]. The use of TCAs is hampered by their side-effect profile and resultant poor tolerability, which are predominantly due to their anticholinergic actions. TCAs also present problems for those on polypharmaceutical regimens due to TCAs' propensity to interact adversely with a number of other medications. This may be especially problematic in older populations.

SSRIs. Fluoxetine and paroxetine demonstrate efficacy in fibromyalgia where citalopram does not [19, 20]. This may reflect the relative selectivity of citalopram, which is highly selective in its inhibition of serotonin reuptake. In contrast, the older SSRIs, such as fluoxetine and paroxetine, are less selective, particularly at higher doses, and also inhibit the reuptake of noradrenaline [21]. This is further demonstrated by the greater efficacy of both serotonin and noradrenaline reuptake inhibitors (SNRIs) and noradrenaline reuptake inhibitors such as esreboxetine [16].

Noradrenaline Reuptake Inhibitors. These agents are less frequently employed. However, esreboxetine has been shown to improve pain and fatigue scores compared with placebo [16].

SNRIs. Dual-acting agents demonstrate as great or greater efficacy than single-acting agents do, such as the SSRIs. Duloxetine has been shown to be effective in a number of clinical trials [22–24], and this is supported by a recent meta-analysis [25]. Milnacipran also demonstrates efficacy [20], although with a higher dosage needed to treat for a 50% pain reduction in comparison with duloxetine. Milnacipran acts as an SNRI but also demonstrates mild N-methyl-D-aspartate antagonism, and this glutamatergic mechanism of action may attenuate central sensitising processes thought to underlie fibromyalgia. Milnacipran is not available in the UK. Venlafaxine is less effective in clinical trials, although the dose employed here is typically 75 mg per day. Doses under 100 mg are usually considered to be predominantly serotonergic, whilst those over 100 mg demonstrate greater noradrenergic effects. This situation may explain these results [18].

α2δ Ligands. α2δ is an auxiliary protein associated with voltage-gated calcium channels. Pregabalin and gabapentin bind to this channel, reducing calcium influx and preventing the synaptic release of noradrenaline, glutamate, and substance P. Two systematic reviews have demonstrated the efficacy of pregabalin [26, 27]. There is, however, a differential dose response for symptoms: 300 mg is effective for sleep alone, whilst 450 mg is effective against pain and poor sleep [18, 28, 29]. An additional benefit has been described, in that pregabalin seems to delay the time to the loss of therapeutic response compared with placebo [29]. Gabapentin demonstrates a similar degree of efficacy as pregabalin [18, 30, 31]. At doses between 1,200 and 2,400 mg, improvements are seen in pain and sleep scores and in scoring on the Fibromyalgia Impact Questionnaire [31].

Nonsteroidal Anti-inflammatory Drugs (NSAIDs), Paracetamol, and Opiates. There is no evidence for the benefit of either NSAIDs or paracetamol. This should be explained to patients early on in treatment. Since these drugs are available over the counter, they are commonly stocked in bathroom cabinets and are often the first analgesics that patients will use. Progressive nonresponse may be associated with dose escalations, which is problematic in terms of upper gastrointestinal bleeds with NSAIDs, worsening of symptoms through chronic headache, and progressive incremental hepatotoxicity with paracetamol. Interestingly, the underlying physiology of fibromyalgia may involve an excess of endogenous opioids, with downregulation and reduced binding capacity at the mu-opioid receptor [32]. This may explain why the use of opiates is without benefit, namely, that they serve as an exogenous factor exacerbating the underlying pathophysiology. Again, nonresponse may result in dose escalation, increased use, progressive tolerance, and ultimately opiate dependence. In spite of their lack of effect in fibromyalgia, these drugs remain in common use, and it is not unusual that the first point of management is a gradual withdrawal of these. This withdrawal may even be met by an improvement in symptoms, as opiates also serve to destabilise affect, which in turn has a detrimental effect on pain scores.

Tramadol. Although conventional opiates are not recommended and may even worsen the condition, tramadol may be a different consideration. In one double-blind randomised control trial using a formulation with paracetamol (Tramacet), tramadol demonstrated efficacy in improving both pain and physical function [33]. This may be because although an agonist of mu-opioid receptors, tramadol is only weakly so, whilst also acting to inhibit the reuptake of serotonin and noradrenaline. Given the lack of an effect seen with traditional opiates, it may be that the latter mechanism of action delivers a benefit.

Zopiclone and Zolpidem. Although not of benefit in the treatment of fibromyalgia per se, these short-acting hypnotics may be useful in the shorter term to relieve poor sleep and the presence of fatigue [20].

Choice of First Agent. Those patients with predominant difficulties in sleep and pain may benefit from an initial trial with a low-dose TCA, such as amitriptyline 25–75 mg. Gabapentin and pregabalin are appropriate alternatives, or indeed additions, especially with the greater dose split being given at night, as these drugs also have a beneficial effect on sleep. In patients in whom anxiety or depression is prominent, a dual-acting antidepressant, such as duloxetine, is often the most sensible first choice. For the especially anxious patient, it may be worth considering pregabalin as a second-line agent or augmentation strategy, given that in the UK, it has an additional license for the treatment of anxiety disorders. Responses to all agents are often idiosyncratic and may be related to tolerability more than to a frank lack of an effect. Common side effects should be explained, taking the approach that forewarned is forearmed and, particularly where antidepressants are concerned, encourages perseverance beyond the initial appearance of side effects, which often results in a more positive outcome. The general principle should be to 'start low and go slow', as this is felt to minimise side effects and maximise tolerance. Early responses to agents, even if small, should be viewed positively but should not be seen as a barrier to further dose increases.

Emerging Pharmacological Treatments

Dopamine Agonists. These drugs may be of particular importance in those patients who have comorbid restless legs syndrome, which is ten times more common than in the general population. Both pramipexole [34] and ropinirole [35] have demonstrated efficacy in randomised clinical trials, but neither has been accepted as mainstream treatment.

Opioid Antagonists. Naltrexone at a low dose (4.5 mg per day) has been examined in a double-blind randomised controlled trial and was found to improve pain and fatigue in fibromyalgia [36]. This will require further exploration, as although emerging neurophysiological understandings of fibromyalgia support the drug's use [32], at a dose this low, it may be that the effects are a consequence of attenuating pro-inflammatory processes, rather than of mu-opioid antagonism.

Sodium Oxybate or Gamma Hydroxybutyrate. This agent seems to be very effective in the treatment of fibromyalgia and is able to reduce fatigue and pain whilst improving sleep [37]. Unfortunately, due to safety concerns, this agent has not made it through to final Food and Drug Administration approval. It has, however, raised interest in the involvement of the GABAergic system.

Substance P Antagonists. Substance P is a neurokinin transmitter active at the level of the dorsal horn of the spinal cord and believed to be involved in the sensitising of the central nervous system that may underlie fibromyalgia. The neurokinin-1 receptor antagonist casopitant, effective in its clinical use against chemotherapy-induced nausea and vomiting, has been examined in a phase II trial of fibromyalgia with comorbid depressive disorder. Although the trial was completed in 2006, the results are yet to be reported or published [38].

Cannabinoids. Early trials have shown promise [39, 40].

Glutamatergic Agents. Early trials have shown promise, although with disappointingly short-lived responses [41].

Nonpharmacological Management

Psychoeducation. This is the simplest form of 'psychological intervention' and is best started during the first consultation at which the diagnosis is discussed. In its barest form, psychoeducation involves the delivery of an understandable definition of the diagnosis, its physiological basis (or as much as is currently understood), the treatments available, the prognosis, and the expected outcome. Psychoeducation should, however, be delivered as an ongoing intervention, rather than as a one-off discussion. Patients will often find that new questions arise during the course of their management programme, and these will need to be answered. This need not be performed by a single member of the team, but rather is more likely to be a team effort. Psychoeducation has been shown to work well when delivered in a group setting, and it may be that the group process provides added benefit [42, 43].

Cognitive-Behavioural Therapy (CBT). CBT has consistently demonstrated a greater effect than other psychotherapies, although the effect sizes reported are small to moderate [44–46]. Benefits are seen for pain, negative mood, and disability, and these are maintained in the longer term in comparison with control conditions (typically 'treatment as usual' or waiting-list groups). It is important that the CBT be directed towards elements of the disorder, rather than dogmatically applying an approach generic to symptoms of anxiety and depression. This may lead to difficulty in finding an appropriate specialist for some services. However, computer delivery of CBT programmes has also been found to be effective [47], so this has potential as a therapeutic alternative.

Exercise and Activity. Overall, regular exercise has been shown to improve tenderness, pain, and well-being compared with no exercise [14, 48]. Different types of exercise have also been examined individually: aerobic exercise appears effective in the reduction of pain, fatigue, and depressive symptoms whilst improving self-rated quality-of-life scores [49, 50]; strength training reduces the severity of fibromyalgia symptoms [51]; and mixed exercise training improves pain and physical function [52]. Aquatic exercise may be useful for pain, quality-of-life scores, physical function, and muscle strength [29, 53–56], but trials are often methodologically flawed [52], and currently, the conclusion is that land-based exercise is more effective [49]. Early investigations have not revealed a benefit of exercise against the cognitive deficits associated with fibromyalgia [57]. A recent Cochrane review [58] advocates 20 minutes of exercise per day, 2–3 days per week, for at least 2.5 weeks.

The central principle of 'prescribed' exercise is similar to suggested principles in prescribing medication: namely, to 'start low and go slow', using a graded approach to exposure to exercise that aims for attainment of moderate intensity [52, 59, 60]. Normally, exercise programmes are delivered in conjunction with other therapies that are aimed at improving symptom management, including medication, self-management education programmes, stress management, relaxation training, and biofeedback. Various combinations of these approaches have demonstrated efficacy [61].

Pain Management and Self-Help Approaches. These approaches have been combined with CBT and psychoeducation to demonstrate efficacy, and combining them with exercise programmes has also demonstrated a beneficial short-term effect [62].

Sleep Hygiene. Given that nonrestorative sleep is a prominent problem for fibromyalgia patients and that even subtle disruptions in sleep may partially explain fatigue and pain, possibly in relation to abnormal sympathetic tone [63], efforts to ensure basic sleep hygiene are important. These may form part of an initial psychoeducational approach.

Acupuncture. Although not widely available and possibly not widely accepted, a recent Cochrane review reports some short-term reductions in pain with acupuncture. However, the methodological quality was poor in most of the studies reviewed, and few measures other than stiffness improved compared with the sham (control) conditions employed [64].

Chronic Fatigue Syndrome

CFS is a disorder comprising chronic idiopathic fatigue, muscle and joint pain, cognitive difficulties, lymph node tenderness, unrefreshing sleep, headaches, sore throat and post-exertional malaise. Depending on the definition used, the prevalence of CFS is between 0.2 and 2.6% worldwide [65]. It affects more women than men and is more common at ages over 40 years [66, 67]. Its clinical similarities with fibromyalgia are striking, and this has led some to question the relevance of considering them as separate entities. However, physiological investigation and treatment responses continue to support their separation, albeit the fact that they are common comorbidities.

The fatigue experienced is debilitating, and sufferers are twice as likely to be unemployed as those with chronic fatigue not meeting the criteria for CFS [68]. Additionally, sufferers are more likely to report functional impairment than those with chronic fatigue alone [68]. The diagnostic nomenclature has proven controversial; having previously been termed 'myalgic encephalomyelitis', the name was changed to 'chronic fatigue syndrome' when research failed to demonstrate evidence for inflammation of the brain or spinal cord. This change has been mistakenly interpreted by some as being representative of the medical community considering the disorder to be one of 'the mind' rather than the brain. This Cartesian division is artificial, and the assumption is far from the truth: some of the more innovative and exciting research conducted on this disorder remains neurophysiological. Definitive treatment of the disorder remains elusive, and to date, the best responses have been demonstrated with cognitive and behavioural interventions [69], which are more likely to result in recovery than other approaches [70]. Rather than reflecting treatment of a disorder of 'the mind', the benefits of these treatments may be related to a positive alteration at the neurophysiological level. Precisely what this change is, or where it occurs, remains unclear.

Diagnosis

CFS is a diagnosis that can only be made once other causes of fatigue have been excluded. As for fibromyalgia, different sets of diagnostic criteria have been developed over the years, some broader and more inclusive than others. Although there has been some discussion as to which are the more appropriate, for the purposes of this chapter, the Center for Disease Control and Prevention (CDC) criteria (1988, revised in 1994) [71] and the Oxford criteria (1991) [72] will be considered; the former focus more on 'physical' symptoms, and the latter focus more on 'mental fatigue', and these criteria are more consistently used in the clinical research that forms the current evidence base. Diagnosis should start with careful history taking and examination. The aim should be not only to identify the symptoms that are most problematic for the patient but also to exclude alternative pathology that could explain the fatigue. Notable clinical findings that might indicate alternative pathology include chest pain, shortness of breath, focal neurological deficits, hallmarks of inflammatory disease, lymphadenopathy, and significant weight loss. This is not an exhaustive list, but it does take into account the recently developed National Institute for Health and Care Excellence guidelines [73].

A comprehensive mental state examination should also be performed in order to rule out all major mental disorders, and especially major depressive, anxiety, and psychotic disorders. The first two have the potential to explain chronic fatigue, whilst the last is an exclusion for the diagnosis. Notwithstanding this, it is equally important to remember that CFS commonly occurs in tandem with anxiety and major depressive disorders. History taking is vital here in determining temporal relationships with fatigue to determine whether it is primary and idiopathic (CFS) or secondary and related to alternative disease processes.

There remains no definitive test for CFS, and although investigations may be useful for the exclusion of alternative diagnoses, they should be kept to a minimum [73, 74]. Current recommendations in this regard include a full blood count, tests for urea and electrolytes, a calcium and bone profile (including phosphate), thyroid function C-reactive protein and urinalysis. A urine drug screen and an autoantibody screen (anti-endomysial antibodies, antinuclear antibodies, and rheumatoid factor) may also be indicated. Although patients often cite infections, and especially viral ones, as precipitating events, viral titres (e.g. Epstein-Barr virus) are not recommended, as they neither rule in nor rule out the diagnosis.

Additional Symptoms and Comorbidities

The most common symptoms reported in addition to fatigue are chronic pain, disturbed sleep, problems concentrating, depression, and anxiety.

Chronic Pain. Pain is a common symptom in CFS that is reported by sufferers as being disabling and as compromising both physical and social function [75]. The CDC criteria include five potential types of pain (muscle pain, joint pain, headache, sore throat, and tender lymph nodes). Muscle pain is the most common, affecting up to 93% of patients [76, 77].

Sleep. CFS patients may overestimate sleep disturbance [78]. However, subtle disruptions may partially explain fatigue and pain, possibly in relation to abnormal sympathetic tone [63]. It has also been suggested that a delayed circadian rhythm may contribute to the symptoms of CFS [79]. In addition, delayed sleep phase disorder may be an important differential diagnosis in some instances.

Cognitive Difficulties. Up to 85% [80] of patients experience significant cognitive difficulties, which include slow thinking, difficulty focussing and poor concentration, confusion, and forgetfulness. These may be the most debilitating symptoms for some patients [81, 82], who may describe thinking as feeling like 'walking through treacle'. Deficits have been proposed in the processing of complex material, with reduced speed and efficiency in the processing of information [83]. Selective deficits have been found in memory processing [84], with working memory deficits being more profound during more complex tasks that require sustained attention [85]. These deficits are not related to comorbid psychopathology, such as anxiety and depressive disorders [86, 87], and are absent in those not reporting 'mental' fatigue [88].

Depression and Anxiety. As in fibromyalgia, depression and anxiety are common comorbidities in CFS. There is an overlap between CFS and MDD [89] and a high lifetime prevalence of MDD in CFS patients [90]. Although just over half of all patients with CFS have no anxiety or depression, 14% have anxiety, 14% have depression, and 18% have both [91]. These pathologies should be excluded at initial assessment as primary causes of chronic fatigue, but in the context of a diagnosis of CFS, they must be adequately and appropriately managed in order to ensure optimal outcomes [73, 74]. The presence of these comorbidities must also be taken into account in the course of psychological interventions, as the cognitions and behaviours thought to perpetuate CFS differ in patients with concomitant anxiety and depressive disorders and as interventions need to be tailored accordingly [91].

Management

Pharmacological Approaches

The discovery of effective medications for the treatment of CFS has been elusive, especially in the treatment of the primary symptom of fatigue. The additional symptoms of chronic pain, difficulties with sleep, and associated comorbidities such as depression and anxiety can and should be actively treated in order to optimise clinical outcomes. Although distinct disorders, this is where the overlap with fibromyalgia may prove helpful, as many of the pharmacological strategies described above might be effective against the symptoms that define this overlap. However, it remains the case that the evidence and, as a consequence, often the licensing of drugs are for fibromyalgia, rather than CFS. Medications that have proven unsuccessful include methylphenidate [92], melatonin [93], SSRIs [94], and galantamine [95].

Sleep. It has been suggested that a delayed circadian rhythm may contribute to the symptoms of CFS [79] and that melatonin supplementation may be of use. However, evidence does not currently support this approach [79, 93], although it may be of use in the treatment of delayed sleep phase disorder. In the UK, this is a prescription-only medication.

Emerging Treatments

D2 Antagonists. Amisulpride proved to be a promising treatment in reducing fatigue and somatic symptoms in a recent pilot study, but this was in comparison to fluoxetine, and further work is required before its use can be recommended [96].

Immunomodulation. Hydrocortisone, fludrocortisone, and antiviral therapies have all been trialled in small samples and poorly designed studies, so there is currently no evidence to support their use [97–99]. Staphylococcus toxoid was used in one study and demonstrated small clinical improvements, providing that it was not discontinued [100]. The authors suggest that the benefit reported stemmed from invigoration of a hypoactive immune system. Its use is not currently recommended.

Nonpharmacological Management

Psychoeducation. Psychoeducation was assessed in CFS in a trial of 'pragmatic rehabilitation'. This involved the psychoeducation of CFS patients by a specialist nurse and the formulation an agreed-upon plan of gradually increasing activity [101]. It is not yet clear whether the efficacy of this approach alone can be sustained.

The most substantial evidence for the successful management of CFS to date comes in the form of two nonpharmacological treatments: CBT and graded exercise therapy (GET). Evidence in this regard comes from older meta-analyses and a recently published and rigorously designed randomised controlled trial, the 'Pacing, graded Activity and Cognitive behaviour therapy: a randomised Evaluation' (PACE) trial. PACE involved an assessment of standard medical care (at least three appointments with a doctor over 12 months) combined with CBT, GET, or adaptive pacing therapy (APT). Fourteen sessions were provided for one of the treatments, which was assigned at initial randomisation and delivered over a period of 23 weeks, with the offer of an additional 'booster' session at 36 weeks. CBT and GET both proved more efficacious when combined with standard medical care than did standard medical care alone or when combined with APT. The PACE trial was not powered to examine differences between CBT and GET. The outcomes examined were treatment effects not only on fatigue but also on the additional domains of work and social adjustment, depression, anxiety, and post-exertional malaise. Patients assessed their outcome at the end of the trial, 52 weeks after initial randomisation, as being 'much' or 'very much' better [69].

CBT. The provision of CBT in PACE was on the basis of the fear avoidance theory of CFS, which regards CFS as a reversible disorder defined by an interaction between physiological, cognitive (fear of engaging in activity), and behavioural (avoidance of activity) processes that contribute to the perpetuation of fatigue and associated symptoms [69]. The aim of treatment was to change the behavioural and cognitive factors assumed to be responsible for this perpetuation of symptoms and the associated disability. In addition to the benefits demonstrated by the primary outcome measures of the PACE trial, the delivery of CBT in this model was also demonstrated as being effective in the reduction of joint and muscle pain in a secondary analysis [102]. The findings of the PACE trial concur with others that were summarised in a meta-analysis performed prior to the availability of the PACE trial results [103] and another performed after the PACE results were published [104]. In adolescents, CBT has also been demonstrated as effective [105], including when delivered using an internet-based model [106]. CBT for CFS may be less effective in group settings [107], and as such, current recommendations are that individual sessions should be used in order to ensure the greatest response to treatment [73].

Exercise and Activity (GET). The PACE trial [69] demonstrated that GET is as effective for fatigue and the same additional associated domains as CBT is, with the exception of depression. GET in the PACE trial was delivered on the basis of deconditioning and exercise intolerance theories of CFS symptoms, which propose that symptoms are perpetuated by reversible physiological changes due to deconditioning and avoidance of activity. The aim of treatment was to facilitate a gradual return to appropriate levels of physical activity and reverse deconditioning in order to reduce fatigue and associated disability. In the PACE trial [69], a goal of 30 minutes of light exercise, five times per week, was set, with the aim being to reach this goal over a period of 52 weeks. A target heart rate was set individually as a means of preventing overexertion. Once this goal was reached, patients then received individual sessions with GET therapists to increase the intensity of activity [69]. GET is thought to work as a behavioural intervention, rather than as an intervention targeting a change in exercise capacity or physical conditioning per se. In this respect, it is more akin to CBT in terms of decreasing symptom-focussed behaviour. GET was also found to be effective in reducing joint and muscle pain and in reducing the frequency of comorbid fibromyalgia in a secondary analysis of the PACE trial [102].

Pacing or APT. Although historically popular among patients, this approach was found to be ineffective in the PACE trial, although some have argued that this was due to an inappropriate definition. In the PACE trial, the definition of pacing was formulated with the assistance of both patients with CFS and CFS-based charities [108, 109], in addition to feedback from clinicians subsequent to a pilot study of a manualised version of pacing (APT). In the context of PACE, APT was based on the envelope theory of CFS [110], which views CFS as an entirely organic disease process that is not reversible by changes in behaviour and that results in a reduced and finite amount of available energy. Pacing therapy was designed to achieve an optimum adaptation to the illness by identifying links between activity and fatigue with avoidance of exacerbations in order to support the best conditions for a natural recovery [108–110].

Support Groups. Membership in support groups was associated with a worse outcome in the PACE trial. This is surprising and conflicts with reports for other disorders, although the reasons for this association are unclear.

Outcome

One of the most important findings in recent years is the confirmation that recovery from CFS is possible [70]. The importance here is in alleviating the adverse effects that have arisen within a culture of therapeutic nihilism. Patients attending National Health Service specialist centres in the UK can expect similar improvements in fatigue, anxiety, and depression to those in the PACE trial [111]. However, service delivery in the real world seems less able to deliver the same improvements in physical function. It is uncertain as to whether this is due to differences in the delivery or content of the treatments offered [111]. Recovery, as defined in the PACE trial by the Chalder Fatigue Questionnaire, the 36-Item Short-Form Health Survey, and case definition (based on the CDC and Oxford criteria) 52 weeks after initial randomisation, is most likely with CBT and GET [70]. However, the effect sizes of these nonpharmacological treatments are moderate, and the interventions rarely lead to complete resolution. Predictors of a poorer response to treatment include poor social adjustment, strong beliefs in an organic cause for fatigue, and current receipt of benefits [112, 113].

Summary

Fibromyalgia and CFS are debilitating conditions that remain poorly understood. Although similar clinical entities, their differential response to pharmacological treatment might suggest that they are separable on a physiological basis, but they are again drawn together by their response to cognitive and behavioural interventions. Whilst remission should always be a goal, complete symptom resolution is not the norm, but 'moderate' improvements are certainly attainable with appropriate management.

References

1 Vincent A, Lahr BD, Wolfe F, et al: Prevalence of fibromyalgia: a population-based study in Olmsted County, Minnesota, utilizing the Rochester Epidemiology Project. Arthritis Care Res (Hoboken) 2013:65:786–792.

2 Wolfe F, Brähler E, Hinz A, et al: Fibromyalgia prevalence, somatic symptom reporting, and the dimensionality of polysymptomatic distress: results from a survey of the general population. Arthritis Care Res (Hoboken) 2013;65:777–785.

3 Wolfe F, Ross K, Anderson J, et al: The prevalence and characteristics of fibromyalgia in the general population. Arthritis Rheum 1995;38:19–28.

4 Wolfe F, Clauw DJ, Fitzcharles MA, et al: The American College of Rheumatology preliminary diagnostic criteria for fibromyalgia and measurement of symptom severity. Arthritis Care Res (Hoboken) 2010;62:600–610.

5 Wolfe F, Clauw DJ, Fitzcharles MA, et al: Fibromyalgia criteria and severity scales for clinical and epidemiological studies: a modification of the ACR Preliminary Diagnostic Criteria for Fibromyalgia. J Rheumatol 2011;38:1113–1122.

6 McKay PG, Duffy T, Martin CR: Are chronic fatigue syndrome and fibromyalgia the same? Implications for the provision of appropriate mental health intervention. J Psychiatr Ment Health Nurs 2009;16:884–894.

7 Sumpton JE, Moulin DE: Fibromyalgia: presentation and management with a focus on pharmacological treatment. Pain Res Manag 2008;13:477–483.

8 Park DC, Glass JM, Minear M, et al: Cognitive function in fibromyalgia patients. Arthritis Rheum 2001;44:2125–2133.

9 Pae CU, Luyten P, Marks DM, et al: The relationship between fibromyalgia and major depressive disorder: a comprehensive review. Curr Med Res Opin 2008;24:2359–2371.

10 Hamilton WT, Gallagher AM, Thomas JM, et al: Risk markers for both chronic fatigue and irritable bowel syndromes: a prospective case-control study in primary care. Psychol Med 2009;39:1913–1921.

11 Dadabhoy D, Clauw DJ: Therapy Insight: fibromyalgia–a different type of pain needing a different type of treatment. Nat Clin Pract Rheumatol 2006;2:364–372.

12 Giesecke T, Williams DA, Harris RE, et al: Subgrouping of fibromyalgia patients on the basis of pressure-pain thresholds and psychological factors. Arthritis Rheum 2003;48:2916–2922.

13 Clauw DJ: Pain management: fibromyalgia drugs are 'as good as it gets' in chronic pain. Nat Rev Rheumatol 2010;6:439–440.

14 Nuesch E, Häuser W, Bernardy K, et al: Comparative efficacy of pharmacological and non-pharmacological interventions in fibromyalgia syndrome: network meta-analysis. Ann Rheum Dis 2013;72:955–962.

15 Fitzcharles MA, Ste-Marie PA, Goldenberg DL, et al: 2012 Canadian Guidelines for the diagnosis and management of fibromyalgia syndrome: executive summary. Pain Res Manag 2013;18:119–126.

16 Hauser W, Bernardy K, Uçeyler N, et al: Treatment of fibromyalgia syndrome with antidepressants: a meta-analysis. JAMA 2009;301:198–209.

17 Arnold LM, Keck PE Jr, Welge JA: Antidepressant treatment of fibromyalgia. A meta-analysis and review. Psychosomatics 2000;41:104–113.

18 Arnold LM, Crofford LJ, Martin SA, et al: The effect of anxiety and depression on improvements in pain in a randomized, controlled trial of pregabalin for treatment of fibromyalgia. Pain Med 2007;8:633–638.

19 Glass JM: Cognitive dysfunction in fibromyalgia and chronic fatigue syndrome: new trends and future directions. Curr Rheumatol Rep 2006;8:425–429.

20 Arnold LM: Biology and therapy of fibromyalgia. New therapies in fibromyalgia. Arthritis Res Ther 2006;8:212.

21 Fishbain D: Evidence-based data on pain relief with antidepressants. Ann Med 2000;32:305–316.

22 Arnold LM, Lu Y, Crofford LJ, et al: A double-blind, multicenter trial comparing duloxetine with placebo in the treatment of fibromyalgia patients with or without major depressive disorder. Arthritis Rheum 2004;50:2974–2984.

23 Arnold LM, Rosen A, Pritchett YL, et al: A randomized, double-blind, placebo-controlled trial of duloxetine in the treatment of women with fibromyalgia with or without major depressive disorder. Pain 2005;119:5–15.

24 Russell IJ, Mease PJ, Smith TR, et al: Efficacy and safety of duloxetine for treatment of fibromyalgia in patients with or without major depressive disorder: results from a 6-month, randomized, double-blind, placebo-controlled, fixed-dose trial. Pain 2008;136:432–444.

25 Lunn MP, Hughes RA, Wiffen PJ: Duloxetine for treating painful neuropathy, chronic pain or fibromyalgia. Cochrane Database Syst Rev 2014;1:CD007115.

26 Üçeyler N, Sommer C, Walitt B, et al: Anticonvulsants for fibromyalgia. Cochrane Database Syst Rev 2013;10:CD010782.

27 Wiffen PJ, Derry S, Moore RA, et al: Antiepileptic drugs for neuropathic pain and fibromyalgia – an overview of Cochrane reviews. Cochrane Database Syst Rev 2013;11:CD010567.

28 Crofford LJ, Rowbotham MC, Mease PJ, et al: Pregabalin for the treatment of fibromyalgia syndrome: results of a randomized, double-blind, placebo-controlled trial. Arthritis Rheum 2005;52:1264–1273.

29 Crofford LJ, Mease PJ, Simpson SL, et al: Fibromyalgia relapse evaluation and efficacy for durability of meaningful relief (FREEDOM): a 6-month, double-blind, placebo-controlled trial with pregabalin. Pain 2008;136:419–431.

30 Hauser W, Bernardy K, Uçeyler N, et al: Treatment of fibromyalgia syndrome with gabapentin and pregabalin – a meta-analysis of randomized controlled trials. Pain 2009;145:69–81.

31 Arnold LM, Goldenberg DL, Stanford SB, et al: Gabapentin in the treatment of fibromyalgia: a randomized, double-blind, placebo-controlled, multicenter trial. Arthritis Rheum 2007;56:1336–1344.

32 Harris RE, Clauw DJ, Scott DJ, et al: Decreased central mu-opioid receptor availability in fibromyalgia. J Neurosci 2007;27:10000–10006.

33 Bennett RM, Kamin M, Karim R, et al: Tramadol and acetaminophen combination tablets in the treatment of fibromyalgia pain: a double-blind, randomized, placebo-controlled study. Am J Med 2003;114:537–545.
34 Holman AJ, Myers RR: A randomized, double-blind, placebo-controlled trial of pramipexole, a dopamine agonist, in patients with fibromyalgia receiving concomitant medications. Arthritis Rheum 2005;52:2495–2505.
35 Holman AJ: Ropinirole, open preliminary observations of a dopamine agonist for refractory fibromyalgia. J Clin Rheumatol 2003;9:277–279.
36 Younger J, Noor N, McCue R, et al: Low-dose naltrexone for the treatment of fibromyalgia: findings of a small, randomized, double-blind, placebo-controlled, counterbalanced, crossover trial assessing daily pain levels. Arthritis Rheum 2013;65:529–538.
37 Russell IJ, Holman AJ, Swick TJ, et al: Sodium oxybate reduces pain, fatigue, and sleep disturbance and improves functionality in fibromyalgia: results from a 14-week, randomized, double-blind, placebo-controlled study. Pain 2011;152:1007–1017.
38 ClinicalTrials.gov: GSK and GW679769; in Fibromyalgia. 2008. http://clinicaltrials.gov/ct2/show/NCT00264628 (accessed March 26, 2014).
39 Lynch ME, Campbell F: Cannabinoids for treatment of chronic non-cancer pain; a systematic review of randomized trials. Br J Clin Pharmacol 2011;72:735–744.
40 Skrabek RQ, Galimova L, Ethans K, et al: Nabilone for the treatment of pain in fibromyalgia. J Pain 2008;9:164–173.
41 Cohen SP, Verdolin MH, Chang AS, et al: The intravenous ketamine test predicts subsequent response to an oral dextromethorphan treatment regimen in fibromyalgia patients. J Pain 2006;7:391–398.
42 Goldenberg DL, Burckhardt C, Crofford L: Management of fibromyalgia syndrome. JAMA 2004;292:2388–2395.
43 Burckhardt CS, Goldenberg DL, American Pain Society: Guideline for the Management of Fibromyalgia Syndrome Pain in Adults and Children. Glenview, IL, American Pain Society (APS), 2005.
44 Vlaeyen JW, Teeken-Gruben NJ, Goossens ME, et al: Cognitive-educational treatment of fibromyalgia: a randomized clinical trial. I. Clinical effects. J Rheumatol 1996;23:1237–1245.
45 Turk DC: Cognitive-behavioral approach to the treatment of chronic pain patients. Reg Anesth Pain Med 2003;28: 573–579.
46 Thieme K, Gracely RH: Are psychological treatments effective for fibromyalgia pain? Curr Rheumatol Rep 2009;11: 443–450.
47 Williams DA, Kuper D, Segar M, et al: Internet-enhanced management of fibromyalgia: a randomized controlled trial. Pain 2010;151:694–702.
48 Fontaine KR, Conn L, Clauw DJ: Effects of lifestyle physical activity on perceived symptoms and physical function in adults with fibromyalgia: results of a randomized trial. Arthritis Res Ther 2010;12:R55.
49 Hauser W, Klose P, Langhorst J, et al: Efficacy of different types of aerobic exercise in fibromyalgia syndrome: a systematic review and meta-analysis of randomised controlled trials. Arthritis Res Ther 2010;12:R79.
50 Dinler M, Diracoglu D, Kasikcioglu E, et al: Effect of aerobic exercise training on oxygen uptake and kinetics in patients with fibromyalgia. Rheumatol Int 2009; 30:281–284.
51 Kingsley JD, McMillan V, Figueroa A: The effects of 12 weeks of resistance exercise training on disease severity and autonomic modulation at rest and after acute leg resistance exercise in women with fibromyalgia. Arch Phys Med Rehabil 2010;91:1551–1557.
52 Busch AJ, Overend TJ, Schachter CL: Fibromyalgia treatment: the role of exercise and physical activity. Int J Clin Rheumatol 2009;4:343–380.
53 Munguia-Izquierdo D, Legaz-Arrese A: Exercise in warm water decreases pain and improves cognitive function in middle-aged women with fibromyalgia. Clin Exp Rheumatol 2007;25:823–830.
54 Tomas-Carus P, Gusi N, Häkkinen A, et al: Eight months of physical training in warm water improves physical and mental health in women with fibromyalgia: a randomized controlled trial. J Rehabil Med 2008;40:248–252.
55 Gusi N, Tomas-Carus P: Cost-utility of an 8-month aquatic training for women with fibromyalgia: a randomized controlled trial. Arthritis Res Ther 2008;10: R24.
56 Tomas-Carus P, Gusi N, Häkkinen A, et al: Improvements of muscle strength predicted benefits in HRQOL and postural balance in women with fibromyalgia: an 8-month randomized controlled trial. Rheumatology (Oxford) 2009;48: 1147–1151.
57 Etnier JL, Karper WB, Gapin JI, et al: Exercise, fibromyalgia, and fibrofog: a pilot study. J Phys Act Health 2009;6: 239–246.
58 Busch AJ, Barber KA, Overend TJ, et al: Exercise for treating fibromyalgia syndrome. Cochrane Database Syst Rev 2007;4:CD003786.
59 Jones KD, Liptan GL: Exercise interventions in fibromyalgia: clinical applications from the evidence. Rheum Dis Clin North Am 2009;35:373–391.
60 Lemos MC, Valim V, Zandonade E, et al: Intensity level for exercise training in fibromyalgia by using mathematical models. BMC Musculoskelet Disord 2010;11:54.
61 Busch AJ, Webber SC, Brachaniec M, et al: Exercise therapy for fibromyalgia. Curr Pain Headache Rep 2011;15:358–367.
62 Hauser W, Bernardy K, Arnold B, et al: Efficacy of multicomponent treatment in fibromyalgia syndrome: a meta-analysis of randomized controlled clinical trials. Arthritis Rheum 2009;61:216–224.
63 Togo F, Natelson BH, Cherniack NS, et al: Sleep structure and sleepiness in chronic fatigue syndrome with or without coexisting fibromyalgia. Arthritis Res Ther 2008;10:R56.
64 Deare JC, Zheng Z, Xue CC, et al: Acupuncture for treating fibromyalgia. Cochrane Database Syst Rev 2013;5: CD007070.
65 Prins JB, van der Meer JW, Bleijenberg G: Chronic fatigue syndrome. Lancet 2006;367:346–355.
66 Bierl C, Nisenbaum R, Hoaglin DC, et al: Regional distribution of fatiguing illnesses in the United States: a pilot study. Popul Health Metr 2004;2:1.
67 Reeves WC, Jones JF, Maloney E, et al: Prevalence of chronic fatigue syndrome in metropolitan, urban, and rural Georgia. Popul Health Metr 2007;5:5.

68 Darbishire L, Ridsdale L, Seed PT: Distinguishing patients with chronic fatigue from those with chronic fatigue syndrome: a diagnostic study in UK primary care. Br J Gen Pract 2003;53:441–445.
69 White PD, Goldsmith KA, Johnson AL, et al: Comparison of adaptive pacing therapy, cognitive behaviour therapy, graded exercise therapy, and specialist medical care for chronic fatigue syndrome (PACE): a randomised trial. Lancet 2011;377:823–836.
70 White PD, Goldsmith K, Johnson AL, et al: Recovery from chronic fatigue syndrome after treatments given in the PACE trial. Psychol Med 2013;43:2227–2235.
71 Reeves WC, Wagner D, Nisenbaum R, et al: Chronic fatigue syndrome – a clinically empirical approach to its definition and study. BMC Med 2005;3:19.
72 Sharpe MC, Archard LC, Banatvala JE, et al: A report – chronic fatigue syndrome: guidelines for research. J R Soc Med 1991;84:118–121.
73 National Collaborating Centre for Primary Care (Great Britain) Royal College of General Practitioners, Chronic Fatigue Syndrome/Myalgic Encephalomyelitis (or Encephalopathy): Diagnosis and Management of Chronic Fatigue Syndrome/Myalgic Encephalomyelitis (or Encephalopathy) in Adults and Children. London, England, National Collaborating Centre for Primary Care, Royal College of General Practitioners, 2007.
74 Fukuda K, Straus SE, Hickie I, et al: The chronic fatigue syndrome: a comprehensive approach to its definition and study. International Chronic Fatigue Syndrome Study Group. Ann Intern Med 1994;121:953–959.
75 Meeus M, Nijs J, Meirleir KD: Chronic musculoskeletal pain in patients with the chronic fatigue syndrome: a systematic review. Eur J Pain 2007;11:377–386.
76 Vercoulen JH, Swanink CM, Fennis JF, et al: Dimensional assessment of chronic fatigue syndrome. J Psychosom Res 1994;38:383–392.
77 King C, Jason LA: Improving the diagnostic criteria and procedures for chronic fatigue syndrome. Biol Psychol 2005;68:87–8106.
78 Majer M, Jones JF, Unger ER, et al: Perception versus polysomnographic assessment of sleep in CFS and non-fatigued control subjects: results from a population-based study. BMC Neurol 2007;7:40.
79 van Heukelom RO, Prins JB, Smits MG, et al: Influence of melatonin on fatigue severity in patients with chronic fatigue syndrome and late melatonin secretion. Eur J Neurol 2006;13:55–60.
80 Komaroff AL: Clinical presentation of chronic fatigue syndrome. Ciba Found Symp 1993;173:43–54; discussion 54–61.
81 Afari N, Buchwald D: Chronic fatigue syndrome: a review. Am J Psychiatry 2003;160:221–236.
82 Jorgensen R: Chronic fatigue: an evolutionary concept analysis. J Adv Nurs 2008;63:199–207.
83 DeLuca J, Johnson SK, Beldowicz D, et al: Neuropsychological impairments in chronic fatigue syndrome, multiple sclerosis, and depression. J Neurol Neurosurg Psychiatry 1995;58:38–43.
84 Grafman J, Schwartz V, Dale JK, et al: Analysis of neuropsychological functioning in patients with chronic fatigue syndrome. J Neurol Neurosurg Psychiatry 1993;56:684–689.
85 Dobbs BM, Dobbs AR, Kiss I: Working memory deficits associated with chronic fatigue syndrome. J Int Neuropsychol Soc 2001;7:285–293.
86 DeLuca J, Johnson SK, Ellis SP, et al: Cognitive functioning is impaired in patients with chronic fatigue syndrome devoid of psychiatric disease. J Neurol Neurosurg Psychiatry 1997;62:151–155.
87 Constant EL, Adam S, Gillain B, et al: Cognitive deficits in patients with chronic fatigue syndrome compared to those with major depressive disorder and healthy controls. Clin Neurol Neurosurg 2011;113:295–302.
88 Capuron L, Welberg L, Heim C, et al: Cognitive dysfunction relates to subjective report of mental fatigue in patients with chronic fatigue syndrome. Neuropsychopharmacology 2006;31:1777–1784.
89 Arnold LM: Understanding fatigue in major depressive disorder and other medical disorders. Psychosomatics 2008;49:185–190.
90 Nater UM, Lin JM, Maloney EM, et al: Psychiatric comorbidity in persons with chronic fatigue syndrome identified from the Georgia population. Psychosom Med 2009;71:557–565.
91 Cella M, White PD, Sharpe M, et al: Cognitions, behaviours and co-morbid psychiatric diagnoses in patients with chronic fatigue syndrome. Psychol Med 2013;43:375–380.
92 Blockmans D, Persoons P, Van Houdenhove B, et al: Does methylphenidate reduce the symptoms of chronic fatigue syndrome? Am J Med 2006;119:167.e23–e30.
93 Williams G, Waterhouse J, Mugarza J, et al: Therapy of circadian rhythm disorders in chronic fatigue syndrome: no symptomatic improvement with melatonin or phototherapy. Eur J Clin Invest 2002;32:831–837.
94 Hartz AJ, Bentler SE, Brake KA, et al: The effectiveness of citalopram for idiopathic chronic fatigue. J Clin Psychiatry 2003;64:927–935.
95 Blacker CV, Greenwood DT, Wesnes KA, et al: Effect of galantamine hydrobromide in chronic fatigue syndrome: a randomized controlled trial. JAMA 2004;292:1195–1204.
96 Pardini M, Guida S, Primavera A, et al: Amisulpride vs. fluoxetine treatment of chronic fatigue syndrome: a pilot study. Eur Neuropsychopharmacol 2011;21:282–286.
97 Cleare AJ, Miell J, Heap E, et al: Hypothalamo-pituitary-adrenal axis dysfunction in chronic fatigue syndrome, and the effects of low-dose hydrocortisone therapy. J Clin Endocrinol Metab 2001;86:3545–3554.
98 Kogelnik AM, Loomis K, Hoegh-Petersen M, et al: Use of valganciclovir in patients with elevated antibody titers against Human Herpesvirus-6 (HHV-6) and Epstein-Barr Virus (EBV) who were experiencing central nervous system dysfunction including long-standing fatigue. J Clin Virol 2006;37(suppl 1):S33–S38.
99 Blockmans D, Persoons P, Van Houdenhove B, et al: Combination therapy with hydrocortisone and fludrocortisone does not improve symptoms in chronic fatigue syndrome: a randomized, placebo-controlled, double-blind, crossover study. Am J Med 2003;114:736–741.

100 Zachrisson O, Regland B, Jahreskog M, et al: Treatment with staphylococcus toxoid in fibromyalgia/chronic fatigue syndrome – a randomised controlled trial. Eur J Pain 2002;6:455–466.
101 Wearden AJ, Dowrick C, Chew-Graham C, et al: Nurse led, home based self help treatment for patients in primary care with chronic fatigue syndrome: randomised controlled trial. BMJ 2010;340:c1777.
102 Bourke JH, Johnson AL, Sharpe M, et al: Pain in chronic fatigue syndrome: response to rehabilitative treatments in the PACE trial. Psychol Med 2014; 44:1545–1552.
103 Price JR, Mitchell E, Tidy E, et al: Cognitive behaviour therapy for chronic fatigue syndrome in adults. Cochrane Database Syst Rev 2008;3:CD001027.
104 Castell BD, Kazantzis N, Moss-Morris RE: Cognitive behavioral therapy and graded exercise for chronic fatigue syndrome: a meta-analysis. Clinical Psychology: Science and Practice 2011; 18:311–324.
105 Stulemeijer M, de Jong LW, Fiselier TJ, et al: Cognitive behaviour therapy for adolescents with chronic fatigue syndrome: randomised controlled trial. BMJ 2005;330:14.
106 Nijhof SL, Bleijenberg G, Uiterwaal CS, et al: Effectiveness of internet-based cognitive behavioural treatment for adolescents with chronic fatigue syndrome (FITNET): a randomised controlled trial. Lancet 2012;379:1412–1418.
107 Bazelmans E, Prins JB, Lulofs R, et al: Cognitive behaviour group therapy for chronic fatigue syndrome: a non-randomised waiting list controlled study. Psychother Psychosom 2005;74:218–224.
108 Cox D, Ludlam S, Mason L, Wagner S, Sharpe M, PACE Trial Management Group: PACE Manual for Therapists: Adaptive Pacing Therapy (APT) for CFS/ME. http://www.pacetrial.org/docs/apt-therapist-manual.pdf (accessed January 7, 2015).
109 National Task Force on CFS/PVFS/ME: Report from the National Task Force on Chronic Fatigue Syndrome (CFS), Post Viral Fatigue Syndrome (PVFS), Myalgic Encephalomyelitis (ME). Bristol, Westcare, 1994.
110 Pesek JR, Jason LA, Taylor RR: An empirical investigation of the envelope theory. J Human Behav Soc Environ 2000;3:59–77.
111 Crawley E, Collin SM, White PD, et al: Treatment outcome in adults with chronic fatigue syndrome: a prospective study in England based on the CFS/ME National Outcomes Database. QJM 2013;106:555–565.
112 Chalder T, Godfrey E, Ridsdale L, et al: Predictors of outcome in a fatigued population in primary care following a randomized controlled trial. Psychol Med 2003;33:283–287.
113 Bentall RP, Powell P, Nye FJ, et al: Predictors of response to treatment for chronic fatigue syndrome. Br J Psychiatry 2002;181:248–252.

Dr. Julius Bourke, MBBS, MRCPsych
The Brain in Pain Study, 3rd floor Dominion House
59 Bartholomew Close
London EC1A 7ED (UK)
E-Mail j.bourke@qmul.ac.uk

Balon R, Wise TN (eds): Clinical Challenges in the Biopsychosocial Interface. Update on Psychosomatics for the 21st Century. Adv Psychosom Med. Basel, Karger, 2015, vol 34, pp 92–108 (DOI: 10.1159/000369088)

Telomeres, Early-Life Stress and Mental Illness

Samuel J. Ridout[a, c] • Kathryn K. Ridout[a, c] • Hung-Teh Kao[b, c] • Linda L. Carpenter[a, c] • Noah S. Philip[a] • Audrey R. Tyrka[a, c] • Lawrence H. Price[a, c]

[a]Mood Disorders Research Program and Laboratory for Clinical and Translational Neuroscience, Butler Hospital, Providence, R.I., [b]Laboratory of Molecular Psychiatry, Butler Hospital, Providence, R.I., [c]Department of Psychiatry and Human Behavior, Alpert Medical School of Brown University, Providence, R.I., USA

Abstract

Telomeres are structures of tandem TTAGGG repeats that are found at the ends of chromosomes and preserve genomic DNA by serving as a disposable buffer to protect DNA termini during chromosome replication. In this process, the telomere itself shortens with each cell division and can consequently be thought of as a cellular 'clock', reflecting the age of a cell and the time until senescence. Telomere shortening and changes in the levels of telomerase, the enzyme that maintains telomeres, occur in the context of certain somatic diseases and in response to selected physical stressors. Emerging evidence indicates that telomeres shorten with exposure to psychosocial stress (including early-life stress) and perhaps in association with some psychiatric disorders. These discoveries suggest that telomere shortening might be a useful biomarker for the overall stress response of an organism to various pathogenic conditions. In this regard, telomeres and their response to both somatic and psychiatric illness could serve as a unifying stress-response biomarker that crosses the brain/body distinction that is often made in medicine. Prospective studies will help to clarify whether this biomarker has broad utility in psychiatry and medicine for the evaluation of responses to psychosocial stressors. The possibility that telomere shortening can be slowed or reversed by psychiatric and psychosocial interventions could represent an opportunity for developing novel preventative and therapeutic approaches.

Introduction

The idea that early-life experiences have enduring sequelae has been at the core of psychiatric theory since the early 20th century. The initial formulations of this idea emphasized the clinical implications, particularly in classical psychoanalytic theory, and there is now ample empirical evidence that childhood adversity increases the risk for major depressive disorder (MDD), bipolar disorder, anxiety disorders, substance disorders, schizophrenia, eating disorders, personality disorders, and suicidality [1]. Risk appears to be dose dependent, and these disorders may be more

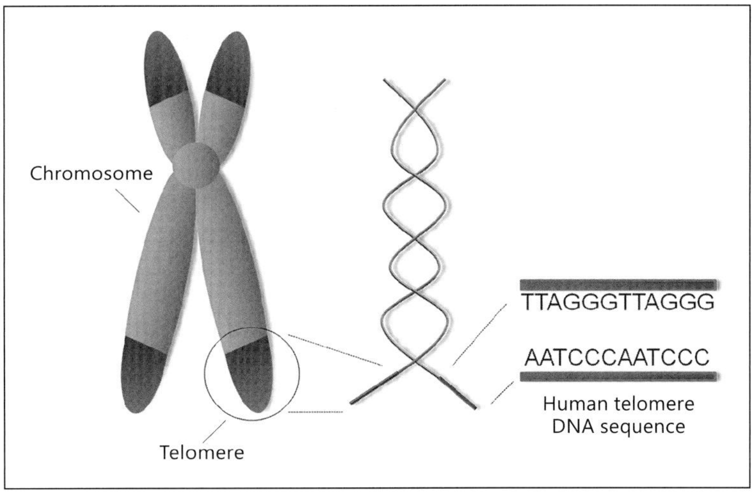

Fig. 1. Chromosome caps and telomeres. Telomeres form the end caps of chromosomes. In humans, telomeres consist of repeated TTAGGG nucleotide sequences ranging from a few to 15 kilobases in length and are found at the end of chromosomal DNA.

resistant to treatment in individuals with a history of childhood maltreatment [1].

In recent years, an etiological role for early-life stress (ELS) has been linked to several prevalent somatic conditions, including irritable bowel syndrome [2], fibromyalgia [3], chronic fatigue syndrome [4], obesity [5], migraine [6], and chronic pain [7]. These disorders have common, but unclear and probably multifactorial, etiology and pathophysiology. However, emerging findings suggest that early environmental factors can impact the risk for conditions generally thought to have a relatively clear pathogenesis, such as cardiovascular disease and type 2 diabetes [8]. Consistent with such findings, individuals with a history of ELS show increased risk for premature death, with one recent study reporting that adults with six or more adverse childhood experiences died nearly 20 years earlier than those without [9].

The hypothalamic-pituitary-adrenal (HPA) axis is a primary system for maintaining homeostasis during physiologic stress, and research on how ELS impacts physiologic function has focused on this system [1]. Other work has demonstrated roles for neuroimmunological, autonomic, oxidative, and non-HPA neuroendocrine responses to stress in linking ELS and disease [10, 11]. Most recently, clinical findings have suggested that telomere biology might offer new insights into the adverse health effects of childhood maltreatment. This chapter, which updates our earlier review [12], examines the current understanding of the relationship between telomeres, illness, and stress and includes key methodological issues.

Basic Concepts of Telomere Biology

Human DNA is sequentially organized into chromosomes, and the DNA sequence must be preserved through cell replication to ensure stability and fidelity of the genome. DNA replication occurs on the lagging strand by utilizing a mechanism of discontinuous synthesis, which would lead to progressive shortening of chromosome ends with each cell replication. To prevent this shortening, chromosome ends contain a specific sequence of nucleotides consisting of tandem TTAGGG repeats ranging from a few to 15 kilobases in length, called telomeres (fig. 1). Telomeres, along with the enzyme telomerase, help elongate and protect the ends of chromosomes so that vital genomic DNA is not lost with each cellular replication [13]. Telomeres are associated with a number of proteins that combine to form a complex that helps preserve the ends of chromosomes from degradation or recognition by DNA repair enzymes, which can trigger repair mechanisms, apoptosis or cellular senescence cascades [14–16].

Telomeres shorten with each cell division [17], and maintenance of telomere function depends on both a minimal length of TTAGGG repeats and telomere-binding proteins [18]. Telomere length is maintained by telomerase, a ribonucleoprotein reverse transcriptase that is mainly expressed in stem cells, germ cells, and regenerating tissues. There is insufficient telomerase in somatic cells to indefinitely maintain telomere length, and most tissues have very low telomerase levels. Consequently, telomeres shorten with age in most somatic tissues, and telomere length can therefore serve as a marker of biological age [19]. Telomere shortening is also influenced by recombination, epigenetic regulation, and genetic factors, as well as by oxidative stress; and the ability of telomerase to counteract these influences is limited. Recently, genome-wide association studies have identified loci that might affect variation in telomere length [20, 21]. In a study of subjects with a history of familial longevity, Lee et al. [20] found that three loci, 4q25, 17q23.2, and 10q11.21, were associated with telomere length. Mangino et al. [21] also identified a locus on chromosome 18q12.2 that was associated with telomere length.

Measurement of Telomere Length

Southern blotting has been the gold standard for measuring telomere length, but limitations to this method include its time-consuming and labor-intensive nature, the large amounts of genomic DNA that are required, the difficulty of deducing telomere length from the resulting smear, and reproducibility. Cawthon [22] developed a method for telomere length measurement that utilizes quantitative polymerase chain reaction (qPCR). Cawthon's method entails separate PCRs to measure telomeres (T), which are normalized to a single copy gene (S), yielding a T/S ratio as a measure of telomere length. qPCR correlates highly with results from Southern blot analyses and is now widely used; in fact, most psychiatric studies examining telomere length have used one of these two methods. However, qPCR has greater measurement error than Southern blotting and can show substantial variability across laboratories [23]. Since individual laboratories internally calibrate their measurements of telomere length, it can be difficult to compare measurements across research groups.

Other methods employ cytometry hybridization techniques [24, 25], which are designed to measure the shortest telomeres and telomeres from specific chromosomes. Once the shortest telomeres are depleted, cells either die or become senescent; therefore, the length of the shortest telomere is a better indicator of cellular aging than the average telomere length. A more detailed discussion of telomere measurement was published by Aubert et al. [26].

Cross-Sectional versus Longitudinal Approaches in Studies of Telomere Length

A major drawback to using telomere length as a clinical measure is its high variability between individuals, which is determined at birth [27, 28]. Moreover, although telomere length is equal between the sexes at birth, shortening with age occurs more rapidly in males than females, and these rates may differ between ethnic groups [29]. These factors limit the power of cross-sectional studies, which utilize measurements at a single time-point. In addition to careful controls for age and sex, such studies require large sample sizes because of the resulting marked variability of telomere length. Aviv et al. [28] estimated that longitudinal studies measuring actual telomere erosion rates within individuals over time would require five-times fewer subjects than cross-sectional studies. Accordingly, longitudinal studies are more powerful than cross-sectional designs for demonstrating causal effects.

Despite these considerations, very few longitudinal telomere studies have been conducted, particularly in psychiatric or stress-related conditions. An alternative approach would be to standardize telomere length in an easily accessible proliferative tissue, which would represent the effects of exposure to the putative causal variable, against telomere length in a postmitotic source because telomere lengths in such tissues change little from birth. However, obtaining samples from postmitotic tissues (i.e., nerves, skeletal muscle, bone) presents practical obstacles. Indeed, even peripheral blood can be difficult to obtain in a longitudinal context.

Source Tissue and Telomere Length

Telomeric DNA in somatic cells shortens with each cell division. Studies comparing telomere length from different source tissues show that intra-individual telomere length is significantly correlated with disparate tissue types in healthy subjects [30]. Due to convenience, most human studies have utilized telomeres derived from peripheral blood leukocytes. However, a possible drawback to this approach is that telomere length may differ among different leukocyte subsets, so that factors favoring predominance of one subset over another can introduce bias [28]. In studies of populations with disease states that exert such effects, such as human immunodeficiency virus infection, telomere length might be more appropriately ascertained in a specific subset of leukocytes. The major determinants of aging, including cell replication, inflammation, and oxidative stress, are all demonstrable in leukocyte telomeres [19, 31, 32]. As a result, controlling for factors that alter leukocyte turnover or subsets (e.g., inflammatory conditions) can help minimize bias. An alternative approach is the use of buccal mucosa cells obtained by oral swab, which is less invasive than venipuncture and therefore useful for studies with children [33–35]; however, there is less experience with this tissue source.

Telomere Length and Dynamics in Somatic Diseases

A number of disease states have been associated with changes in telomere length, including diabetes mellitus, obesity, and heart disease. However, there is, as yet, no clear unitary mechanism to account for telomere shortening across these various conditions. One common factor is that they all entail physiologic stress or a state of disequilibrium. Genome-wide association studies have identified sites associated with telomere shortening during physiologic stress in various patient populations and in several disease states. This is a first step toward developing a mechanistic understanding of how telomere shortening can be observed as a common outcome of physiologic disequilibrium due to multiple etiologies. The recent findings of several diseases that are of major public health concern are discussed below.

Diabetes Mellitus

Diabetes mellitus has been consistently correlated with shortened leukocyte telomere length [36]. Moreover, pancreatic beta cell telomere length is inversely correlated with the hemoglobin A1c (HbA1c) level, which is a measure of diabetes control [37]. Even gestational diabetes, which reflects intra-uterine exposure to stress, has been associated with shorter fetal telomere length [38]. Gene variants in subpopulations may link telomere length with diabetes [39]. Saxena et al. [39] reported that variants in the casein kinase II gene were associated with telomere length in diabetics of Punjabi Sikh heritage. Liu et al. [40], in a study comparing 71 patients with newly diagnosed type II diabetes and 52 controls, found that depressive symptoms were associated with diabetes and that telomere length correlated negatively with depressive symptoms, age, HbA1c levels, and measures of insulin resistance.

Obesity

Obesity is associated with significantly shortened leukocyte telomere length, even when controlling for covariates such as age, smoking, C-reactive protein, diabetes, and hypertension [41]. Severely obese patients demonstrated shorter relative telomere length at baseline and 1 year after bariatric surgery, irrespective of whether they also had metabolic syndrome [42]. Indeed, in the setting of the accelerated catabolic state immediately after bariatric surgery, telomere length attrition was accelerated [42]. It is unclear whether beneficial effects of bariatric surgery on telomere length and telomerase activity might become evident further out from the point of the surgery, especially in patients who maintain weight loss for several years.

Heart Disease

The rate of telomere length attrition has been correlated with cardiovascular damage in middle-aged adults, even after adjustment for traditional cardiovascular risk factors [43]. In cross-sectional studies, leukocyte telomere length was inversely associated with carotid intima medial thickness, a marker of cardiovascular disease risk and atherosclerotic damage, in obese men [44]. In a longitudinal study, telomere length correlated negatively with cardiovascular disease risk, incident carotid artery plaques, and plaque progression [45].

A study examining cardiovascular health and telomere length in young men with a history of intra-uterine growth restriction (IUGR) reported higher cardiovascular risk factors in the IUGR group compared to control men, as expected; however, the IUGR group unexpectedly had longer leukocyte telomere length [46]. The authors acknowledged that this finding contradicted the large body of existing data on telomere length, disease risk, and progression. Noting that age and telomere length were inversely correlated in the IUGR group, they suggested that accelerated telomere shortening might occur in the IUGR men as they aged further, which would be consistent with their apparent increased risk for cardiovascular disease. These findings underscore the perils of cross-sectional assessment of telomere length as a predictor of disease risk in specific patient populations and demonstrate the importance of study designs that can capture dynamic changes in telomere length over time.

Asthma and Pulmonary Disease

Lifelong asthma was associated with reduced leukocyte telomere length in a study cohort of individuals aged 26–38 years (n = 1,037) [47]. This reduction was correlated with blood eosinophil counts, suggesting a contributing role of inflammation, and these findings persisted even after adjusting for obesity and smoking status. There was no association between telomere length and asthma only in childhood or adolescent/adult-onset asthma. In a large study of 934 chronic obstructive pulmonary disease cases, 2,834 asthma cases and 15,846 control subjects, Albrecht et al. [48] found that telomeres were shorter in asthmatics and patients with chronic obstructive pulmonary disease after adjusting for age, sex and smoking status. Additionally, they found that the results of tests of lung function (forced expiratory volume in 1 second, forced vital capacity, and their ratio) were positively associated with telomere length, indicating that better lung function within the diseased population was associated with longer telomeres; the same association was evident, although weaker, in healthy controls. The authors suggested that cellular senescence might contribute to the pathogenesis of lung disease, with decrements in lung function observed in the general population due to intrinsic processes associated with aging.

Telomeres in Somatic Diseases: Summary

While telomere length in these conditions could be merely a disease marker (i.e., an indicator of ongoing disease), other evidence implicates telomere length as a risk marker (i.e., a predictor of the likelihood of disease despite current clinical health). For example, in a study on healthy older adults, Cawthon et al. [49] found telomere length highly predictive of eventual mortality, even though the cause of death was variable. Other studies implicate telomere length as a risk marker for cancer [50, 51] and hypertension [52]. Furthermore, reports of reduced telomere length in association with smoking [53], obesity [54], and alcohol abuse [55] are consistent with these conditions as risk factors for increased mortality.

Telomere dysfunction can play a causal role in disease, and telomerase deficiency has been causally linked with the genetic disorders dyskeratosis congenita, familial idiopathic pulmonary fibrosis, and familial bone marrow failure syndromes [19]. Progeroid syndromes, which are characterized by clinical manifestations of accelerated aging and molecular evidence of defective DNA repair, may also reflect the causal involvement of telomeres [19]. One report suggests an increased rate of neuropsychiatric disorders in dyskeratosis congenita [56]. At this point, it would be premature to exclude an etiologic contribution of telomere dysfunction in other conditions.

Telomere Length and Dynamics in Psychiatric Conditions

Most of the findings implicating telomeres in psychiatry have involved mood disorders, independent of stress. In an initial epidemiological study (n = 433), Lung et al. [57] reported an association between reduced leukocyte telomere length and the high-activity allele of the monoamine oxidase A promoter polymorphism, which has been linked to aggression and impulsivity; this association was later found to be mediated by MDD [58]. Simon et al. [59] demonstrated shorter telomeres in patients with MDD (n = 15) or bipolar disorder (type I or II not stated) (n = 29) compared with healthy controls (n = 44) [59]. This result was replicated by Hartmann et al. [60], who found no effect of illness duration or severity or of the nature or intensity of treatment on telomere length in a study comparing MDD patients (n = 54) with controls (n = 20). Similarly, Karabatsiakis et al. [61] reported that a history of depression (n = 44), regardless of the current symptomatology or disease severity, was associated with shortened telomeres in the main effector populations of the adaptive immune system compared to controls (n = 50). In a cohort study by Verhoeven et al. [62] that involved 1,095 MDD patients, 802 remitted patients, and 510 control subjects, patients with MDD had shorter telomeres, and higher symptom severity and longer symptom duration in the last 4 years were associated with shorter telomeres, suggesting a dose-response relationship. The telomere shortening in MDD was not entirely state dependent, as the effect was even evident in remitted patients. In the prospective Dunedin Study (n = 1,037) [63], one of the few studies to evaluate telomere length at two time points, persistent internalizing disorders predicted greater telomere shortening at the 38-year time point in a dose-response manner. This was particularly true in men and was independent of other covariates that were often associated with telomere shortening (e.g., childhood maltreatment, tobacco use, low socioeconomic status).

Elvsåshagen et al. [64], who described reduced telomere length in bipolar II patients (n = 28) compared with controls (n = 28), detected an association with lifetime number of depressive episodes, but not with illness duration. Wikgren et al. [65], who reported shorter telomeres in MDD patients (n = 91) vs. controls (n = 451), also noted an association with hypocortisolism in both groups. However, Wolkowitz et al. [66] found no difference in telomere length between unmedicated MDD (n = 18) and control (n = 17) subjects but did find inverse correlations with lifetime depression exposure and measures of oxidative stress and inflammation. These authors also reported increased telomerase activity in unmedicated MDD patients vs. controls, with superior antidepressant responses in patients showing the greatest further increases [67]. In an epidemiological study of 952 patients with coronary heart disease, Hoen et al. [68] found an association between MDD and shorter telomeres. In the only study reviewed in this section that did not utilize leukocytes, no differences in telomere length in the occipital cortex of patients with MDD (n = 24) [69] or in cerebellar gray matter of patients with MDD (n = 15), bipolar disorder (n = 46), or schizophrenia (n = 46) were found compared to controls [70]. Zhang et al. [71] found reduced telomere length in soldiers with posttraumatic stress disorder (PTSD) (n = 84) compared to age-matched non-PTSD controls (n = 566). Similarly, Jergović et al. [72] reported shorter telomere length in 30 middle-aged war veterans with current PTSD compared to 17 age-matched healthy controls, but they found no difference in telomerase activity. Martinsson et al. [73] found that long-term lithium treatment for bipolar disorder (n = 256) was associated with longer telomeres and that an increasing number of depressive episodes was associated with shorter telomeres compared to healthy controls (n = 139).

Shorter leukocyte telomeres have been reported in schizophrenia [74] (with one study failing to replicate this finding [75]), schizophrenia with lower global assessment of functioning [76], obstructive sleep apnea [77], migraine [78], mild cognitive impairment [79], and Alzheimer's disease [80] (with one study failing to replicate the latter two findings [81]). Reduced telomere length was also correlated with decreased mental health in chronic heart failure [82] (but not in community-dwelling elderly men [83]), poorer cognition in community-dwelling elders [84] and healthy women [85], unspecified poor sleep quality in healthy women [86], and pessimism in postmenopausal women [87]. It is still unclear whether the shorter telomeres observed in these conditions reflect a specific or nonspecific pre-existing marker of illness vulnerability, a specific or nonspecific marker of ongoing disease, or an entirely nonspecific sequela of psychosocial stress or lifestyle factors (e.g., smoking, obesity) with which these conditions are associated.

Telomere Length and Dynamics with Psychosocial Stressors

Telomere dynamics are impacted by biophysical stress and stressors (e.g., radiation, toxins) [88, 89]. The first evidence that psychosocial stress might also have such effects was from a study by Epel et al. [90] that compared highly stressed mothers caring for a chronically ill child (n = 39) and low-stress mothers with a healthy child (n = 19). Mothers in the highest quartile of perceived stress had shorter telomeres and lower telomerase activity than mothers in the lowest quartile. In a follow-up study of 62 women, these investigators found that reduced telomere length correlated with increased nocturnal urinary cortisol and catecholamines, while low telomerase activity correlated with increased nocturnal urinary epinephrine and greater decreases in heart rate variability during the Trier Social Stress Test (TSST) [91]. Subsequent studies have examined telomere length and telomerase activity in various stress-related contexts. Damjanovic et al. [92] reported shorter telomeres and increased telomerase activity in caregivers of Alzheimer's disease patients (n = 41) compared with controls (n = 41). Kiefer et al. [93], in a study of 56 women, observed reduced telomere length with greater dietary restraint, defined as chronic preoccupation with weight and attempts at restricting food intake leading to chronic psychological stress. In an epidemiological study of 647 sisters of women with breast cancer, Parks et al. [94] found that reduced telomere length correlated with perceived stress, especially in women who were >55 years old, had a recent major loss, or had higher morning urinary epinephrine levels. Humphreys et al. [95] detected shorter telomeres in women exposed to intimate partner violence (n = 61) compared with controls (n = 41). In a study of female caregivers of dementia partners (n = 14) and controls (n = 9), Tomiyama et al. [96] found that shorter telomeres were associated with greater salivary cortisol responses to the TSST and higher overnight urinary free cortisol. In an expanded sample from this study (n = 22 caregivers, n = 22 controls), telomerase activity was lower at baseline in caregivers but rose in both groups during the TSST [97]; and in another expanded sample (n = 27 caregivers, n = 23 controls), reduced telomere length correlated with higher anticipatory threat appraisal, which in turn, correlated with caregiver status, even though telomere length did not differ between the two groups [98].

Kroenke et al. [33] found that buccal telomere length was inversely correlated with heart rate and cortisol reactivity in 78 children during mildly stressful laboratory challenge tasks. Malan et al. [99] observed shorter telomeres in women who developed PTSD following rape (n = 9) compared with those who did not (n = 53). In a study of patients with (n = 18) and without (n = 18) chronic osteoarthritis pain, Sibille et al. [100] found reduced telomere length in those with chronic pain and high stress vs. those with no pain and low stress. Reasoning that hostility correlates with heightened stress reactivity, Brydon et al. [101] found that hostility was inversely correlated with telomere length and positively correlated with telomerase activity in men, but not in women, in an epidemiological sample of 434 adults. Supporting these observational findings in humans, Kotrschal et al. [102] showed that 6-month exposure to reproductive stress in female mice and crowding stress in male mice induced telomere shortening compared with unstressed control mice. In a study of 333 healthy men and women aged 54–76 years, Zalli et al. [103] demonstrated that shorter telomere length and increased telomerase activity were associated with reduced social support, lower optimism, higher hostility, and greater early-life adversity in men, but not in women. Finally, reduced telomere length has been correlated with sociodemographic variables thought to be proxies for sustained psychosocial stress, including lower socioeconomic status [34, 104], African-American ethnicity [29], lower educational attainment [105, 106], and current and long-term work schedule [107].

Telomeres and Early-Life Stress

The first evidence linking ELS with reduced telomere length came from a study by Tyrka et al. [108] on healthy adults with (n = 10) or without (n = 21) a reported history of childhood maltreatment. Other studies have since examined this issue, including the Twins United Kingdom study, which detected no difference in telomere length between individuals who endorsed childhood sexual (n = 34) or physical abuse (n = 20) and those who did not (n = 516 and n = 520, respectively; Glass et al. [109]). Similarly, Jodczyk et al. [110] reported that leukocyte telomere length in participants aged 28–30 years (n = 677) did not correlate with 26 measures of life course adversity, stress that occurred prior to 25 years of age, or with the summary risk scores for each developmental domain. However, Kananen et al. [111] confirmed an association between shorter telomere length and increasing number of reported childhood adverse life events in 974 adults in the Finnish Health 2000 project, even when a relationship with current psychological distress or DSM-IV anxiety disorder diagnosis was absent. Similarly, in a study of 215 older adults recalling ELS, Savolainen et al. [112] found that although temporary separation from parents or a self-reported history of trauma were not associated with telomere length, participants reporting both experiences had shorter telomeres, suggesting an additive effect of stress and traumatic events on telomere length.

Kiecolt-Glaser et al. [113], in a study comprising dementia family caregivers (n = 58) and control subjects (n = 74), reported that shorter telomeres were associated with multiple childhood adversities. Surtees et al. [114], who studied 4,441 women in the United Kingdom European Prospective Investigation into Cancer-Norfolk database, found that shorter telomeres correlated with increased reported childhood adversity experiences, but not with current social adversity or emotional health. Consistent with the results of Malan et al. [99], O'Donovan et al. [115] observed reduced telomere length in adults with chronic PTSD (n = 43) vs. healthy control subjects (n = 47); this was accounted for by those PTSD subjects reporting multiple categories of childhood trauma (n = 18).

In the first study to show effects of early adversity on telomere length in children, Drury et al. [116] found that greater time spent in institutional care correlated with reduced buccal cell telomere length in 100 children aged 6–10 years who participated in the prospective Bucharest Early Intervention Project. Drury et al. [117] reported that buccal cell telomere length was significantly shorter in children with higher exposure to family violence and disruption and that witnessing family violence had an especially potent impact on telomere length in girls, but not in boys, in a population of children aged 5–15 years (n = 80). Entringer et al. [118] demonstrated that the experience of severe psychosocial stress by mothers during pregnancy was associated with shorter telomeres in young adult offspring (n = 45) vs. control subjects (n = 49), suggesting that telomere vulnerability to ELS could extend even to the antenatal period. In the first prospective longitudinal study to determine telomere length at two time points, which involved 236 children tested at age 5 years and again at age 10 years, Shalev et al. [35] found greater buccal cell telomere shortening in children exposed to >2 forms of violence (n = 39) compared with those that were unexposed (n = 128) or less exposed (n = 69). The social environment to which a child is exposed has also been shown to have an effect on telomere length. Theall et al. [119], in a study of neighborhood stress, found that salivary telomere length in 99 children aged 4–14 years was significantly shorter in children exposed to highly disordered neighborhood environments. Similarly, Mitchell et al. [120] found reduced telomere length in 40 9-year-old African American boys associated with low income, low maternal education, unstable family structure, and harsh parenting. This effect was moderated by genetic variants in the serotonergic and dopaminergic pathways, suggesting interplay between telomere length and genetic sensitivity to environmental exposure. Emerging data suggests that early intervention with at-risk children may have a beneficial impact on telomere length. Asok et al. [121], in a study of 89 children, found that parental responsiveness to their child's cues moderated the association between ELS and telomere length, resulting in longer telomeres, even with exposure to ELS, which suggested that there could be measures that provide protective effects, if implemented early. Taken together, these studies support a relationship between ELS and reduced telomere length and suggest that this effect is dose dependent and might be susceptible to amelioration or reversal with appropriate intervention.

Potential Mechanisms Mediating Telomere Length in Early-Life Stress

Wolkowitz et al. [122] observed that many of the biochemical derangements in depression and chronic stress result in cellular effects that are indistinguishable from aging. Indeed, one interpretation of the high comorbidity of depression with diseases of aging, such as cardiovascular disease, cerebrovascular disease, and metabolic syndrome, might be that stress-engendered depression is itself such a disease. In this conceptualization, telomere shortening would be an expected concomitant and/or consequence of the HPA axis dysregulation, enhanced glutamatergic excitotoxicity, increased oxidative stress, impaired neurotrophin function, and immune dysregulation that are reported in chronic stress and depression. Supporting this is evidence suggesting that cortisol can reduce telomerase activity [96, 123]. Further supporting the interaction between stress response and telomere length, Zalli et al. [103] reported that shorter telomeres and increased telomerase activity were associated with impaired physiologic stress responses, such as blunted post-stress systolic blood pressure recovery, heart rate variability, and cortisol. Revesz et al. [124] showed that inflammation, as measured by C-reactive protein and IL-6 levels, a high awakening cortisol response, and an increased heart rate were associated with shorter telomere length. Szebeni et al. [125] demonstrated that oligodendrocytes in post-mortem brains of patients with MDD had shorter telomeres compared to normal controls and that the levels of telomerase reverse transcriptase was lower in MDD patients. The expression of enzymes involved in oxidative stress, such as oligodendrocyte superoxide dismutase, catalase, and glutathione peroxidase, were also lower in oligodendrocytes from the MDD patients. Szebeni et al. hypothesized that blunted responses to oxidative stress, as well as reduced telomerase activity, might contribute to telomere shortening in depression. Furthermore, animal models support the idea that oxidative stress can shorten telomeres, as evidenced by the direct effects of oxidizing substances and antioxidants on telomere length [126].

A review of the biochemistry of aging and telomere dynamics [19, 31, 32, 88, 89] is beyond the present scope, but it is notable that there has yet to be direct demonstration of these mechanisms in affected human subjects. Although attention has turned to the role of epigenetics as a major transductive mechanism for adult sequelae of ELS [127, 128], there are still no direct studies of telomere dynamics in this regard. Lifestyle factors, such as smoking, obesity, and alcohol abuse, are frequent sequelae of ELS, and these factors also affect telomere length. While most studies have controlled for such influences, it is possible that these or other factors could account for the association between reduced telomere length and ELS in cohort studies.

Telomeres and Early-Life Stress: Methodological Issues

Nearly all human studies examining the health implications of telomere length have been cross-sectional in design *with respect to telomere assessment*, which has limited the ability to draw causal inferences about telomere shortening; the same is true for all but one [35] of the 15 studies addressing the effects of ELS. Analogously, *assessment of ELS* can be either prospective or retrospective; all but three [35, 116, 121] studies in this area have been retrospective.

The limitations of cross-sectional vs. longitudinal measurement of telomere length have been discussed. The retrospective determination of ELS is highly variable across studies, and more systematic and comprehensive approaches are likely to compensate for the bias toward false negatives [129]. Several studies have correlated the number of discrete childhood adversities to telomere length, suggesting that early stressors may have additive effects. Ideally, assessment tools should have good psychometric properties; short of that, ascertainment methods requiring the least amount of judgment or interpretation could be more reliable. Such considerations may explain why Glass et al. [109] and Jodczyk et al. [110] failed to replicate an association between ELS and reduced telomere length; however, timing and type of ELS and the impact of mitigating psychosocial or genetic factors ('resilience') [130] could also affect these findings.

Effects of Therapeutic Stress Reduction on Telomeres

Therapeutic interventions designed to mitigate the adverse effects of psychosocial stress (e.g., threat appraisal, rumination, negative affect, stress arousal) might promote telomere maintenance [131]. Supporting this idea, Puterman et al. [132] showed that vigorous exercise attenuated the correlation between perceived stress and reduced telomere length in a sample of 63 healthy women. In a prospective study, Jacobs et al. [133] found that a 3-month intensive meditation retreat increased telomerase activity in participants (n = 30) compared with controls (n = 30); this effect was mediated by increased perceived control and decreased neuroticism. Daubenmier et al. [134] found that decreased chronic stress, anxiety, dietary restraint, dietary fat intake, cortisol, and glucose were correlated with increased telomerase activity both in overweight women receiving a 4-month mindfulness-based intervention for stress eating (n = 47) and in wait-list controls (n = 47). Lin et al. [135] summarized studies examining the effects of lifestyle interventions on telomere length and general health status.

Preliminary data suggest that increases in telomere length due to lifestyle intervention may be durable, as demonstrated in a 5-year follow-up study by Ornish et al. [136]. In a small group of men with low-risk prostate cancer who were undergoing active surveillance, one group (n = 10) received diet, activity, stress management and social support intervention, while the controls (n = 25) received only standard active surveillance. They found that telomere length after 5 years was associated with adherence to the lifestyle intervention, and there was a statistically significant increase in telomere length and preservation of telomerase activity in the intervention group. Positive results in a small sample study such as this are intriguing, as they support the idea that telomere length could serve as an objective measure for evaluating intervention efficacy that can be tracked over time as well as serve as a marker of health and disease. Lengacher et al. [137] provided preliminary evidence that mindfulness-based stress reduction over 12 weeks increased telomerase activity in peripheral blood mononuclear cells from 142 breast cancer survivors.

Summary and Implications

In recent years, the number of papers published on telomeres has more than tripled from roughly 5,000 articles in 2008 [19] to nearly 16,000 to date, and most studies on the relationship between telomere length, psychosocial stress, and psychiatric illness have been published during this brief period. At present, support is strongest for an association between reduced telomere length and psychosocial stress and depression. Given the relationship between stress and depression, this is not surprising, but the mechanisms underlying this effect are still unknown.

The emerging association of reduced telomere length with ELS presents new opportunities for understanding the relationship between stress and psychiatric illness. As proposed by Wolkowitz et al. [122], the downstream consequences of early adversity could be conceptualized as accelerated aging, as it is associated with adverse health outcomes in adults. ELS could also be thought of as predisposition to dysregulated homeostasis/allostatic load [138]. Alternatively, it is possible that ELS does not cause reduced telomere length, but is rather a pre-existing (risk) or acquired (disease) marker for those individuals who subsequently *characterize* their early-life experiences as stressful. At this point, it is still unclear what components of ELS are responsible for its observed association with reduced telomere length.

Research also points to a role of telomerase in understanding telomere dynamics in ELS. Telomerase maintains telomere length, and its activity might be expected to strongly correlate with telomere shortening, suggesting that the effects of chronic stress on this enzyme, rather than on the telomere itself, are important. However, to date, results do not support a simple relationship between telomere length and telomerase activity, with some findings suggesting that telomerase activity might compensatorily increase in response to stress and/or telomere shortening. These uncertainties, in conjunction with the technical difficulty associated with the telomerase assay, may limit the utility of telomerase activity for informing our understanding in this area.

As in most rapidly emerging areas, publication bias in favor of positive findings could be a factor overstating the robustness of the association of ELS with reduced telomere length. Additionally, many publications to date are based on secondary analyses from studies originally designed for other purposes, and most use banked blood specimens to determine telomere length. It is clear that telomere length is affected by many factors, including genetic susceptibility, cellular replication, and oxidative stress. However, cross-sectional measurements of telomere length reflect the interplay of these factors, making it difficult to establish the causal effects of specific experiential exposures. Indeed, such cross-sectional measurements must be recognized as a second-order proxy for the true variable of interest, *change* in telomere length, which can only be directly assessed by measuring telomere length before and after an exposure. This consideration, in conjunction with the great variability in telomere length between individuals, will make it very difficult to develop telomere length as a clinical biomarker of ELS.

Despite these limitations, the findings reviewed here suggest that telomere length has real potential as a biomarker for use in studies aimed at clarifying the sequelae of ELS and perhaps in studies designed to identify future vulnerability and evaluate intervention efficacy. Well-designed prospective studies will determine whether telomere length and dynamics will serve merely as an additional biomarker of general health or as a primary target to evaluate severity of disease and treatment efficacy.

References

1 Heim C, Newport DJ, Mletzko T, Miller AH, Nemeroff CB: The link between childhood trauma and depression: insights from HPA axis studies in humans. Psychoneuroendocrinology 2008;33:693–710.

2 Barreau F, Ferrier L, Fioramonti J, Bueno L: New insights in the etiology and pathophysiology of irritable bowel syndrome: contribution of neonatal stress models. Pediatr Res 2007;62:240–245.

3 Schweinhardt P, Sauro KM, Bushnell MC: Fibromyalgia: a disorder of the brain? Neuroscientist 2008;14:415–421.

4 Heim C, Nater UM, Maloney E, Boneva R, Jones JF, Reeves WC: Childhood trauma and risk for chronic fatigue syndrome: association with neuroendocrine dysfunction. Arch Gen Psychiatry 2009;66:72–80.

5 Charmandari E, Kino T, Souvatzoglou E, Chrousos GP: Pediatric stress: hormonal mediators and human development. Horm Res 2003;59:161–179.

6 Tietjen GE, Peterlin BL: Childhood abuse and migraine: epidemiology, sex differences, and potential mechanisms. Headache 2011;51:869–879.

7 Jones GT, Power C, Macfarlane GJ: Adverse events in childhood and chronic widespread pain in adult life: results from the 1958 British Birth Cohort Study. Pain 2009;143:92–96.

8 Gluckman PD, Hanson MA: Living with the past: evolution, development, and patterns of disease. Science 2004;305:1733–1736.

9 Brown DW, Anda RF, Tiemeier H, Felitti VJ, Edwards VJ, Croft JB, Giles WH: Adverse childhood experiences and the risk of premature mortality. Am J Prev Med 2009;37:389–396.

10 Graham JE, Christian LM, Kiecolt-Glaser JK: Stress, age, and immune function: toward a lifespan approach. J Behav Med 2006;29:389–400.

11 Walker AJ, Kim Y, Price JB, Kale RP, McGillivray JA, Berk M, Tye SJ: Stress, inflammation, and cellular vulnerability during early stages of affective disorders: biomarker strategies and opportunities for prevention and intervention. Front Psychiatry 2014;5:34.

12 Price LH, Kao HT, Burgers DE, Carpenter LL, Tyrka AR: Telomeres and early-life stress: an overview. Biol Psychiatry 2013;73:15–23.

13 Blackburn EH, Greider CW, Szostak JW: Telomeres and telomerase: the path from maize, Tetrahymena and yeast to human cancer and aging. Nat Med 2006;12:1133–1138.

14 de Lange T: Shelterin: the protein complex that shapes and safeguards human telomeres. Genes Dev 2005;19:2100–2110.
15 Degerman S, Siwicki JK, Osterman P, Lafferty-Whyte K, Keith WN, Roos G: Telomerase upregulation is a postcrisis event during senescence bypass and immortalization of two Nijmegen breakage syndrome T cell cultures. Aging Cell 2010;9:220–235.
16 Kishi S, Lu KP: A critical role for Pin2/TRF1 in ATM-dependent regulation. Inhibition of Pin2/TRF1 function complements telomere shortening, radiosensitivity, and the G(2)/M checkpoint defect of ataxia-telangiectasia cells. J Biol Chem 2002;277:7420–7429.
17 Blackburn EH: Telomeres and telomerase: their mechanisms of action and the effects of altering their functions. FEBS Lett 2005;579:859–862.
18 Blackburn EH: Telomeres: structure and synthesis. J Biol Chem 1990;265:5919–5921.
19 Aubert G, Lansdorp PM: Telomeres and aging. Physiol Rev 2008;88:557–579.
20 Lee JH, Cheng R, Honig LS, Feitosa M, Kammerer CM, Kang MS, Schupf N, Lin SJ, Sanders JL, Bae H, Druley T, Perls T, Christensen K, Province M, Mayeux R: Genome wide association and linkage analyses identified three loci-4q25, 17q23.2, and 10q11.21-associated with variation in leukocyte telomere length: the Long Life Family Study. Front Genet 2013;4:310.
21 Mangino M, Richards JB, Soranzo N, Zhai G, Aviv A, Valdes AM, Samani NJ, Deloukas P, Spector TD: A genome-wide association study identifies a novel locus on chromosome 18q12.2 influencing white cell telomere length. J Med Genet 2009;46:451–454.
22 Cawthon RM: Telomere measurement by quantitative PCR. Nucleic Acids Res 2002;30:e47.
23 Aviv A, Hunt SC, Lin J, Cao X, Kimura M, Blackburn E: Impartial comparative analysis of measurement of leukocyte telomere length/DNA content by Southern blots and qPCR. Nucleic Acids Res 2011;39:e134.
24 Lauzon W, Sanchez Dardon J, Cameron DW, Badley AD: Flow cytometric measurement of telomere length. Cytometry 2000;42:159–164.
25 Slijepcevic P: Telomere length measurement by Q-FISH. Methods Cell Sci 2001; 23:17–22.
26 Aubert G, Hills M, Lansdorp PM: Telomere length measurement-caveats and a critical assessment of the available technologies and tools. Mutat Res 2012;730: 59–67.
27 Takubo K, Izumiyama-Shimomura N, Honma N, Sawabe M, Arai T, Kato M, Oshimura M, Nakamura K: Telomere lengths are characteristic in each human individual. Exp Gerontol 2002;37:523–531.
28 Aviv A, Valdes AM, Spector TD: Human telomere biology: pitfalls of moving from the laboratory to epidemiology. Int J Epidemiol 2006;35:1424–1429.
29 Geronimus AT, Hicken MT, Pearson JA, Seashols SJ, Brown KL, Cruz TD: Do US black women experience stress-related accelerated biological aging?: A novel theory and first population-based test of black-white differences in telomere length. Hum Nat 2010;21:19–38.
30 Gramatges MM, Bertuch AA: Measuring relative telomere length: is tissue an issue? Aging 2010;2:756–757.
31 Oeseburg H, de Boer RA, van Gilst WH, van der Harst P: Telomere biology in healthy aging and disease. Pflugers Arch 2010;459:259–268.
32 von Zglinicki T, Martin-Ruiz C: Telomeres as biomarkers for ageing and age-related diseases. Curr Mol Med 2005;5: 197–203.
33 Kroenke CH, Epel E, Adler N, Bush NR, Obradovic J, Lin J, Blackburn E, Stamperdahl JL, Boyce WT: Autonomic and adrenocortical reactivity and buccal cell telomere length in kindergarten children. Psychosom Med 2011;73:533–540.
34 Needham BL, Fernandez JR, Lin J, Epel ES, Blackburn EH: Socioeconomic status and cell aging in children. Soc Sci Med 2012;74:1948–1951.
35 Shalev I, Moffitt TE, Sugden K, Williams B, Houts RM, Danese A, Mill J, Arseneault L, Caspi A: Exposure to violence during childhood is associated with telomere erosion from 5 to 10 years of age: a longitudinal study. Mol Psychiatry 2012; 18:576–581.
36 Zhao J, Miao K, Wang H, Ding H, Wang DW: Association between telomere length and type 2 diabetes mellitus: a meta-analysis. PloS One 2013;8:e79993.
37 Tamura Y, Izumiyama-Shimomura N, Kimbara Y, Nakamura KI, Ishikawa N, Aida J, Chiba Y, Mori S, Arai T, Aizawa T, Araki A, Takubo K, Ito H: Beta cell telomere attrition in diabetes: inverse correlation between HbA1c and telomere length. J Clin Endocrinol Metab 2014;99:2771–2777.
38 Xu J, Ye J, Wu Y, Zhang H, Luo Q, Han C, Ye X, Wang H, He J, Huang H, Liu Y, Dong M: Reduced fetal telomere length in gestational diabetes. PloS One 2014; 9:e86161.
39 Saxena R, Bjonnes A, Prescott J, Dib P, Natt P, Lane J, Lerner M, Cooper JA, Ye Y, Li KW, Maubaret CG, Codd V, Brackett D, Mirabello L, Kraft P, Dinney CP, Stowell D, Peyton M, Ralhan S, Wander GS, Mehra NK, Salpea KD, Gu J, Wu X, Mangino M, Hunter DJ, De Vivo I, Humphries SE, Samani NJ, Spector TD, Savage SA, Sanghera DK: Genome-wide association study identifies variants in casein kinase II (CSNK2A2) to be associated with leukocyte telomere length in a Punjabi Sikh diabetic cohort. Circ Cardiovasc Genet 2014;7:287–295.
40 Liu Z, Zhang J, Yan J, Wang Y, Li Y: Leucocyte telomere shortening in relation to newly diagnosed type 2 diabetic patients with depression. Oxid Med Cell Longev 2014;2014:673959.
41 Chen S, Yeh F, Lin J, Matsuguchi T, Blackburn E, Lee ET, Howard BV, Zhao J: Short leukocyte telomere length is associated with obesity in American Indians: the Strong Heart Family study. Aging 2014;6:380–389.
42 Formichi C, Cantara S, Ciuoli C, Neri O, Chiofalo F, Selmi F, Tirone A, Colasanto G, Di Cosmo L, Vuolo G, Pacini F: Weight loss associated with bariatric surgery does not restore short telomere length of severe obese patients after 1 year. Obes Surg 2014;24:2089–2093.
43 Masi S, D'Aiuto F, Martin-Ruiz C, Kahn T, Wong A, Ghosh AK, Whincup P, Kuh D, Hughes A, von Zglinicki T, Hardy R, Deanfield JE, on behalf of the NSHD scientific and data collection teams: Rate of telomere shortening and cardiovascular damage: a longitudinal study in the 1946 British Birth Cohort. Eur Heart J 2014;35:3296–3303.

44 O'Donnell CJ, Demissie S, Kimura M, Levy D, Gardner JP, White C, D'Agostino RB, Wolf PA, Polak J, Cupples LA, Aviv A: Leukocyte telomere length and carotid artery intimal medial thickness: the Framingham Heart Study. Arterioscler Thromb Vasc Biol 2008;28: 1165–1171.
45 Chen S, Lin J, Matsuguchi T, Blackburn E, Yeh F, Best LG, Devereux RB, Lee ET, Howard BV, Roman MJ, Zhao J: Short leukocyte telomere length predicts incidence and progression of carotid atherosclerosis in American Indians: the Strong Heart Family Study. Aging 2014; 6:414–427.
46 Laganovic M, Bendix L, Rubelj I, Kirhmajer MV, Slade N, Lela IV, Premuzic V, Nilsson PM, Jelakovic B: Reduced telomere length is not associated with early signs of vascular aging in young men born after intrauterine growth restriction: a paradox? J Hypertens 2014;32:1613–1620.
47 Belsky DW, Shalev I, Sears MR, Hancox RJ, Harrington H, Houts R, Moffitt TE, Sugden K, Williams B, Poulton R, Caspi A: Is chronic asthma associated with shorter leukocyte telomere length at midlife? Am J Respir Crit Care Med 2014;190:384–391.
48 Albrecht E, Sillanpaa E, Karrasch S, Alves AC, Codd V, Hovatta I, Buxton JL, Nelson CP, Broer L, Hagg S, Mangino M, Willemsen G, Surakka I, Ferreira MA, Amin N, Oostra BA, Backmand HM, Peltonen M, Sarna S, Rantanen T, Sipila S, Korhonen T, Madden PA, Gieger C, Jorres RA, Heinrich J, Behr J, Huber RM, Peters A, Strauch K, Wichmann HE, Waldenberger M, Blakemore AI, de Geus EJ, Nyholt DR, Henders AK, Piirila PL, Rissanen A, Magnusson PK, Vinuela A, Pietilainen KH, Martin NG, Pedersen NL, Boomsma DI, Spector TD, van Duijn CM, Kaprio J, Samani NJ, Jarvelin MR, Schulz H: Telomere length in circulating leukocytes is associated with lung function and disease. Eur Respir J 2014; 43:983–992.
49 Cawthon RM, Smith KR, O'Brien E, Sivatchenko A, Kerber RA: Association between telomere length in blood and mortality in people aged 60 years or older. Lancet 2003;361:393–395.
50 Wu X, Amos CI, Zhu Y, Zhao H, Grossman BH, Shay JW, Luo S, Hong WK, Spitz MR: Telomere dysfunction: a potential cancer predisposition factor. J Natl Cancer Inst 2003;95:1211–1218.
51 Ma H, Zhou Z, Wei S, Liu Z, Pooley KA, Dunning AM, Svenson U, Roos G, Hosgood HD, 3rd, Shen M, Wei Q: Shortened telomere length is associated with increased risk of cancer: a meta-analysis. PloS One 2011;6:e20466.
52 Yang Z, Huang X, Jiang H, Zhang Y, Liu H, Qin C, Eisner GM, Jose PA, Rudolph L, Ju Z: Short telomeres and prognosis of hypertension in a Chinese population. Hypertension 2009;53:639–645.
53 Morla M, Busquets X, Pons J, Sauleda J, MacNee W, Agusti AG: Telomere shortening in smokers with and without COPD. Eur Respir J 2006;27:525–528.
54 Valdes AM, Andrew T, Gardner JP, Kimura M, Oelsner E, Cherkas LF, Aviv A, Spector TD: Obesity, cigarette smoking, and telomere length in women. Lancet 2005;366:662–664.
55 Pavanello S, Hoxha M, Dioni L, Bertazzi PA, Snenghi R, Nalesso A, Ferrara SD, Montisci M, Baccarelli A: Shortened telomeres in individuals with abuse in alcohol consumption. Int J Cancer 2011; 129:983–992.
56 Rackley S, Pao M, Seratti GF, Giri N, Rasimas JJ, Alter BP, Savage SA: Neuropsychiatric conditions among patients with dyskeratosis congenita: a link with telomere biology? Psychosomatics 2012; 53:230–235.
57 Lung FW, Fan PL, Chen NC, Shu BC: Telomeric length varies with age and polymorphisms of the MAOA gene promoter in peripheral blood cells obtained from a community in Taiwan. Psychiatr Genet 2005;15:31–35.
58 Lung FW, Chen NC, Shu BC: Genetic pathway of major depressive disorder in shortening telomeric length. Psychiatr Genet 2007;17:195–199.
59 Simon NM, Smoller JW, McNamara KL, Maser RS, Zalta AK, Pollack MH, Nierenberg AA, Fava M, Wong KK: Telomere shortening and mood disorders: preliminary support for a chronic stress model of accelerated aging. Biol Psychiatry 2006;60:432–435.
60 Hartmann N, Boehner M, Groenen F, Kalb R: Telomere length of patients with major depression is shortened but independent from therapy and severity of the disease. Depress Anxiety 2010;27: 1111–1116.
61 Karabatsiakis A, Kolassa IT, Kolassa S, Rudolph KL, Dietrich DE: Telomere shortening in leukocyte subpopulations in depression. BMC Psychiatry 2014;14: 192.
62 Verhoeven JE, Revesz D, Epel ES, Lin J, Wolkowitz OM, Penninx BW: Major depressive disorder and accelerated cellular aging: results from a large psychiatric cohort study. Mol Psychiatry 2014; 19:895–901.
63 Shalev I, Moffitt TE, Braithwaite AW, Danese A, Fleming NI, Goldman-Mellor S, Harrington HL, Houts RM, Israel S, Poulton R, Robertson SP, Sugden K, Williams B, Caspi A: Internalizing disorders and leukocyte telomere erosion: a prospective study of depression, generalized anxiety disorder and post-traumatic stress disorder. Mol Psychiatry 2014;19:1163–1170.
64 Elvsashagen T, Vera E, Boen E, Bratlie J, Andreassen OA, Josefsen D, Malt UF, Blasco MA, Boye B: The load of short telomeres is increased and associated with lifetime number of depressive episodes in bipolar II disorder. J Affect Disord 2011;135:43–50.
65 Wikgren M, Maripuu M, Karlsson T, Nordfjall K, Bergdahl J, Hultdin J, Del-Favero J, Roos G, Nilsson LG, Adolfsson R, Norrback KF: Short telomeres in depression and the general population are associated with a hypocortisolemic state. Biol Psychiatry 2012;71:294–300.
66 Wolkowitz OM, Mellon SH, Epel ES, Lin J, Dhabhar FS, Su Y, Reus VI, Rosser R, Burke HM, Kupferman E, Compagnone M, Nelson JC, Blackburn EH: Leukocyte telomere length in major depression: correlations with chronicity, inflammation and oxidative stress–preliminary findings. PloS One 2011;6:e17837.
67 Wolkowitz OM, Mellon SH, Epel ES, Lin J, Reus VI, Rosser R, Burke H, Compagnone M, Nelson JC, Dhabhar FS, Blackburn EH: Resting leukocyte telomerase activity is elevated in major depression and predicts treatment response. Mol Psychiatry 2012;17:164–172.
68 Hoen PW, de Jonge P, Na BY, Farzaneh-Far R, Epel E, Lin J, Blackburn E, Whooley MA: Depression and leukocyte telomere length in patients with coronary heart disease: data from the heart and soul study. Psychosom Med 2011; 73:541–547.
69 Teyssier JR, Ragot S, Chauvet-Gelinier JC, Trojak B, Bonin B: Expression of oxidative stress-response genes is not activated in the prefrontal cortex of patients with depressive disorder. Psychiatry Res 2011;186:244–247.

70 Zhang D, Cheng L, Craig DW, Redman M, Liu C: Cerebellar telomere length and psychiatric disorders. Behav Genet 2010; 40:250–254.

71 Zhang L, Hu XZ, Benedek DM, Fullerton CS, Forsten RD, Naifeh JA, Li X, Li H, Benevides KN, Smerin S, Le T, Choi K, Ursano RJ: The interaction between stressful life events and leukocyte telomere length is associated with PTSD. Mol Psychiatry 2014;19:856–857.

72 Jergovic M, Tomicevic M, Vidovic A, Bendelja K, Savic A, Vojvoda V, Rac D, Lovric-Cavar D, Rabatic S, Jovanovic T, Sabioncello A: Telomere shortening and immune activity in war veterans with posttraumatic stress disorder. Prog Neuropsychopharmacol Biol Psychiatry 2014;54:275–283.

73 Martinsson L, Wei Y, Xu D, Melas PA, Mathe AA, Schalling M, Lavebratt C, Backlund L: Long-term lithium treatment in bipolar disorder is associated with longer leukocyte telomeres. Transl Psychiatry 2013;3:e261.

74 Kao HT, Cawthon RM, Delisi LE, Bertisch HC, Ji F, Gordon D, Li P, Benedict MM, Greenberg WM, Porton B: Rapid telomere erosion in schizophrenia. Mol Psychiatry 2008;13:118–119.

75 Nieratschker V, Lahtinen J, Meier S, Strohmaier J, Frank J, Heinrich A, Breuer R, Witt SH, Nothen MM, Rietschel M, Hovatta I: Longer telomere length in patients with schizophrenia. Schizophr Res 2013;149:116–120.

76 Yu WY, Chang HW, Lin CH, Cho CL: Short telomeres in patients with chronic schizophrenia who show a poor response to treatment. J Psychiatry Neurosci 2008;33:244–247.

77 Barcelo A, Pierola J, Lopez-Escribano H, de la Pena M, Soriano JB, Alonso-Fernandez A, Ladaria A, Agusti A: Telomere shortening in sleep apnea syndrome. Respir Med 2010;104: 1225–1229.

78 Ren H, Collins V, Fernandez F, Quinlan S, Griffiths L, Choo KH: Shorter telomere length in peripheral blood cells associated with migraine in women. Headache 2010;50:965–972.

79 Grodstein F, van Oijen M, Irizarry MC, Rosas HD, Hyman BT, Growdon JH, De Vivo I: Shorter telomeres may mark early risk of dementia: preliminary analysis of 62 participants from the nurses' health study. PloS One 2008;3:e1590.

80 Hochstrasser T, Marksteiner J, Humpel C: Telomere length is age-dependent and reduced in monocytes of Alzheimer patients. Exp Gerontol 2012;47:160–163.

81 Zekry D, Herrmann FR, Irminger-Finger I, Graf C, Genet C, Vitale AM, Michel JP, Gold G, Krause KH: Telomere length and ApoE polymorphism in mild cognitive impairment, degenerative and vascular dementia. J Neurol Sci 2010; 299:108–111.

82 Huzen J, van der Harst P, de Boer RA, Lesman-Leegte I, Voors AA, van Gilst WH, Samani NJ, Jaarsma T, van Veldhuisen DJ: Telomere length and psychological well-being in patients with chronic heart failure. Age Ageing 2010; 39:223–227.

83 Rius-Ottenheim N, Houben JM, Kromhout D, Kafatos A, van der Mast RC, Zitman FG, Geleijnse JM, Hageman GJ, Giltay EJ: Telomere length and mental well-being in elderly men from the Netherlands and Greece. Behav Genet 2012;42:278–286.

84 Yaffe K, Lindquist K, Kluse M, Cawthon R, Harris T, Hsueh WC, Simonsick EM, Kuller L, Li R, Ayonayon HN, Rubin SM, Cummings SR: Telomere length and cognitive function in community-dwelling elders: findings from the Health ABC Study. Neurobiol Aging 2011;32: 2055–2060.

85 Valdes AM, Deary IJ, Gardner J, Kimura M, Lu X, Spector TD, Aviv A, Cherkas LF: Leukocyte telomere length is associated with cognitive performance in healthy women. Neurobiol Aging 2010; 31:986–992.

86 Prather AA, Puterman E, Lin J, O'Donovan A, Krauss J, Tomiyama AJ, Epel ES, Blackburn EH: Shorter leukocyte telomere length in midlife women with poor sleep quality. J Aging Res 2011;2011:721390.

87 O'Donovan A, Lin J, Dhabhar FS, Wolkowitz O, Tillie JM, Blackburn E, Epel E: Pessimism correlates with leukocyte telomere shortness and elevated interleukin-6 in post-menopausal women. Brain Behav Immun 2009;23:446–449.

88 Blasco MA: Telomeres and human disease: ageing, cancer and beyond. Nat Rev Genet 2005;6:611–622.

89 Holt SE, Shay JW: Role of telomerase in cellular proliferation and cancer. J Cell Physiol 1999;180:10–18.

90 Epel ES, Blackburn EH, Lin J, Dhabhar FS, Adler NE, Morrow JD, Cawthon RM: Accelerated telomere shortening in response to life stress. Proc Natl Acad Sci U S A 2004;101:17312–17315.

91 Epel ES, Lin J, Wilhelm FH, Wolkowitz OM, Cawthon R, Adler NE, Dolbier C, Mendes WB, Blackburn EH: Cell aging in relation to stress arousal and cardiovascular disease risk factors. Psychoneuroendocrinology 2006;31:277–287.

92 Damjanovic AK, Yang Y, Glaser R, Kiecolt-Glaser JK, Nguyen H, Laskowski B, Zou Y, Beversdorf DQ, Weng NP: Accelerated telomere erosion is associated with a declining immune function of caregivers of Alzheimer's disease patients. J Immunol 2007;179:4249–4254.

93 Kiefer A, Lin J, Blackburn E, Epel E: Dietary restraint and telomere length in pre- and postmenopausal women. Psychosom Med 2008;70:845–849.

94 Parks CG, Miller DB, McCanlies EC, Cawthon RM, Andrew ME, DeRoo LA, Sandler DP: Telomere length, current perceived stress, and urinary stress hormones in women. Cancer Epidemiol Biomarkers Prev 2009;18:551–560.

95 Humphreys J, Epel ES, Cooper BA, Lin J, Blackburn EH, Lee KA: Telomere shortening in formerly abused and never abused women. Biol Res Nurs 2012;14: 115–123.

96 Tomiyama AJ, O'Donovan A, Lin J, Puterman E, Lazaro A, Chan J, Dhabhar FS, Wolkowitz O, Kirschbaum C, Blackburn E, Epel E: Does cellular aging relate to patterns of allostasis?: An examination of basal and stress reactive HPA axis activity and telomere length. Physiol Behav 2012;106:40–45.

97 Epel ES, Lin J, Dhabhar FS, Wolkowitz OM, Puterman E, Karan L, Blackburn EH: Dynamics of telomerase activity in response to acute psychological stress. Brain Behav Immun 2010;24:531–539.

98 O'Donovan A, Tomiyama AJ, Lin J, Puterman E, Adler NE, Kemeny M, Wolkowitz OM, Blackburn EH, Epel ES: Stress appraisals and cellular aging: A key role for anticipatory threat in the relationship between psychological stress and telomere length. Brain Behav Immun 2012;26:573–579.

99 Malan S, Hemmings S, Kidd M, Martin L, Seedat S: Investigation of telomere length and psychological stress in rape victims. Depress Anxiety 2011;28:1081–1085.

100 Sibille KT, Langaee T, Burkley B, Gong Y, Glover TL, King C, Riley JL, 3rd, Leeuwenburgh C, Staud R, Bradley LA, Fillingim RB: Chronic pain, perceived stress, and cellular aging: an exploratory study. Mol Pain 2012;8:12.

101 Brydon L, Lin J, Butcher L, Hamer M, Erusalimsky JD, Blackburn EH, Steptoe A: Hostility and cellular aging in men from the Whitehall II cohort. Biol Psychiatry 2012;71:767–773.

102 Kotrschal A, Ilmonen P, Penn DJ: Stress impacts telomere dynamics. Biol Lett 2007;3:128–130.

103 Zalli A, Carvalho LA, Lin J, Hamer M, Erusalimsky JD, Blackburn EH, Steptoe A: Shorter telomeres with high telomerase activity are associated with raised allostatic load and impoverished psychosocial resources. Proc Natl Acad Sci U S A 2014;111:4519–4524.

104 Cherkas LF, Aviv A, Valdes AM, Hunkin JL, Gardner JP, Surdulescu GL, Kimura M, Spector TD: The effects of social status on biological aging as measured by white-blood-cell telomere length. Aging Cell 2006;5:361–365.

105 Steptoe A, Hamer M, Butcher L, Lin J, Brydon L, Kivimaki M, Marmot M, Blackburn E, Erusalimsky JD: Educational attainment but not measures of current socioeconomic circumstances are associated with leukocyte telomere length in healthy older men and women. Brain Behav Immun 2011;25:1292–1298.

106 Surtees PG, Wainwright NW, Pooley KA, Luben RN, Khaw KT, Easton DF, Dunning AM: Educational attainment and mean leukocyte telomere length in women in the European Prospective Investigation into Cancer (EPIC)-Norfolk population study. Brain Behav Immun 2012;26:414–418.

107 Parks CG, DeRoo LA, Miller DB, McCanlies EC, Cawthon RM, Sandler DP: Employment and work schedule are related to telomere length in women. Occup Environ Med 2011;68:582–589.

108 Tyrka AR, Price LH, Kao HT, Porton B, Marsella SA, Carpenter LL: Childhood maltreatment and telomere shortening: preliminary support for an effect of early stress on cellular aging. Biol Psychiatry 2010;67:531–534.

109 Glass D, Parts L, Knowles D, Aviv A, Spector TD: No correlation between childhood maltreatment and telomere length. Biol Psychiatry 2010;68:e21–22; author reply e23–e24.

110 Jodczyk S, Fergusson DM, Horwood LJ, Pearson JF, Kennedy MA: No association between mean telomere length and life stress observed in a 30 year birth cohort. PloS One 2014;9:e97102.

111 Kananen L, Surakka I, Pirkola S, Suvisaari J, Lonnqvist J, Peltonen L, Ripatti S, Hovatta I: Childhood adversities are associated with shorter telomere length at adult age both in individuals with an anxiety disorder and controls. PloS One 2010;5:e10826.

112 Savolainen K, Eriksson JG, Kananen L, Kajantie E, Pesonen AK, Heinonen K, Raikkonen K: Associations between early life stress, self-reported traumatic experiences across the lifespan and leukocyte telomere length in elderly adults. Biol Psychol 2014;97:35–42.

113 Kiecolt-Glaser JK, Gouin JP, Weng NP, Malarkey WB, Beversdorf DQ, Glaser R: Childhood adversity heightens the impact of later-life caregiving stress on telomere length and inflammation. Psychosom Med 2011;73:16–22.

114 Surtees PG, Wainwright NW, Pooley KA, Luben RN, Khaw KT, Easton DF, Dunning AM: Life stress, emotional health, and mean telomere length in the European Prospective Investigation into Cancer (EPIC)-Norfolk population study. J Gerontol A Biol Sci Med Sci 2011;66:1152–1162.

115 O'Donovan A, Epel E, Lin J, Wolkowitz O, Cohen B, Maguen S, Metzler T, Lenoci M, Blackburn E, Neylan TC: Childhood trauma associated with short leukocyte telomere length in posttraumatic stress disorder. Biol Psychiatry 2011;70:465–471.

116 Drury SS, Theall K, Gleason MM, Smyke AT, De Vivo I, Wong JY, Fox NA, Zeanah CH, Nelson CA: Telomere length and early severe social deprivation: linking early adversity and cellular aging. Mol Psychiatry 2012;17:719–727.

117 Drury SS, Mabile E, Brett ZH, Esteves K, Jones E, Shirtcliff EA, Theall KP: The association of telomere length with family violence and disruption. Pediatrics 2014;134:e128–e137.

118 Entringer S, Epel ES, Kumsta R, Lin J, Hellhammer DH, Blackburn EH, Wust S, Wadhwa PD: Stress exposure in intrauterine life is associated with shorter telomere length in young adulthood. Proc Natl Acad Sci U S A 2011;108:E513–E518.

119 Theall KP, Brett ZH, Shirtcliff EA, Dunn EC, Drury SS: Neighborhood disorder and telomeres: connecting children's exposure to community level stress and cellular response. Soc Sci Med 2013;85:50–58.

120 Mitchell C, Hobcraft J, McLanahan SS, Siegel SR, Berg A, Brooks-Gunn J, Garfinkel I, Notterman D: Social disadvantage, genetic sensitivity, and children's telomere length. Proc Natl Acad Sci U S A 2014;111:5944–5949.

121 Asok A, Bernard K, Roth TL, Rosen JB, Dozier M: Parental responsiveness moderates the association between early-life stress and reduced telomere length. Dev Psychopathol 2013;25:577–585.

122 Wolkowitz OM, Epel ES, Reus VI, Mellon SH: Depression gets old fast: do stress and depression accelerate cell aging? Depress Anxiety 2010;27:327–338.

123 Choi J, Fauce SR, Effros RB: Reduced telomerase activity in human T lymphocytes exposed to cortisol. Brain Behav Immun 2008;22:600–605.

124 Revesz D, Verhoeven JE, Milaneschi Y, de Geus EJ, Wolkowitz OM, Penninx BW: Dysregulated physiological stress systems and accelerated cellular aging. Neurobiol Aging 2014;35:1422–1430.

125 Szebeni A, Szebeni K, DiPeri T, Chandley MJ, Crawford JD, Stockmeier CA, Ordway GA: Shortened telomere length in white matter oligodendrocytes in major depression: potential role of oxidative stress. Int J Neuropsychopharmacol 2014;17:1579–1589.

126 Ludlow AT, Spangenburg EE, Chin ER, Cheng WH, Roth SM: Telomeres shorten in response to oxidative stress in mouse skeletal muscle fibers. J Gerontol A Biol Sci Med Sci 2014;69:821–830.

127 Low FM, Gluckman PD, Hanson MA: Developmental plasticity and epigenetic mechanisms underpinning metabolic and cardiovascular diseases. Epigenomics 2011;3:279–294.

128 Tyrka AR, Price LH, Marsit C, Walters OC, Carpenter LL: Childhood adversity and epigenetic modulation of the leukocyte glucocorticoid receptor: preliminary findings in healthy adults. PloS One 2012;7:e30148.

129 Hardt J, Rutter M: Validity of adult retrospective reports of adverse childhood experiences: review of the evidence. J Child Psychol Psychiatry 2004; 45:260–273.
130 Nugent NR, Tyrka AR, Carpenter LL, Price LH: Gene-environment interactions: early life stress and risk for depressive and anxiety disorders. Psychopharmacology (Berl) 2011;214: 175–196.
131 Epel E, Daubenmier J, Moskowitz JT, Folkman S, Blackburn E: Can meditation slow rate of cellular aging? Cognitive stress, mindfulness, and telomeres. Ann N Y Acad Sci 2009;1172: 34–53.
132 Puterman E, Lin J, Blackburn E, O'Donovan A, Adler N, Epel E: The power of exercise: buffering the effect of chronic stress on telomere length. PloS One 2010;5:e10837.
133 Jacobs TL, Epel ES, Lin J, Blackburn EH, Wolkowitz OM, Bridwell DA, Zanesco AP, Aichele SR, Sahdra BK, MacLean KA, King BG, Shaver PR, Rosenberg EL, Ferrer E, Wallace BA, Saron CD: Intensive meditation training, immune cell telomerase activity, and psychological mediators. Psychoneuroendocrinology 2011;36:664–681.
134 Daubenmier J, Lin J, Blackburn E, Hecht FM, Kristeller J, Maninger N, Kuwata M, Bacchetti P, Havel PJ, Epel E: Changes in stress, eating, and metabolic factors are related to changes in telomerase activity in a randomized mindfulness intervention pilot study. Psychoneuroendocrinology 2012;39: 917–928.
135 Lin J, Epel E, Blackburn E: Telomeres and lifestyle factors: Roles in cellular aging. Mutat Res 2012;730:85–89.
136 Ornish D, Lin J, Chan JM, Epel E, Kemp C, Weidner G, Marlin R, Frenda SJ, Magbanua MJ, Daubenmier J, Estay I, Hills NK, Chainani-Wu N, Carroll PR, Blackburn EH: Effect of comprehensive lifestyle changes on telomerase activity and telomere length in men with biopsy-proven low-risk prostate cancer: 5-year follow-up of a descriptive pilot study. Lancet Oncol 2013;14: 1112–1120.
137 Lengacher CA, Reich RR, Kip KE, Barta M, Ramesar S, Paterson CL, Moscoso MS, Carranza I, Budhrani PH, Kim SJ, Park HY, Jacobsen PB, Schell MJ, Jim HS, Post-White J, Farias JR, Park JY: Influence of mindfulness-based stress reduction (MBSR) on telomerase activity in women with breast cancer (BC). Biol Res Nurs 2014; 16:438–447.
138 McEwen BS, Stellar E: Stress and the individual. Mechanisms leading to disease. Arch Intern Med 1993;153: 2093–2101.

Lawrence H. Price, MD
Butler Hospital
345 Blackstone Blvd.
Providence, RI 02906 (USA)
E-Mail Lawrence_Price_MD@Brown.edu

Balon R, Wise TN (eds): Clinical Challenges in the Biopsychosocial Interface. Update on Psychosomatics for the 21st Century. Adv Psychosom Med. Basel, Karger, 2015, vol 34, pp 109–122 (DOI: 10.1159/000369089)

Coping with Losses, Grief, and Mourning in Prostate Cancer

Daniela Wittmann

Department of Urology, University of Michigan, Ann Arbor, Mich., USA

Abstract

Prostate cancer is a highly prevalent disease with a high likelihood of survival. If treated, survivors live with significant and lasting treatment-related side effects. Surgical treatment is associated with urinary incontinence and erectile dysfunction, and radiation leads to urinary and bowel irritability as well as erectile dysfunction. Patients who undergo hormonal treatment cope with sexual dysfunction, bone density loss, hot flashes, mood symptoms, and cardiac and metabolic disorders. Functional losses have a significant impact on patients and their partners' quality of life and are associated with distress and psychosocial morbidity. Psychosocial treatment is largely unavailable in usual care, but has been shown to reduce distress, to increase positive reappraisal of the illness, and to contribute to the recovery of sexual intimacy. Treatment for grief and mourning, typical reactions to loss, has not been introduced into psychosocial interventions but is increasingly recognized as a path toward a 'new normal' after prostate cancer treatment.

Introduction

Although some have dubbed prostate cancer 'the good cancer' because the majority of men survive it for long periods [1], it is a perspective that perhaps overlooks the profound impact that prostate cancer and its treatment have on men's lives and on the lives of their partners over many years. According to the most recent statistics, one in six American men has a lifetime chance of being diagnosed with prostate cancer. If the man is African American, the chance increases to one in five. If the man has a father or brother already diagnosed with prostate cancer, his chance becomes one in three [2]. The United States has one of the highest incidences of prostate cancer; Norway and France are the world leaders, with Western Europe, United States, and Australia following closely behind [3]. Thus, when we speak about the effect of prostate cancer and its treatment on men and their partners, we are describing a high-level population impact.

Screening for prostate cancer through prostate-specific antigen (PSA) testing has led to the cancer being detected early, while it is still localized. Men with nonaggressive localized prostate treatment have the option of choosing either active surveillance with recurrent PSA testing and biopsies or watchful waiting, which enables them to opt for treatment when progression of their prostate cancer becomes clear through symptoms.

A recent guideline on PSA screening, which remains controversial [4, 5], has cautioned against over-treatment, which may result in unnecessary post-treatment morbidity. Between 20% and 32% of men choose active surveillance or watchful waiting, partially driven by counseling by their physicians, who anticipate a slow cancer course, and partially because of their awareness that all definitive treatments will have side effects with a potentially significant impact on the quality of their lives [6, 7]. However, many men opt for definitive treatment once they realize that they have cancer, regardless of how aggressive it is. Definitive treatment for localized prostate cancer usually means either surgical removal of the prostate or irradiation of the prostate, both using a variety approaches. For men with more aggressive prostate cancer, androgen deprivation therapy or chemotherapy is added to surgical or radiation treatment. For metastatic disease, a systemic approach, including androgen deprivation therapy or chemotherapy, is used alone [8].

The impact of prostate cancer treatment on patients' functional status has been well described over the past 2 decades [9–14]. Based on interest in understanding the impact of cancer treatments on the quality of patients' lives, a variety of measures were developed to capture functional morbidity and validated in cohorts or prostate cancer survivors. Some examples of widely used measures are the UCLA Prostate Cancer Index [15] and the Expanded Prostate Cancer Index Composite [16, 17]. Treatment for localized prostate cancer tends to result in specific side effects; some are time limited, while others persist. Treatment for advanced prostate cancer has more profound effects on physical function and brings about the realization of a shortened lifespan. Both localized and advanced prostate cancers lead to changes that can be and usually are experienced by prostate cancer survivors as losses. As a result, survivors must adjust and cope not only physically but also psychologically. Clinical care therefore must address both aspects of the survivor's experience.

Functional Losses after Prostate Cancer Treatment

Urinary Incontinence and Irritability

Urinary incontinence is associated with surgical treatment for prostate cancer [18]. The length of time during which the patient has to cope with this side effect has diminished with improvements in surgical technique, particularly with nerve-sparing and, to some degree, with robotic surgery, which allows for better viewing of the operative field. Approximately 1–40% of men complain of urinary incontinence, and about 10% remain incontinent 1 year after surgery [19]. While attainment of urinary continence is possible for the majority, urinary incontinence is very bothersome to men, particularly if they are not aware that it will get better over time. Urinary incontinence has the effect of making men feel particularly regressed and infantile, which is a major assault on their masculinity and sense of control over their body. Urinary irritability, also defined as urethral pain, urgency, and frequency, can be associated with radiation treatment. These symptoms can be temporary or persistent [20]. While bothersome in themselves, they can lead to sufficient pelvic discomfort to have a negative impact on psychological health as well as on sexual desire and arousal [21].

Bowel Irritability
Frequency, urgency, and overall bowel problems have been reported by patients treated with radiation therapy in studies of quality of life [22]. As many as 11% of patients experience rectal incontinence and bleeding. Bowel problems lead to significant distress in the patient who, like the patient with urinary incontinence, experiences loss of control over his body, with concomitant embarrassment and loss of confidence in social situations [23]. The effect of bowel problems on sexual function and confidence has not been studied in prostate cancer, although studies on colorectal cancer suggest that loss of control over bowels leads to sexual dysfunction [24].

Sexual Dysfunction
Sexuality is a complex phenomenon. An optimal sexual encounter requires intact physiologic sexual function, sexual confidence and undistracted focus, and a sense of uninhibited mutuality in an interaction with a similarly functionally intact and emotionally present partner. At its best, the biological (physical function), psychological (confidence and focus), and social (relationship) components of sexuality work together to create a vital human experience. The importance of attending to all of the aspects of the multidimensional nature of sexuality was first proposed by Surgeon General David Satcher, who described it as is '… an integral part of human life. It (sexuality) carries the awesome potential to create new life. It can foster intimacy and bonding as well as shared pleasure in our relationships. It fulfills a number of personal and social needs, and we value the sexual part of our being for the pleasure and benefits it affords …' [25]. In 2002, the World Health Organization [26] defined sexual health as '… a state of physical, emotional, mental and social well-being in relation to sexuality …'

Although approximately 25% of men come to prostate cancer treatment with already suboptimal erectile function [27], most of them are able to use phosphodiesterase-5 inhibitors. After prostatectomy, men learn how much function they will have recovered over the course of the 2 years after treatment, although some continue to recover even after that. It is currently impossible to predict how well an individual man will recover erectile function, but factors such as nerve-sparing, age, and pre-operative erectile function have been shown to be influential [28, 29]. Studies have shown that the majority of men need some treatment for erectile dysfunction (ED) after prostatectomy. Radiation treatment can temporarily result in irritation of the urethra, which may make sex unpleasant. Sexual function gradually declines over 2 years. Most men have some degree of ED after radiation treatment [30]. Men who are treated with androgen deprivation lose not only erectile function but also the hormonally driven desire for sex [31]. Feminization due to the loss of testosterone may result in gynecomastia, which interferes with men's self-image as men [32].

Research on the effect of treatment-related ED on a man's psychology has unequivocally documented patients' suffering and difficulty in coming to terms with it. Using the Expanded Prostate Cancer Index Composite's measure of a man's psychological response to the sexual side effect, called 'bother,' studies have reported that men are bothered by their impaired sexual function, even when the rest of their lives are happy and going well and even when their erection recovery is relatively successful [33]. This is not surprising, given the fact that culturally, men conflate sexuality with masculinity and fear rejection if unable to perform sexually [34, 35]. Studies in which men were interviewed about the sexual side effect of prostate cancer treatment led to increasing recognition that men experience feelings of loss, lack of viability as men, and helplessness about how to cope [36–40]. Surgery and radiation treatment result in ED, but hormonal treatment leads to feminization of the man's body as well. Such changes represent tremendous losses in all aspects of sexuality. Studies have shown that beyond the loss of sexual function, men experience a disturbance in their body image, with a resulting sense of loss of masculinity [41–43]. Rarely mentioned is the fact that some heterosexual men grieve the loss of ejaculation as an aspect of their orgasm experience. For gay men, the loss of ejaculate as a part of their sensory sexual experience after surgery is an additional loss of pleasure that may lead to grief and depression in the wake of prostate cancer treatment [44–46].

Partners also report experiencing losses in a number of areas, which include sexuality, emotional intimacy, and partnership. As they cope, they typically focus on mourning the relationship changes, although they may continue to have sexual needs that they either forego or meet individually [47–50]. As time moves forward, partners are at risk for feeling dissatisfied in the relationship [51].

Understanding couples' challenges is important because patients and partners face the patient's treatment-related side effect together. Barriers to their recovery can be contextual and preexisting or based on the sexual losses engendered by prostate cancer treatment [52]. Some research suggests that men and their partners have different needs as they face the recovery of sexual intimacy [53]. An understanding of the kind of support that couples need requires that both the patient's and the partner's needs are appreciated so that mutuality can be fostered.

Long-term studies focused on the side effects of prostate cancer treatment have shown that treatment-related ED in men who survive prostate cancer persists over time [14]. There are virtually no long-term studies that have focused on the impact of those side effects on men, their partners, and their relationships. However, studies by Galbraith and Tanner [40, 49] eloquently show that the psychological impact persists as well. Thus, the functional, psychological, and relationship losses become permanent.

Losses in Advanced and Metastatic Prostate Cancer

The diagnosis of advanced prostate cancer brings about awareness that treatment will significantly alter physical function and that functional changes may be permanent. It also leads some men to reckon with mortality. Particularly for younger men, the consideration of significant symptoms and mortality can come as a shock. Regardless of the method of coping, advanced prostate cancer is emblematic of loss, grief, and coming to terms with a shortened lifespan. In her study of men with advanced cancer, Jonsson et al. [43], after describing the ways in which men saw the impact of the diagnosis on their lives, concluded that an overriding wish reported by all was to return to a normal life, even if for a short while. Encapsulated in this modest wish is both the desire to deny the forthcoming losses and the recognition that they are inevitable.

Physical Changes

The effect of hormonal treatment on men's bodies varies from patient to patient. It is also affected by the preparatory and sustained physical conditioning that patients engage in during treatment. The profound loss of testosterone alters patients' body mass and shifts the areas in which body fat accumulates. Patients notice weight gain, greater girth, and loss of muscle mass. Concurrently, they experience loss of body and facial hair. They begin to look more feminine and less fit. In some patients, gynecomastia, or breast enlargement, becomes evident [31]. The alteration of physical appearance affects the patient's body image because he has lost the look with which he is familiar. For many men, this is an upsetting prospect before treatment and an unhappy transition. Many become embarrassed, even in front of their partners and family members [54]. The reactions of others in their environment can increase this self-consciousness. Unless they are offered support and find a way to come to terms with these changes, patients can experience themselves as demasculinized, and their self-esteem plummets [32].

Loss of Function due to Androgen Deprivation
Similar to other treatments for prostate cancer, hormonal treatment induces functional losses. In this case, the functions that are targeted are sexual function, mood, and vitality [55]. The loss of testosterone leads men to lose sexual desire and erectile function. The ability to stimulate to orgasm can diminish. Low testosterone can also contribute to irritability and loss of cognitive acuity. Finally, it affects the patient's energy level. In sum, patients can experience a loss of vitality that makes it difficult for them to function effectively in their roles in their lives.

Comorbidities
Men treated with hormonal therapy acquire a risk of additional conditions, such as metabolic syndrome and diabetes, heart disease, osteoporosis, and cognitive changes [56]. The treatments required to control those conditions add to the already significant number of treatment effects on vitality, sexual function, mood, and the ability to fulfill social roles.

The Impact of Advanced or Metastatic Cancer on Relationships
The partners of men with advanced or metastatic cancer report feelings of grief about the men that they lost because of the challenging adjustment to many functional changes [57]. The losses that they enumerate are multiple and profound. While they can easily identify the typical physical and functional losses, the ones that are more painful are the frequent inability to effectively communicate with the patient about the changes, the changes in role function, and a lack of hope that these changes could be reversed or modified.

Death
In the last stages of metastatic prostate cancer, it is no longer the losses of function or even relationships that are experienced most acutely. For patients who are nearing the end of their life, the world is shrinking, and their focus is narrowing. From interviews with 2 dying men, Lindqvist and colleagues [42] report that their conversation about the past was only centered on the past of the illness, and not on their lives. In the present, the men found their no longer functioning bodies bothersome, and their future reference point was death and beyond. However, it is important not to overlook that there are individual differences and preferences. Blagbrough [58] describes the role of sexuality in patients with advanced cancer with compassion. Men and their partners often turn to each other for support and comfort and derive strength from each other at a time of crisis or hardship. The comfort may be emotional and physical, even including sexual closeness. While the focus is narrow and loss is the overarching experience, the need for human connection remains to the end.

Theoretical Models of the Impact of Cancer on the Individual's Psychology and on Couples' Emotional and Sexual Intimacy

Recovery from or mitigation of the side effects of prostate cancer treatment is strenuous and requires expertise on the part of the care provider, who can skillfully evaluate and treat or refer to a specialist. This process also requires commitment on the part of the patient. Coordination of care, which is currently often lacking, is critical. Physiologic treatments are necessary to redress functional decline, and psychosocial treatments help the patient and partner, if available, to cope with physiologic changes and rehabilitation. The importance of offering physiologic and psychosocial rehabilitation in concert with each other cannot be overstated. Too often, physiologic treatments without psychological support have failed.

Theoretical models attempting to describe the impact of cancer on survivors' lives began to appear in the research literature nearly 10 years after the side effects of cancer began to be documented. In 2001, Wilmoth [59] wrote about sexual losses in breast cancer. In interviews with survivors, she identified 4 major themes: missing parts, loss of bleeding (becoming old), loss of sexual sensations, and loss of womanhood. She called the aftermath of breast cancer 'the altered sexual self.' It is uncanny how easily this description fits the man after prostate cancer treatment: missing prostate, loss of ejaculate (becoming old), loss of sexual sensation, and loss of manhood. Wilmoth's model speaks eloquently to the recognition that cancer treatment can result not only in loss of sexual function but also in the person's experience of loss of a familiar body image, the ability to create life, pleasure, and identity.

Manne was the earliest advocate of a broader approach. She proposed that beyond the impact of cancer and its treatment on the individual's psychology, or perhaps because of it, couples' communication is also affected, and particularly the willingness to talk about difficult, cancer-related topics [60]. She described this reluctance as 'protective buffering,' a concept adopted from the cardiology literature [61]. In examining cancer survivors' communication, she found that 'protective buffering' was damaging to couples in more satisfying relationships. She developed a model of couples' adaptation to cancer that proposed that openness, reciprocity, and self-disclosure by both members of the couple would lead to better psychological and relationship adaptation.

Proponents of later models integrated the physiologic impacts with the psychosocial ones into a biopsychosocial approach to prostate cancer. They saw the biopsychosocial paradigm as being most clearly observable in the impact of cancer on the biopsychosocial dimensions of sexuality.

Tierney [62] suggested that patients respond to the loss of function, such as sexual function or fertility, with distress, grief, anxiety, or depression. She also suggested that sexual relationships were bound to be affected when patients' function was altered and when they were affected emotionally. Wittmann and colleagues [63] similarly applied the biopsychosocial concept to prostate cancer, adding grief and mourning as the processes through which men and their partners recover from the losses engendered by prostate cancer treatment.

Bober and Varela [64], echoing the previous models, added religious beliefs, cultural values, and social norms to indicate that sexual losses in cancer are experienced in a wider social milieu, which has its own effect on that experience. Although these models of the impact of cancer on sexuality have not been fully translated into interventions, they can be helpful for clinicians, who can use them to guide their discussions with patients concerned about sexual dysfunction or generally about the way in which prostate cancer and its treatment altered them, their relationships, and their lives. By asking questions from a biopsychosocial perspective, the clinician can discover whether he/she will be the main treatment provider or whether a specialized referral is necessary.

Galbraith [40], in his study of men's reflections on surviving prostate cancer, provided a model that has a biopsychosocial perspective on the changes/losses that men experience as a result of prostate cancer and its treatment. This model is based on the men's recognition that these changes/losses are permanent. The men studied also recognized that they had unmet needs with regard to their psychological and emotional adaptation, their relationships, and their healthcare. Galbraith did not specifically postulate a process, but he described the men's recognition that they have to adapt to a 'new normal.'

A Biopsychosocial Approach to the Care of Prostate Cancer Survivors

Physiologic Rehabilitation for the Side Effects of Localized Prostate Cancer Treatments
A recently published guideline by the American Cancer Society for prostate cancer survivorship care has detailed methods through which patients can be encouraged to maintain optimal biopsychosocial functionality [65].

Urinary Incontinence and Urinary Irritability
After prostatectomy, men can engage in pelvic floor rehabilitation to recover bladder control. This may include several visits to a qualified physical therapist and daily exercises to strengthen the pelvic floor until continence is achieved [66]. Studies have shown that engagement in pelvic floor rehabilitation before and after surgery for prostate cancer increases the likelihood of early recovery of bladder control [67–69]. Urinary irritability, present after both prostatectomy and radiation treatment, can be managed with pelvic floor rehabilitation and medications. Frequency responds well to 'timed' voiding: delaying voiding while tensing the pelvic floor helps to expand the bladder's capacity and leads to a decrease in frequency. Relief of incontinence and bladder spasms can come from medications as well [65].

Erectile Dysfunction
Early intervention for ED has been termed 'penile rehabilitation.' The goal of penile rehabilitation is to prevent fibrosis of the penile corpora after prostatectomy and to encourage, through blood flow and regular stimulation, compensation for the lack of activity of the neurovascular bundles that govern erections. Even if they were spared during surgery, these bundles do not perform their function reliably for up to 2 years. The notion of penile rehabilitation is gaining acceptance, but it remains an emerging rather than evidence-based practice. Penile rehabilitation methodologies have been developing for the past 10 years [70–72]. A recent review by Fode et al. [73] described the empirical evidence that underlies approaches to penile rehabilitation, such as a daily low dose of phosphodiesterase-5 inhibitors, alprostadil injections, and vacuum devices. The evidence is weak. Penile rehabilitation has not been well tested in randomized clinical trials, and the duration of rehabilitation has not been established. We can therefore conclude that penile rehabilitation has shown promise but that well-designed clinical trials are needed to provide solid evidence for its effectiveness. Regardless of the approach, penile rehabilitation can have the benefit of engaging patients in the recovery process, thus encouraging self-care and self-efficacy. Although well established in the literature, penile rehabilitation is not routinely offered in usual care. Advocates suggest that it should become an integral component of prostate cancer survivorship care after definitive treatment for localized prostate cancer. Penile rehabilitation has not typically been offered to patients after radiation treatment or to those on hormonal treatment, but could be easily implemented to promote the health of penile tissues and offer patients an opportunity for self-management.

If testosterone was low prior to definitive treatment or was dropped afterward, testosterone supplementation is sometimes considered for a selected group of patients whose prostate cancer pathological findings reveal a slow-growing cancer and whose PSA remains undetectable for a period of several months. The treatment remains somewhat controversial because studies have raised the possibility that it might increase the risk of prostate cancer progression and result in cardiac morbidity [74–77]. A vigorous debate is in process.

For men who experience ED, treatments can be prescribed empirically until the patient finds the one that suits him and his partner best. Phosphodiesterase-5 inhibitors; alprostadil administered through penile suppositories or intracavernosal injections; and a mixture of papaverine and alprostadil, also administered through an injection, and vacuum devices, can be effective [78]. These treatments can be used by patients either alone or in combination under medical supervision. For men with persistent ED who wish to have penetrative sex, penile implants become an option that they can discuss with their providers [79–81]. Some men have incorporated strap-on dildos into their sexual repertoire to provide their partners with penetrative sex without undergoing surgery themselves [82]. Men have been shown to not use erectile aids consistently, perhaps because their expectations of the outcomes are overly optimistic and dispose them toward becoming discouraged and unable to pursue rehabilitation effectively. Counseling support may add the necessary dimension to help men to accept and implement penile rehabilitation because without it, men's uptake of aids to erectile function has been minimal [83, 84].

Physiologic Rehabilitation for the Side Effects of Advanced and Metastatic Prostate Cancer Treatments

The American Cancer Society provides detailed guidance for the treatment of the side effects of advanced and metastatic prostate cancer [65]. Men on hormonal therapy are encouraged to pursue exercise strategies that strengthen muscles and bones. Hot flashes can be addressed with SSRIs. Treatment for comorbidities, such as metabolic syndrome and heart disease, is typically managed by specialists.

Psychosocial Care

Psychosocial interventions are generally not available in usual care. They have been explored and tested only in academic institutions. The earliest psychosocial interventions in prostate cancer were often directed toward the recovery of men's erectile function after localized treatment because this is an area in which men readily acknowledge distress and are likely to pursue help [33, 85]. The interventions generally provide a psychoeducational component that alerts men and their partners to the sexual side effects of prostate cancer treatment and methodologies for restoring the man's erectile function. Some interventions also incorporate sexual health information for post-menopausal partners. Interventions have used psychoeducational approaches [86], efforts to reduce distress with a psychoeducational component [87], and counseling to improve sexual function or adherence to ED treatment [84]. Sexual function was also the variable of interest in interventions in which partners were included as participants. These interventions included psychoeducation about the impact of prostate cancer on the man's sexual function and rehabilitation options for ED, along with rehabilitation for female post-menopausal sexuality. They also provided psychosocial support in the form of both cognitive-behavioral strategies to help men and their partners overcome their dislike of erectile aids and pointers for improving communication about sexual issues [88, 89].

Two psychosocial researchers have focused on couples' coping without specifically focusing on sexual dysfunction. Northouse and colleagues developed a nurse-led intervention for dyads during all phases of the trajectory of the illness, having identified early that couples have different needs, based on age and the phase of illness [57]. The researchers developed and tested an intervention that can be tailored to those needs in a person-to-person home visit as well as in a web-based format [90, 91]. The intervention led to decreased distress and a more positive appraisal of the illness, particularly on the part of the partners. Based on her model, which emphasized the negative role of 'protective buffering' in couples' adaptation after prostate cancer treatment [60], Manne [92] developed an intervention for couples to enhance emotional intimacy, as represented by mutual openness and transparency regarding cancer-related concerns. Manne hypothesized that such an approach would decreases couples' distress and, in fact, did find that to be the case in couples with fewer psychological resources. Her recognition of the need to reduce distress through couple connectedness reflected her understanding of the complex psychological nature of the recovery of couples' emotional equilibrium after the patient's treatment for prostate cancer.

Loss and Grief

Despite the recognition in the prostate cancer-related psychosocial research literature that men and their partners experience losses and grieve them, in usual care or in research interventions, patients and partners are not typically educated to regard the side effects of prostate cancer treatment as losses that can be addressed and distress that can be alleviated with guided grief work. However, this conceptualization can help patients, partners, and even healthcare providers to feel less helpless and frustrated. Grief helps the process of coming to terms with a less-than-desirable outcome and opens the way to a new, heretofore unimagined adaptation.

Explicit attention to loss and grief in the context of helping patients and partners to cope with the sequelae of prostate cancer is emerging, although it has been mentioned in most of the psychosocial literature on prostate cancer. A theoretical model that incorporates grief and mourning into the recovery of sexual intimacy for men treated with surgery for prostate cancer and their partners was proposed by Wittmann and colleagues [63]. They applied concepts from the bereavement literature, in which the death of a spouse unalterably changes the world of the bereaved spouse [93]. No longer able to rely on the familiarity of a life that included the deceased spouse, the surviving spouse must grieve the loss. Without setting aside the memory of the previous life, the surviving spouse creates a new life in which the life space previously occupied by the deceased is meaningfully filled anew. Similarly, existential and functional losses in prostate cancer have to be grieved, and a meaningful new way of functioning individually and with others has to be developed. Wittmann and colleagues proposed that grief work be included in helping couples to recover their sexual relationship. This methodology is applicable to other losses as well.

Because functional outcomes are often uncertain for a long time after prostate cancer treatments, it is admittedly difficult to counsel with a sense of clarity about what the future holds. In her work on ambiguous loss, Boss describes the way in which moving into the grief process can be resisted because of this uncertainty of outcomes [94]. In a further exploration of this issue for women with breast cancer, Pilai-Friedman and Ashline [95] proposed that sexual losses in cancer (and these can be extrapolated to other functional losses) can be experienced as 'disenfranchised' because they do not rise to the same level of importance as pain or death [95]. As a consequence, prostate cancer survivors may not feel that their long-term prostate cancer treatment-related effects are a legitimate topic of discussion with their providers and may not seek help. Feeling unhappy about physical or sexual problems is stigmatized in our culture [96, 97], and men will be reticent to speak up. While we can clearly understand this about patients, we may want to recognize that this resistance may reside among healthcare providers as well. Trained to provide solutions, healthcare providers may not feel comfortable witnessing grief about losses that may not be fully overcome. Addressing sexual issues is particularly uncomfortable for providers, as has been documented in several studies [98, 99]. For patients, an inability to cope with loss may be at the core of a lack of engagement with rehabilitation activities. Conversely, the ability to grieve leads to a new adaptation and can provide the patient and partner with the emotional strength to accept functional changes and to creatively problem solve toward a new adaptation, as has been described in the literature on another chronic illness [100]. It is therefore important for healthcare providers to be familiar with grief as a normal reaction to loss of function in prostate cancer, so that patients can work toward maximal return of functioning.

Grief is an animating emotional process, unlike depression, which can become immobilizing. Based on a model developed by Warden, for normal grief to proceed, patients with prostate cancer must engage in four tasks of grief and mourning: (1) acknowledge that functional losses have taken place, (2) experience the emotions associated with those losses, (3) memorialize the kind of functioning that you had previously, and (4) develop a new way of being in a world with altered functioning [101]. It is a process that can be facilitated by psychosocial providers, such as social workers, psychologists, psychiatrists, or nurses, who are familiar with these concepts and with grief intervention. Pillai-Friedman and Ashline suggested that encouraging patients to grieve through telling and re-telling, ritual, or formal or alternative treatments that are designed to facilitate grief can lead to diminution of the intensity of the feelings about the losses and an ability to be open to a path toward re-eroticizing their differently functioning bodies. Involving partners, who experience their own grief and mourning about the patient's cancer diagnosis, functional losses, and changed relationship, can be particularly helpful and meaningful because re-defining a new level of functioning as a 'team' creates a common goal as well as greater emotional and sexual intimacy.

Patients who are unable to grieve existential and functional losses may develop a complicated grief reaction, defined by Prigerson in the context of bereavement as 'intense yearning, difficulty accepting the death, excessive bitterness, numbness, emptiness and feeling uneasy moving on with future looking bleak' [102]. What is often conceptualized in medical practices as depression and treated with antidepressants, with variable success, may be complicated grief in which the patient or family member cannot bear the feelings of grief and builds defenses against them. Resisting grief is exhausting and unproductive. Unlike depression, which can arise without a precipitant, complicated grief is dense with meaning. Complicated grief may symptomatically respond to antidepressants but, like trauma, is better treated with grief counseling or psychotherapy [103]. In this way, the patient or family member has an opportunity to develop insight into the unalterable changes that prostate cancer created in his/her life with someone neutral, sympathetic, and well versed in grief work who can help them to understand that his/her resistance to normal grief holds him/her back and can be overcome. Overcoming resistance to complicated grief leads to engagement in normal grief, which, as stated above, can lead to empowerment and the development of meaning in the context of coping with cancer.

Conclusion

Successful coping with cancer can lead to a more positive appraisal of the illness experience, and even to growth, an outcome that has been described both in prostate cancer and in other cancer populations [104–106]. Alerting patients and families to the likelihood that they will become distressed, will experience losses, and may need to grieve them can paradoxically reduce their distress and prepare them for the necessary grief work [107]. Attending to losses and fostering grief work allow patients and family members move from experiencing the shock and loss of prostate cancer diagnosis and treatment to a greater sense of control, which comes from no longer feeling overwhelmed and is likely to lead to other positive health outcomes associated with preventing or reducing distress, anxiety, and depression. Working collaboratively with multidisciplinary providers who can help prostate cancer survivors to cope with the side effects of the illness, such as physical therapists, sex therapists, endocrinologists, and cardiologists, will alleviate their symptom burden. Including mental health specialists with expertise in facilitating prostate cancer survivors' grief work in the team will foster the survivors' and family members' psychological resilience, which is necessary for successful navigation of the prostate cancer experience.

References

1 Maliski SL, Heilemann MV, McCorkle R: From 'death sentence' to 'good cancer': couples' transformation of a prostate cancer diagnosis. Nurs Res 2002;51:391–397.

2 Siegel R, DeSantis C, Virgo K, et al: Cancer treatment and survivorship statistics, 2012. CA Cancer J Clin 2012;62:220–241.

3 Ferlay J, Soerjomataram I, Ervik M, et al: GLOBOCAN 2012 v1.0, Cancer Incidence and Mortality Worldwide: IARC Cancer Base No. 11. Lyon, International Agency for Research on Cancer, 2013.

4 Qaseem A, Barry MJ, Denberg TD, Owens DK, Shekelle P: Screening for prostate cancer: a guidance statement from the Clinical Guidelines Committee of the American College of Physicians. Ann Intern Med 2013;158:761–769.

5 Prasad SM, Drazer MW, Huo D, Hu JC, Eggener SE: 2008 US Preventive Services Task Force recommendations and prostate cancer screening rates. JAMA 2012;307:1692–1694.

6 Weiner AB, Patel SG, Etzioni R, Eggener SE: National trends in the management of low- and intermediate-risk prostate cancer in the United States. J Urol 2014 DOI: 10.1016/j.juro.2014.07.111.

7 Knight SJ, Latini DM: Sexual side effects and prostate cancer treatment decisions: patient information needs and preferences. Cancer J 2009;15:41–44.

8 Delongchamps NB: Prostate cancer: review in 2014. Diagn Interv Imaging 2014;95:739–742.

9 Hollenbeck BK, Dunn RL, Wei JT, Sandler HM, Sanda MG: Sexual health recovery after prostatectomy, external radiation, or brachytherapy for early stage prostate cancer. Curr Urol Rep 2004;5:212–219.

10 Schaake W, Wiegman EM, de Groot M, et al: The impact of gastrointestinal and genitourinary toxicity on health related quality of life among irradiated prostate cancer patients. Radiother Oncol 2014;110:284–290.

11 Kumar RJ, Barqawi A, Crawford ED: Adverse events associated with hormonal therapy for prostate cancer. Rev Urol 2005;7(suppl 5)S37–S43.

12 Namiki S, Saito S, Tochigi T, Ioritani N, Terai A, Arai Y: Impact of salvage therapy for biochemical recurrence on health-related quality of life following radical prostatectomy. Int J Urol 2007;14:186–191.

13 Pinkawa M, Fischedick K, Asadpour B, et al: Health-related quality of life after adjuvant and salvage postoperative radiotherapy for prostate cancer – a prospective analysis. Radiother Oncol 2008;88:135–139.

14 Resnick MJ, Koyama T, Fan KH, et al: Long-term functional outcomes after treatment for localized prostate cancer. N Engl J Med 2013;368:436–445.

15 Litwin MS, Hays RD, Fink A, Ganz PA, Leake B, Brook RH: The UCLA Prostate Cancer Index: development, reliability, and validity of a health-related quality of life measure Med Care 1998;36:1002–1012.

16 Wei JT, Dunn RL, Litwin MS, Sandler HM, Sanda MG: Development and validation of the expanded prostate cancer index composite (EPIC) for comprehensive assessment of health-related quality of life in men with prostate cancer. Urology 2000;56:899–905.

17 Wheat JC, Hedgepeth RC, He C, Zhang L, Wood DP Jr: Clinical interpretation of the Expanded Prostate Cancer Index Composite-Short Form sexual summary score. J Urol 2009;182:844–849.

18 Penson DF, McLerran D, Feng Zet al: 5-year urinary and sexual outcomes after radical prostatectomy: results from the Prostate Cancer Outcomes Study. J Urol 2008;179:S40–S44.

19 Huang KH, Carter SC, Shih YC, Hu JC: Robotic and standard open radical prostatectomy: oncological and quality-of-life outcomes. J Comp Eff Res 2013;2:293–299.

20 Chen RC, Zhang Y, Chen MH, et al: Patient-reported quality of life during radiation treatment for localized prostate cancer: results from a prospective phase II trial. BJU Int 2012;110:1690–1695.

21 Namiki S, Litwin MS, Kwan L, et al: Association of lower urinary tract symptoms with sexual dysfunction: a cross-cultural study between Japanese and American men with localized prostate cancer. BJU Int 2009;104:1071–1076.

22 Hamstra DA, Conlon AS, Daignault S, et al: Multi-institutional prospective evaluation of bowel quality of life after prostate external beam radiation therapy identifies patient and treatment factors associated with patient-reported outcomes: the PROSTQA experience. Int J Radiat Oncol Biol Phys 2013;86:546–553.

23 Namiki S, Kwan L, Kagawa-Singer M, et al: Distress and social dysfunction following prostate cancer treatment: a longitudinal cross-cultural comparison of Japanese and American men. Prostate Cancer Prostatic Dis 2009;12:67–71.

24 Gornicki A, Richter P, Polkowski W, et al: Anorectal and sexual functions after preoperative radiotherapy and full-thickness local excision of rectal cancer. Eur J Surg Oncol 2014;40:723–730.

25 Satcher D: The Surgeon General's call to action to promote sexual health and responsible sexual behavior. http://www.surgeongeneral.gov/library/sexual-health/call.htm 2001 (accessed July 7, 2014).

26 World Health Organization: Defining sexual health: a report of a technical consultation on sexual health 28–31 January 2002. Geneva, World Health Organization, Sexual Health Document Series, 2002.
27 Walz J, Perrotte P, Suardi N, et al: Baseline prevalence of erectile dysfunction in a prostate cancer screening population. J Sex Med 2008;5:428–435.
28 Dubbelman YD, Dohle GR, Schroder FH: Sexual function before and after radical retropubic prostatectomy: a systematic review of prognostic indicators for a successful outcome. Eur Urol 2006; 50:711–718; discussion 718–720.
29 Capitanio U, Briganti A, Gallina A, et al: Predictive models before and after radical prostatectomy. Prostate 2010;70: 1371–1378.
30 Incrocci L: Sexual function after external-beam radiotherapy for prostate cancer: what do we know? Crit Rev Oncol Hematol 2006;57:165–173.
31 Gomella LG: Contemporary use of hormonal therapy in prostate cancer: managing complications and addressing quality-of-life issues. BJU Int 2007; 99(suppl 1):25–29; discussion 30.
32 Wassersug RJ, Oliffe JL: The social context for psychological distress from iatrogenic gynecomastia with suggestions for its management. J Sex Med 2009;6: 989–1000.
33 Sanda MG, Dunn RL, Michalski J, et al: Quality of life and satisfaction with outcome among prostate-cancer survivors. N Engl J Med 2008;358:1250–1261.
34 Hyde A, Drennan J, Howlett E, Brady D: Young men's vulnerability in constituting hegemonic masculinity in sexual relations. Am J Mens Health 2009;3: 238–251.
35 Stamogiannou I, Grunfeld EA, Denison K, Muir G: Beliefs about illness and quality of life among men with erectile dysfunction. Int J Impot Res 2005;17: 142–147.
36 Bokhour BG, Clark JA, Inui TS, Silliman RA, Talcott JA: Sexuality after treatment for early prostate cancer: exploring the meanings of 'erectile dysfunction. J Gen Intern Med 2001;16:649–655.
37 Katz A: Quality of life for men with prostate cancer. Cancer Nurs 2007;30: 302–308.
38 Katz A: What happened? Sexual consequences of prostate cancer and its treatment. Can Fam Physician 2005;51:977–982.
39 Hedestig O, Sandman PO, Tomic R, Widmark A: Living after radical prostatectomy for localized prostate cancer: a qualitative analysis of patient narratives. Acta Oncol 2005;44:679–686.
40 Galbraith ME, Hays L, Tanner T: What men say about surviving prostate cancer: complexities represented in a decade of comments. Clin J Oncol Nurs 2012;16:65–72.
41 Ervik B, Asplund K: Dealing with a troublesome body: a qualitative interview study of men's experiences living with prostate cancer treated with endocrine therapy. Eur J Oncol Nurs 2012;16:103–108.
42 Lindqvist O, Rasmussen BH, Widmark A, Hyden LC: Time and bodily changes in advanced prostate cancer: talk about time as death approaches. J Pain Symptom Manage 2008;36:648–656.
43 Jonsson A, Aus G, Bertero C: Men's experience of their life situation when diagnosed with advanced prostate cancer. Eur J Oncol Nurs 2009;13:268–273.
44 Hart TL, Coon DW, Kowalkowski MA, et al: Changes in sexual roles and quality of life for gay men after prostate cancer: challenges for sexual health providers. J Sex Med 2014;11:2308–2317.
45 Hart SL, Coon DW, Kowalkowski MA, Latini DM: Gay men with prostate cancer report significantly worse HRQOL than heterosexual men. J Urol 2011; 185:e68–e69 (abstract).
46 Hartman ME, Irvine J, Currie KL, et al: Exploring gay couples' experience with sexual dysfunction after radical prostatectomy: a qualitative study. J Sex Marital Ther 2014;40:233–253.
47 Bruun P, Pedersen BD, Osther PJ, Wagner L: The lonely female partner: a central aspect of prostate cancer. Urol Nurs 2011;31:294–299.
48 Couper JW, Bloch S, Love A, Macvean M, Duchesne GM, Kissane D: Psychosocial adjustment of female partners of men with prostate cancer: a review of the literature. Psychooncology 2006;15: 937–953.
49 Tanner T, Galbraith M, Hays L: From a woman's perspective: life as a partner of a prostate cancer survivor. J Midwifery Womens Health 2011;56:154–160.
50 Wittmann D, Carolan M, Given B, et al: Exploring the role of the partner in couples' sexual recovery after surgery for prostate cancer. Support Care Cancer 2014;22:2509–2215.
51 Couper JW, Bloch S, Love A, Duchesne G, Macvean M, Kissane DW: The psychosocial impact of prostate cancer on patients and their partners. Med J Aust 2006;185:428–432.
52 Wittmann D, Northouse L, Crossley H, et al: A pilot study of potential pre-operative barriers to couples' sexual recovery after radical prostatectomy for prostate cancer. J Sex Marital Ther 2015;41:155–168.
53 Sanders S, Pedro LW, Bantum EO, Galbraith ME: Couples surviving prostate cancer: Long-term intimacy needs and concerns following treatment. Clin J Oncol Nurs 2006;10:503–508.
54 Aucoin MW, Wassersug RJ: The sexuality and social performance of androgen-deprived (castrated) men throughout history: implications for modern day cancer patients. Soc Sci Med 2006;63: 3162–3173.
55 Nguyen PL, Alibhai SM, Basaria S, et al: Adverse effects of androgen deprivation therapy and strategies to mitigate them. Eur Urol 2014 DOI: 10.1016/j.eururo.2014.07.010.
56 Casey RG, Corcoran NM, Goldenberg SL: Quality of life issues in men undergoing androgen deprivation therapy: a review. Asian J Androl 2012;14:226–231.
57 Harden J, Northouse L, Cimprich B, Pohl JM, Liang J, Kershaw T: The influence of developmental life stage on quality of life in survivors of prostate cancer and their partners. J Cancer Surviv 2008; 2:84–94.
58 Blagbrough J: Importance of sexual needs assessment in palliative care. Nurs Stand 2010;24:35–39.
59 Wilmoth MC: The aftermath of breast cancer: an altered sexual self. Cancer Nurs 2001;24:278–286.
60 Manne S, Ostroff J, Rini C, Fox K, Goldstein L, Grana G: The interpersonal process model of intimacy: the role of self-disclosure, partner disclosure, and partner responsiveness in interactions between breast cancer patients and their partners. J Fam Psychol 2004;18:589–599.
61 Coyne JC, Smith DA: Couples coping with a myocardial infarction: a contextual perspective on wives' distress. J Pers Soc Psychol 1991;61:404–412.
62 Tierney DK: Sexuality: a quality-of-life issue for cancer survivors. Semin Oncol Nurs 2008;24:71–79.

63 Wittmann D, Foley S, Balon R: A biopsychosocial approach to sexual recovery after prostate cancer surgery: the role of grief and mourning. J Sex Marital Ther 2011;37:130–144.
64 Bober SL, Varela VS: Sexuality in adult cancer survivors: challenges and intervention. J Clin Oncol 2012;30:3712–3719.
65 Skolarus TA, Wolf AM, Erb NL, et al: American Cancer Society prostate cancer survivorship care guidelines. CA Cancer J Clin 2014;64:225–249.
66 MacDonald R, Fink HA, Huckabay C, Monga M, Wilt TJ: Pelvic floor muscle training to improve urinary incontinence after radical prostatectomy: a systematic review of effectiveness. BJU Int 2007;100:76–81.
67 Prota C, Riberio LS, Gomes CM, et al: Early pelvic floor biofeedback training promotes improvement of erectile function after radical prostatectomy. J Urol 2009;181:524–525.
68 Rajkowska-Labon E, Bakula S, Kucharzewski M: Efficacy of physiotherapy for urinary incontinence following prostate cancer surgery. 2014;2014:785263.
69 Dieperink KB, Johansen C, Hansen S, et al: The effects of multidisciplinary rehabilitation: RePCa-a randomised study among primary prostate cancer patients. Biomed Res Int 2013;109:3005–3013.
70 Tal R, Teloken P, Mulhall JP: Erectile function rehabilitation after radical prostatectomy: practice patterns among AUA members. J Sex Med 2011;8:2370–2376.
71 Mazzola C, Mulhall JP: Penile rehabilitation after prostate cancer treatment: outcomes and practical algorithm. Urol Clin North Am 2011;38:105–118.
72 Mulhall JP, Morgentaler A: Penile rehabilitation should become the norm for radical prostatectomy patients. J Sex Med 2007;4:538–543.
73 Fode M, Ohl DA, Ralph D, Sonksen J: Penile rehabilitation after radical prostatectomy: what the evidence really says. BJU Int 2013;112:998–1008.
74 Khera M: Androgens and erectile function: a case for early androgen use in postprostatectomy hypogonadal men. J Sex Med 2009;6(suppl 3):234–238.
75 Kava BR: To treat or not to treat with testosterone replacement therapy: a contemporary review of management of late-onset hypogonadism and critical issues related to prostate cancer. Curr Urol Rep 2014;15:422.
76 Kaplan AL, Trinh QD, Sun M, et al: Testosterone replacement therapy following the diagnosis of prostate cancer: outcomes and utilization trends. J Sex Med 2014;11:1063–1070.
77 Trost LW, Hellstrom WJ: Testosterone deficiency, supplementation, and prostate cancer: maintaining a balanced perspective. J Sex Med 2013;10:2879–2881.
78 Matthew AG, Goldman A, Trachtenberg J, et al: Sexual dysfunction after radical prostatectomy: prevalence, treatments, restricted use of treatments and distress. J Urol 2005;174:2105–2110.
79 Ramsawh HJ, Morgentaler A, Covino N, Barlow DH, DeWolf WC: Quality of life following simultaneous placement of penile prosthesis with radical prostatectomy. J Urol 2005;174:1395–1398.
80 Akin-Olugbade O, Parker M, Guhring P, Mulhall J: Determinants of patient satisfaction following penile prosthesis surgery. J Sex Med 2006;3:743–748.
81 Hamilton Z, Mirza M: Post-prostatectomy erectile dysfunction: contemporary approaches from a US perspective. Res Rep Urol 2014;6:35–41.
82 Warkentin KM, Gray RE, Wassersug RJ: Restoration of satisfying sex for a castrated cancer patient with complete impotence: a case study. J Sex Marital Ther 2006;32:389–399.
83 Miller DC, Wei JT, Dunn RL, et al: Use of medications or devices for erectile dysfunction among long-term prostate cancer treatment survivors: potential influence of sexual motivation and/or indifference. Urology 2006;68:166–71.
84 Titta M, Tavolini IM, Moro FD, Cisternino A, Bassi P: Sexual counseling improved erectile rehabilitation after non-nerve-sparing radical retropubic prostatectomy or cystectomy–results of a randomized prospective study. J Sex Med 2006;3:267–273.
85 Schover LR, Fouladi RT, Warneke CL, et al: Seeking help for erectile dysfunction after treatment for prostate cancer. Arch Sex Behav 2004;33:443–454.
86 Davison BJ, Elliott S, Ekland M, Griffin S, Wiens K: Development and evaluation of a prostate sexual rehabilitation clinic: a pilot project. BJU Int 2005;96:1360–1364.
87 Molton IR, Siegel SD, Penedo FJ, et al: Promoting recovery of sexual functioning after radical prostatectomy with group-based stress management: the role of interpersonal sensitivity. J Psychosom Res 2008;64:527–536.
88 Canada AL, Neese LE, Sui D, Schover LR: Pilot intervention to enhance sexual rehabilitation for couples after treatment for localized prostate carcinoma. Cancer 2005;104:2689–2700.
89 Schover LR, Canada AL, Yuan Y, et al: A randomized trial of internet-based versus traditional sexual counseling for couples after localized prostate cancer treatment. Cancer 2012;118:500–509.
90 Northouse LL, Mood DW, Schafenacker A, et al: Randomized clinical trial of a family intervention for prostate cancer patients and their spouses. Cancer 2007;110:2809–2818.
91 Northouse L, Schafenacker A, Barr KL, et al: A tailored web-based psychoeducational intervention for cancer patients and their family caregivers. Cancer Nurs 2014;37:321–330.
92 Manne SL, Kissane DW, Nelson CJ, Mulhall JP, Winkel G, Zaider T: Intimacy-enhancing psychological intervention for men diagnosed with prostate cancer and their partners: a pilot study. J Sex Med 2011;8:1197–1209.
93 Parkes CM: Psycho-social transitions: a field for study. Soc Sci Med 1971;5:101–115.
94 Boss P: Ambiguous Loss: Learning to Live with Unresolved Grief. Cambridge, MA, Harvard Press, 1999.
95 Pillai-Friedman T, Ashline JL: Women, breast cancer survivorship, sexual losses, and disenfranchised grief – a treatment model for clinicians. Sex Relatsh Ther 2014;29:436–453.
96 Gray RE, Fitch M, Phillips C, Labrecque M, Fergus K: To tell or not to tell: patterns of disclosure among men with prostate cancer. Psychooncology 2000;9:273–282.
97 Wassersug RJ, Oliffe JL: The social context for psychological distress from iatrogenic gynecomastia with suggestions for its management. J Sex Med 2009;6:989–1000.
98 Marwick C: Survey says patients expect little physician help on sex. JAMA 1999;281:2173–2174.

99 Nichols CM, Barrett K: Female sexual dysfunction: a survey of Ob/Gyn resident education and experience. Program of the Annual International Society for the Study of Women's Sexual Health, October 2005.
100 Wittmann D, Keshavan M: Grief and mourning in schizophrenia. Psychiatry 2007;70:154–166.
101 Worden JW: Children and Grief: When a Parent Dies. New York, Guilford, 1996.
102 Prigerson HG, Frank R, Kasl SV, et al: Complicated grief and bereavement-related depression as distinct disorders: preliminary empirical validation in elderly bereaved spouses. Am J Psychiatry 1995;152:22–30.
103 Forbes D, Creamer M, Phelps A, et al: Australian guidelines for the treatment of adults with acute stress disorder and post-traumatic stress disorder. Aust N Z J Psychiatry 2007;41:637–648.
104 Zebrack BJ, Stuber ML, Meeske KA, et al: Perceived positive impact of cancer among long-term survivors of childhood cancer: a report from the childhood cancer survivor study. Psychooncology 2012;21:630–639.
105 Ruini C, Vescovelli F, Albieri E: Post-traumatic growth in breast cancer survivors: new insights into its relationships with well-being and distress. J Clin Psychol Med Settings 2013;20: 383–391.
106 Morris BA, Wilson B, Chambers SK: Newfound compassion after prostate cancer: a psychometric evaluation of additional items in the Posttraumatic Growth Inventory. Support Care Cancer 2013;21:3371–3378.
107 Abelson JL, Khan S, Liberzon I, Erickson TM, Young EA: Effects of perceived control and cognitive coping on endocrine stress responses to pharmacological activation. Biol Psychiatry 2008;64:701–107.

Daniela Wittmann, PhD, MSW, Clinical Assistant Professor
Department of Urology, University of Michigan
2800 Plymouth Road, Bldg 16, Rm 115W
Ann Arbor MI 48109–2800 (USA)
E-Mail dwittman@med.umich.edu

Balon R, Wise TN (eds): Clinical Challenges in the Biopsychosocial Interface. Update on Psychosomatics for the 21st Century. Adv Psychosom Med. Basel, Karger, 2015, vol 34, pp 123–134 (DOI: 10.1159/000369090)

Psychodermatology

Gabrielle E. Brown[a, b] • Mona Malakouti[b, d] • Eric Sorenson[b, c] • Rishu Gupta[e] • John Y.M. Koo[b]

[a]University of Arizona, College of Medicine, Tucson, Ariz., [b]Department of Dermatology, University of California, San Francisco, and [c]University of Southern California, Los Angeles, Calif., [d]Chicago Medical School, Rosalind Franklin University of Medicine and Science, North Chicago, and [e]MacNeal Hospital, Berywn, Ill., USA

Abstract

Psychodermatology is an underappreciated field that studies psychocutaneous disorders, which are conditions that have both dermatologic and psychiatric characteristics. Underlying psychiatric comorbidity is estimated to occur in up to one-third of dermatologic patients, and psychiatric illness may either be the cause or the consequence of dermatologic disease. Psychodermatologic patients lack insight and often do not recognize a psychiatric etiology for their symptoms and therefore comprise some of the most challenging cases to treat. Herein, we discuss the background and clinical presentation of the most commonly encountered psychodermatologic conditions, including delusional infestation, neurotic excoriations, factitial dermatitis, trichotillomania and body dysmorphic disorder, followed by practical diagnostic and therapeutic recommendations.

Introduction

Although dermatology and psychiatry are two seemingly different specialties, there is significant overlap in many dermatologic and psychiatric conditions. Psychodermatology is an underappreciated field that studies psychocutaneous disorders, which are diseases that have both dermatologic and psychiatric characteristics. Patients with psychocutaneous disorders are more likely to seek the help of dermatologists rather than psychiatrists since they are often unable to recognize a psychiatric etiology for their condition or are embarrassed by the stigma associated with psychiatric illness. However, surveys administered to physicians revealed that only 18% of dermatologists and 21% of psychiatrists have a clear understanding of the field of psychodermatology [1, 2]. Psychiatric disease may either be the cause or the result of dermatologic disease, and an underlying psychiatric disease is estimated to be present in one-third of dermatology patients [3, 4]. The classic example of a psychiatric disease resulting in cutaneous signs is delusional infestation (DI), in which patients endorse a fixed, false belief that they are infested with living organisms or inanimate objects in the absence of objective evidence. The cutaneous lesions in these patients are the result of self-inflicted excoriations from their futile efforts to remove the imaginary insects. Conversely, psychiatric disease may be the consequence of a disfiguring skin disease such as psoriasis or acne vulgaris, since patients may experience psychosocial difficulties that are severe enough to result in clinical depression. While many cases, such as the latter example, are manageable and those patients are easy to empathize with, other patients, such as those with DI, comprise some of the most challenging cases for dermatologists to manage. With the increasing importance of patient satisfaction in the United States with regard to physician ratings and value-based reimbursement, it is essential that providers be prepared to skillfully manage patients with psychodermatologic disorders. First, we will introduce psychodermatologic conditions in a logical categorization scheme. Then, we will further discuss the most commonly encountered conditions, including DI, neurotic excoriations, factitial dermatitis, trichotillomania (TTM) and body dysmorphic disorder (BDD), and provide practical recommendations for optimal therapeutic approaches to successfully manage psychodermatologic patients.

Classification of Psychodermatologic Disorders

Psychodermatologic conditions are grouped into four broad categories: primary psychiatric disorders, secondary psychiatric disorders, psychophysiologic disorders and cutaneous sensory disorders (CSDs) (table 1) [5]. It is important for providers to be able to distinguish between the various categories, as the distinction will often help guide the choice of the optimal therapeutic approach. While most cases can be categorized using the above-mentioned classification scheme, the separate categories are not mutually exclusive. For example, psoriasis is often exacerbated by stress and is therefore considered a psychophysiologic condition. However, the physical appearance of psoriasis may have a negative impact on psychosocial functioning and quality of life, resulting in secondary psychiatric disorders such as anxiety and depression. While psychodermatology is composed of heterogeneous disorders of various presentations and etiologies, the underlying psychiatric component is an important aspect that providers managing dermatologic patients should be prepared to address.

Primary Psychiatric Disorders

The primary psychiatric disorders include conditions in which the psychiatric component is primary and all skin manifestations are secondary and self-induced. The skin problem is solely reflective of an underlying psychiatric condition and is not explained by a primary skin pathophysiology. Examples of common primary psychiatric disorders include DI, neurotic excoriations, factitial dermatitis, TTM, BDD, onychotillomania and onychophagia.

Secondary Psychiatric Disorders

Psychiatric conditions that are the consequence of the adverse psychosocial and emotional effects of disfiguring skin disease are referred to as secondary psychiatric disorders. Depression, anxiety, and social phobia are some of the more commonly observed psychiatric disorders resulting from cutaneous disease. The dermatologic diseases that are potentially disfiguring include psoriasis, atopic dermatitis, acne vulgaris, vitiligo and alopecia areata; however, all skin disorders can be disfiguring and potentially devastating to the patient.

Treatment of dermatological disease and the resulting clinical improvement can improve psychological function. Isotretinoin, an oral medication used in the treatment of nodulocystic acne vulgaris, was initially thought to increase the risk of depression and suicidality; however, multiple studies have refuted this theory [6–8]. Rather, isotretinoin has been shown to improve reported mood in patients suffering from severe acne [7–9].

Table 1. Categorization of psychodermatologic disorders

Categories	Examples of psychodermatologic conditions
Primary psychiatric disorders	Delusional infestations Neurotic excoriations Factitial dermatitis Trichotillomania Body dysmorphic disorder Onychotillomania Onychophagia Psychogenic pruritus
Secondary psychiatric disorders	Depression Anxiety Social phobia
Psychophysiologic disorders	Psoriasis Atopic dermatitis Hyperhydrosis Acne vulgaris Lichen simplex chronicus Seborrheic dermatitis
Cutaneous sensory disorders	Glossodynia Vulvodynia

Psychophysiologic Disorders

Psychophysiologic disorders are true skin conditions that are characteristically susceptible to psychological factors such as stress, anxiety or emotional volatility in terms of disease precipitation or exacerbation. However, psychological exacerbation is not observed in all patients; therefore, patients may be divided into two groups, stress responders and nonstress responders. Examples of psychophysiologic disorders include psoriasis, atopic dermatitis, acne vulgaris, rosacea, lichen simplex chronicus, seborrheic dermatitis and hyperhidrosis. A significant proportion of patients with these disorders are known to be 'stress-responders', meaning the presence of stressors in these patients frequently results in exacerbation of disease activity.

Psychophysiologic disorders such as psoriasis, atopic dermatitis, and acne have been associated with comorbid psychiatric illness, including depression, anxiety, and suicidal ideation [10–12]. In psoriasis patients, psychological interventions and antidepressant medications have been shown to improve the patient's perception of symptom severity, compliance with treatment, and overall quality of life independent of any changes in clinical severity [13]. Therefore, patients with psychophysiologic disorders may benefit from a holistic approach that addresses both the dermatologic condition as well as the psychological status. Selective serotonin reuptake inhibitors (SSRIs) are the first-line treatment for depression in dermatologic disorders [14], and the antihistamine effects of tricyclic antidepressants (TCAs) confer an additional benefit for dermatologic conditions associated with pruritus [14]. Conversely, some psychotropic medications, such as mood stabilizers, are known to induce cutaneous reactions or exacerbate dermatologic conditions, for example, the well-recognized, lithium-induced, psoriasis exacerbation phenomenon [15]. Table 2 provides

Table 2. Dermatologic side effects of psychotropic medications

Dermatologic side effect	Medication class	Associated psychotropic medications
Acneiform eruption	Mood stabilizers SSRIs	Lithium Citalopram, fluoxetine, fluvoxamine, paroxetine, sertraline
Alopecia	Mood stabilizers Neuroleptics SSRIs TCAs Atypical antidepressants	Carbamazepine, lithium, valproic acid Haloperidol, quetiapine Citalopram, fluoxetine, fluvoxamine, paroxetine, sertraline Amitriptyline, clomipramine, imipramine Venlafaxine
Angioedema	Mood stabilizers TCAs Atypical antidepressants	Carbamazepine Amitriptyline, clomipramine, desipramine, imipramine Bupropion, trazodone
Eczema	Mood stabilizers	Carbamazepine, lithium
Erythema multiforme	Mood stabilizers SSRIs Atypical antidepressants	Carbamazepine, lithium Paroxetine, sertraline Bupropion, trazodone
Exanthem	Neuroleptics Sedative hypnotics SSRIs TCAs Atypical antidepressants	Risperidone Alprazolam, clobazam, clorazepate, flurazepam, tetrazepam Citalopram, fluoxetine, fluvoxamine, paroxetine, sertraline Amitriptyline, desipramine, imipramine Bupropion, trazodone
Hyperhidrosis	SSRIs Atypical antidepressants	Citalopram, fluoxetine Venlafaxine
Hyperpigmentation	Neuroleptics SSRIs TCAs	Aripiprazole, chlorproethazine, chlorpromazine, clozapine, haloperidol, olanzapine, quetiapine, risperidone, thioridazine, trifluoperazine, ziprasidone Citalopram, fluoxetine, fluvoxamine, paroxetine, sertraline Clomipramine, desipramine, imipramine
Lichenoid eruption	Mood stabilizers	Carbamazepine
Photosensitivity	SSRIs Mood stabilizers Neuroleptics TCAs	Citalopram, fluoxetine, fluvoxamine, paroxetine, sertraline Carbamazepine Aripiprazole, chlorpromazine, haloperidol, olanzapine, quetiapine, risperidone, thioridazine, trifluoperazine, ziprasidone Amitriptyline, imipramine
Psoriasiform eruption	Mood stabilizers SSRIs Atypical antidepressants	Lithium Fluoxetine, paroxetine Trazodone, venlafaxine
Stevens-Johnson Syndrome	Mood stabilizers Atypical antidepressants	Carbamazepine, lamotrigine Venlafaxine
Toxic epidermal necrolysis	Mood stabilizers Sedative hypnotics	Carbamazepine, lamotrigine Clobazam, flurazepam
Urticaria	Mood stabilizers Neuroleptics SSRIs TCAs Atypical antidepressants	Lithium Chlorpromazine Citalopram, fluoxetine, fluvoxamine, paroxetine, sertraline Clomipramine, imipramine Trazodone

further information regarding the dermatological reactions observed when taking psychotropic medications.

Cutaneous Sensory Disorders

CSDs are conditions in which the patient experiences unpleasant cutaneous sensory disturbances, such as pain (allodynia) or burning, itching, or stinging sensations. The symptoms occur with or without an established psychiatric diagnosis and are not known to be due to a primary skin disorder or any known underlying neurologic or medical condition. CSDs are often confined to a specific anatomical location and most frequently involve the face, scalp, and perineum. Examples of CSDs include stomatodynia, glossodynia, vulvodynia, and scrotodynia [16].

The presence of a comorbid psychiatric disorder, such as depression, anxiety, or body image disturbances, can contribute to a heightened awareness of abnormal cutaneous sensations such as pruritus and pain [17]. Therefore, the CSD will often improve following treatment of the psychiatric disorder [16]. Patients with no identifiable psychiatric comorbidity may also benefit from psychotropic medications that provide analgesic and antipruritic effects, such as the TCAs doxepin and amitriptyline [16]. Nonpharmacologic approaches, such as cognitive behavioral therapy, have been shown to improve symptoms of glossodynia [18] and vulvodynia [19].

Primary Psychiatric Disorders in Psychodermatology

The background, epidemiology, typical clinical presentation, and recommended diagnostic and therapeutic approaches for the more common primary psychiatric disorders in psychodermatology are outlined below.

Delusional Infestations

DIs, also known as delusions of parasitosis, are a type of monosymptomatic hypochondriacal psychosis characterized by a false, fixed belief that one is infested with living organisms or inanimate materials in the absence of objective proof. Delusional patients are among the most difficult cases to successfully manage since they are often distrusting of the provider and resistant to accepting treatment. Since they typically lack insight, patients primarily seek care from a dermatologist rather than a psychiatrist. It is estimated that the average dermatologist will encounter two to three patients every 5 years [5]. There is a bimodal age distribution for this disease, with peaks observed between ages 20 and 30 and again in patients over 50 years old [20]. While there is an equal gender distribution in patients younger than 50 years old, there is a female predominance observed in those over the age of 50 [20].

Clinical Presentation and Diagnosis

Patients with DI experience sensations of formication, including crawling, biting, or stinging, and they believe that these symptoms represent a cutaneous infestation and may attempt to pick the imagined parasites out of their skin. Upon physical examination, evidence of self-mutilation may vary from minor excoriations to deep, gouged-out ulcers. Patients with DI frequently collect specimens they claim to have extracted from their skin, which may include scabs, skin flakes, hair, clothing fibers and even insects. The patient will store the specimens in various containers, such as in an empty matchbox or mint tin, which is referred to as the 'matchbox sign', 'ziplock sign' or 'specimen sign' [20]. Patients may even go to the lengths of consulting entomologists and exterminators in order to identify and eradicate the imagined cutaneous parasite [21].

Most importantly, a real infestation with parasites, such as scabies incognito, must be excluded

[21]. The symptoms of formication that are observed in DI may be secondary to a variety of medical conditions or the use of illicit substances and medications; therefore, a differential diagnosis should be considered. Medical conditions associated with pruritus or paresthesia include certain infections, endocrine disorders (diabetes mellitus, hypothyroidism), and vitamin deficiency (B1, niacin, folic acid, B12), among other etiologies [20]. Basic laboratory tests, including complete blood count, thyroid function, and vitamin B12 levels, can effectively rule out medical etiologies. In contrast, substance-induced DI can result from the use of illicit substances, such as cocaine, methamphetamine, or narcotics, as well as from the use of prescribed medications [20]. Therefore, a urine toxicology screen may be helpful to rule out common substance-related causes of formication. In the absence of any primary skin disease, it may be difficult to justify performing a biopsy; however, there is merit in biopsies as a means of providing further objective evidence against an infestation and to optimize trust and therapeutic rapport with the patient.

Therapeutic Approach

There is value to early intervention in DI, as patients with a shorter duration of an active delusion have been shown to have an increased probability of achieving remission following treatment [22]. Furthermore, patients left untreated have been observed to further isolate themselves and subsequently progress into a more severe delusional state [23]. There are two main considerations to managing DI: developing a therapeutic rapport and prescribing antipsychotic medication.

The provider's therapeutic approach when managing these difficult patients is important because the patient is unlikely to agree to psychiatric referral. Even pharmacologic intervention is unlikely to be accepted by the patient unless a well-established and trusting relationship has developed. Therefore, the crucial supportive role that the dermatologist serves by simply listening cannot be overstated.

The desperation to be relieved from symptoms may override the need for validation; therefore, the patient may be receptive to pharmacologic treatment (table 3). The typical antipsychotic agent pimozide (Orap®) is the most studied pharmacologic agent for the treatment of DI [24]. The utility of pimozide in DI was illustrated in a review of 53 patients with DI who received pimozide, in which 50 (94%) achieved partial or complete remission from delusional symptoms [24]. It is believed that at low doses, the dopamine-blocking effects of pimozide address psychotic symptoms, while its opioid antagonism effects alleviate cutaneous crawling sensations [25]. Risperidone (Risperdal®) is the most-studied atypical antipsychotic agent for DI, and it has been shown to be efficacious in DI; of 35 patients receiving risperidone for DI, 24 (69%) achieved partial or complete remission [26]. Other reportedly efficacious antipsychotic medications include olanzapine (Zyprexa®) and aripiprazole (Abilify®) [26]. When the patient begins to experience the clinical benefit of an antipsychotic, adherence to the medication will generally increase.

Neurotic Excoriations

Neurotic excoriations, also referred to as psychogenic excoriations, is a disorder characterized by self-induced cutaneous lesions resulting from the uncontrollable impulse to excessively pick, rub, or scratch the skin in the absence of a primary skin disorder. Patients with neurotic excoriations may openly acknowledge that the lesions are self-induced. Psychiatric comorbidity, such as mood and anxiety disorders, is commonly observed in patients with neurotic excoriations, and the skin-picking behavior is a manifestation of the underlying psychopathology [27]. The picking episodes may be triggered by a variety of factors such as stress, anxiety, or localized pruritus, or they may

Table 3. Psychopharmacologic agents used in the management of primary psychodermatologic conditions (Disclaimer: not a complete discussion; please consult Physicians' Desk Reference and other sources for further guidance)

Medication	Class	Indication	Dermatologic dosage	Usual maximum dermatologic dosage	Adverse reactions	Contraindications
Pimozide (Orap®)	Typical antipsychotic	Delusional infestations, factitial dermatitis	Start at 0.5 mg/day and titrate every 2–4 weeks in 0.5- to 1-mg increments	5 mg/day	Sedation, arrhythmias (QTc prolongation, torsades de pointes), seizures, orthostatic hypotension, EPS, NMS, leukopenia, neutropenia	Arrhythmia history, hypomagnesemia, hypokalemia, SSRIs, TCAs, macrolide antibiotics, fluoroquinolones, azole antifungal agents
Risperidone (Risperdal®)	Atypical antipsychotic	Delusional infestations, factitial dermatitis	Start at 0.5 mg/day then titrate by 0.5-mg increments every 2–4 weeks	4–6 mg/day	Sedation, weight gain, galactorrhea, hyperglycemia, seizures, EPS, NMS, leukopenia, neutropenia, QT prolongation	
Olanzapine (Zyprexa®)	Atypical antipsychotic	Delusional infestations, factitial dermatitis	Start at 2.5 mg/day then titrate to 5–10 mg/day	20 mg/day	Weight gain, diabetes, hyperglycemia, seizures, hyperlipidemia, EPS, NMS, neutropenia, anemia,	
Aripiprazole (Abilify®)	Atypical antipsychotic	Delusional infestations, factitial dermatitis	Start at 2–5 mg/day then titrate to 10–15 mg/day	30 mg/day	Akathisia, headache, agitation, seizures, diabetes, hypertension, neutropenia	
Fluoxetine (Prozac®)	SSRI	Neurotic excoriations, trichotillomania, body dysmorphic disorder	Start at 10 mg and titrate to 20–80 mg/day	80 mg/day	Nausea, diarrhea, dyspepsia, headache, anorgasmia, suicidality, QT prolongation	
Sertraline (Zoloft®)	SSRI	Neurotic excoriations, factitial dermatitis, trichotillomania, body dysmorphic disorder	Start at 25 mg/day then titrate to 50–200 mg/day	200 mg/day	Nausea, diarrhea, dyspepsia, headache, anorgasmia, suicidality, hyponatremia	
Fluvoxamine (Luvox®)	SSRI	Neurotic excoriations, factitial dermatitis, trichotillomania, body dysmorphic disorder	Start at 50 mg/day then titrate to 50–100 mg BID	300 mg/day	Nausea, diarrhea, dyspepsia, headache, anorgasmia, suicidality, hyponatremia	
Doxepin (Sinequan®)	TCA	Neurotic excoriations, trichotillomania	Start at 10 mg/day and titrate to therapeutic dose	300 mg/day	Sedation, xerostomia, constipation, increased appetite, anticholinergic effects, QT prolongation, seizures, suicidality	Glaucoma, acute MI, urinary retention, prostatic hypertrophy, gastrointestinal or genitourinary obstruction
Clomipramine (Anafranil®)	TCA	Trichotillomania	Start at 25 mg/day then titrate to 150–250 mg/day	250 mg/day	Headache, constipation, orthostatic hypotension, anticholinergic effects, QT prolongation, seizures, suicidality	Acute MI

EPS = extrapyramidal symptoms; NMS = neuroleptic malignant syndrome.

occur as a result of an unconscious tendency. Although neurotic excoriations are believed to be underreported, it is estimated to occur in 2% of dermatology patients [28]. The patient population is predominantly female, with the typical age of onset ranging between 15 and 45 years old [29].

Clinical Presentation and Diagnosis

The clinical presentation of a patient with neurotic excoriations provides important clues to the diagnosis. The self-inflicted insults are morphologically heterogeneous, with a combination of excoriations, scabbing, erosions, and crusts in active lesions and atrophic, hyperpigmented or hypopigmented scars and lichenification characteristics of older lesions. The most common site of excoriation is the face, although other reachable body sites, such as the arms and legs, are also commonly observed, particularly on the extensor surfaces [27]. The 'butterfly sign' describes the characteristic area of sparing the unreachable areas of the back in the interscapular area, which resembles the shape of a butterfly [28, 29]. A thorough history and physical exam supplemented by appropriate laboratory tests should be performed in order to rule out any potential medical or psychiatric causes. Medical explanations for pruritus are broad and include urticaria, uremia, hepatitis, xerosis and cutaneous dysesthesia. Pruritus resulting from psychiatric causes may include anxiety, depression, hypochondriasis of somatoform disorders, or self-mutilation behavior in borderline personality disorder.

Therapeutic Approach

First and foremost, psychosocial factors and the emotional well being of the patient must be evaluated and addressed in order to achieve a successful outcome [30]. If the patient has a comorbid psychiatric disorder such as anxiety, depression, obsessive-compulsive disorder (OCD), or psychosis, it should be treated accordingly, regardless of whether they are considered to be the etiology for neurotic excoriations. Even if psychiatric illness is not the etiologic factor, it may contribute by exacerbating the tendency for skin picking. Unlike delusional patients, those with neurotic excoriations frequently acknowledge responsibility for self-inducing the lesions; therefore, they often agree to an intervention or a referral to a psychiatrist. With nonpharmacologic therapy, such as habit-reversal therapy or psychotherapy, the compulsive symptoms and any psychosocial stressors can be identified and addressed. If the patient is receptive to pharmacologic therapy, SSRIs such as fluoxetine (Prozac®), sertraline (Zoloft®), and fluvoxamine (Fluvox®), are thought to decrease the compulsive tendencies that are frequently associated with this disorder (table 3) [28]. The TCA doxepin (Sinequan®) is useful for neurotic excoriations due to its antipruritic properties, and topical treatment, such as topical corticosteroids or antipruritic lotions, can provide further relief from pruritus. The lesions should be evaluated for secondary infections and treated with topical or oral antibiotics if necessary.

Factitial Dermatitis

Factitial dermatitis, or dermatitis artefacta, is characterized by self-induced injury using more than fingernails – e.g., instruments such as cigarette lighters, sharp objects or irritating, corrosive chemicals. In contrast to patients with neurotic excoriations or TTM, who freely acknowledge the self-inflicted nature of their disorder, those with factitial dermatitis deny complicity. Self-injurious behavior is often triggered by a psychosocial stressor and represents an outlet for expressing anger or satisfying internal emotional needs. Often, patients report a history of physical, emotional, or sexual abuse in conjunction with an underlying personality disorder with borderline features [31]. Although the incidence of this disease is difficult to assess, in a study evaluating 35 psychodermatology patients, nearly one-third were diagnosed with factitial dermatitis [32]. Similar to other factitious disorders, a female predominance is observed.

Clinical Presentation and Diagnosis

Lesions are found on physically reachable areas of the body such as the face, upper trunk, and extremities, and they lack recognizable characteristics of primary dermatoses and have an atypical morphology, often with well-demarcated and angulated borders [31]. Dermatologic differential diagnoses include pyoderma gangrenosum, collagen vascular disorder, vasculitis, and arthropod bites [33], and psychiatric differential diagnoses include DI, OCD or Munchausen's syndrome.

Therapeutic Approach

The provider should avoid confronting the patient's physical role in producing the lesions and rather focus on mediating stress and other factors instigating the self-harming behavior. Treatment should address the dermatologic lesions, such as wound irrigation, debridement, and topical or oral antibiotics, as needed, and covering the wounds with occlusive dressings might discourage the patient from further self-mutilation. Adjuvant psychiatric therapy should include both pharmacologic and nonpharmacologic interventions, and high-dose SSRIs could help to decrease underlying compulsive tendencies (table 3). As dopaminergic dysfunction is believed to contribute to self-injurious behavior, antipsychotic drugs, such as pimozide and risperidone, might decrease the self-induced injuries observed in factitial dermatitis [31]. Patients with more severe presentations or comorbid borderline personality disorder could benefit from intensive psychotherapy [34].

Trichotillomania

TTM is the impulsive, repetitive action of pulling out hair, resulting in significant hair loss. Any region of the body with hair is susceptible to hair pulling, with the eyebrows, eyelashes, and scalp comprising the most common sites. The patient experiences built tension prior to pulling hair and will often feel pleasure, relief, or gratification following hair removal. Patients often admit their complicity; however, some patients are unwilling or ashamed to acknowledge their role. The prevalence of TTM is controversial, with survey studies reporting prevalence rates ranging from 0.6 to 13.3% [35, 36]. TTM is predominantly observed in females, with an early age of onset averaging between 10.7 and 13 years [37, 38].

Clinical Presentation and Diagnosis

Upon exam, alopecia is generally irregular and nonscarring, with associated broken, sparse hair and often with a background of excoriations. Hairs are broken at different lengths on the scalp, and biopsy findings of melanin pigment casts, increased number of catagen hairs, and traumatized hair bulbs in the absence of perifollicular inflammation (trichomalacia) are suggestive of the diagnosis. While similar behaviors are observed in a patient subset with OCD, these patients do not experience gratification from pulling hair, in contrast to the pleasure experienced in TTM. However, making such fine distinction between TTM and OCD may or may not be useful to a practicing dermatologist. Dermatologic differential diagnoses include alopecia areata, androgenic alopecia, alopecia mucinosa, tinea capitis, lichen planopilaris, folliculitis decalvans, and discoid lupus erythematosus. Tinea capitis may be ruled out by the absence of scaling and negative fungal culture [39].

Therapeutic Approach

Topical corticosteroids can reduce the inflammation resulting from trauma due to the act of hair pulling, and hair growth supplements may be prescribed to accelerate hair regrowth. The first-line pharmaceutical approach depends on the nature of the involved underlying psychopathology. Frequently, these patients are treated with an antidepressant, such as a high-dose SSRI or a TCA (table 3). The TCA clomipramine (Anafranil®) is the most-studied medication for TTM, and it has been shown to reduce the frequency of hair-pulling urges [40]. Behavioral therapy focused on habit-reversal training is an effective nonpharmacologic intervention to decrease the repetitive, self-inflicted behaviors observed in TTM [41]. The combination of clomipramine and habit-reversal training is effective in decreasing the frequency of hair pulling [39], and any underlying psychiatric comorbidity, such as anxiety, depression, or psychosis, should be treated accordingly.

Body Dysmorphic Disorder

BDD is a somatoform condition characterized by the preoccupation with a nonexistent or minor physical flaw. An individual with BDD experiences significant social and occupational distress as a result of fixation on the imagined or minor physical defect. BDD is relatively common and is estimated to affect around 1.8–2.4% of the general population [42, 43]. Patients with BDD experience embarrassment and deliberately avoid confiding in the provider; therefore, these figures likely underestimate the true prevalence of this disease [44]. With regard to gender, there is a slightly higher prevalence of this disease in women compared to men [42, 43]. BDD can appear as early as childhood, with a mean age of onset of 16 years old [45].

Clinical Presentation and Diagnosis

Individuals with BDD fixate on a specific aspect of their appearance that they find to be unattractive or 'deformed'. The face is commonly involved; however, body parts such as the hips, breasts, abdomen and buttocks are frequently the focus of concern. Patients will present to a dermatologist or plastic surgeon with a complaint regarding the skin (wrinkles, scarring, color, etc.), hair (excessive facial or body hair, loss of hair, etc.), or part of the body (breasts, hips, abdomen, buttocks, etc.) [46]. While the alleged defects cause overwhelming anxiety and distress, the site of complaint is unremarkable in appearance. The distress manifests by the patient spending excessive time thinking about the defect and attempting to conceal it. BDD may not be diagnosed if the condition is better explained by a different disorder. For instance, if the preoccupation is limited to concerns about weight, anorexia nervosa or bulimia nervosa should be considered.

Therapeutic Approach

Many patients with BDD seek cosmetic correction for their perceived physical flaws [47, 48]. However, cosmetic intervention generally does not result in patient satisfaction with BDD symptoms, as 81% of patients in a cross-sectional survey study reported dissatisfaction with the outcome of the consultation or surgery [48]. High-dose SSRIs have been shown to be efficacious in BDD [49, 50], and the nonpharmacologic approach to treating BDD includes cognitive-behavioral therapy, which has also been shown to be effective [51]. Interpersonal psychotherapy has shown promising results as an alternative therapy for patients who discontinue cognitive-behavioral therapy; however, further empirical support is needed [52]. The poor insight that is characteristic of BDD leads to poor adherence to the aforementioned interventions; therefore, it may be difficult to motivate such patients for treatment [52].

Conclusion

Psychodermatology is a fascinating yet underappreciated field that is characterized by complex disorders containing both dermatologic and psychiatric elements. Adopting a systematic approach that utilizes psychopharmacologic and nonpharmacologic interventions will result in successful management of psychodermatologic patients.

References

1 Jafferany M, Stoep AV, Dumitrescu A, et al: Psychocutaneous disorders: a survey study of psychiatrists' awareness and treatment patterns. South Med J 2010; 103:1199–1203.
2 Jafferany M, Vander Stoep A, Dumitrescu A, et al: The knowledge, awareness, and practice patterns of dermatologists toward psychocutaneous disorders: results of a survey study. Int J Dermatol 2010;49:784–789.
3 Gupta MA: Commentary: psychodermatology. Clin Dermatol 2013;31:1–2.
4 Gordon-Elliott JS, Muskin PR: Managing the patient with psychiatric issues in dermatologic practice. Clin Dermatol 2013;31:3–10.
5 Koo J, Lee CS: Delusions of parasitosis. A dermatologist's guide to diagnosis and treatment. Am J Clin Dermatol 2001;2: 285–290.
6 Cohen J, Adams S, Patten S: No association found between patients receiving isotretinoin for acne and the development of depression in a Canadian prospective cohort. Can J Clin Pharmacol 2007;14:e227–e233.
7 Nevoralova Z, Dvorakova D: Mood changes, depression and suicide risk during isotretinoin treatment: a prospective study. Int J Dermatol 2013;52: 163–168.
8 Wolverton SE, Harper JC: Important controversies associated with isotretinoin therapy for acne. Am J Clin Dermatol 2013;14:71–76.
9 McGrath EJ, Lovell CR, Gillison F, et al: A prospective trial of the effects of isotretinoin on quality of life and depressive symptoms. Br J Dermatol 2010; 163:1323–1329.
10 Kurd SK, Troxel AB, Crits-Christoph P, et al: The risk of depression, anxiety, and suicidality in patients with psoriasis: a population-based cohort study. Arch Dermatol 2010;146:891–895.
11 Halvorsen JA, Lien L, Dalgard F, et al: Suicidal ideation, mental health problems, and social function in adolescents with eczema: a population-based study. J Invest Dermatol 2014;134:1847–1854.
12 Purvis D, Robinson E, Merry S, et al: Acne, anxiety, depression and suicide in teenagers: a cross-sectional survey of New Zealand secondary school students. J Paediatr Child Health 2006;42:793–796.
13 D'Erme AM, Zanieri F, Campolmi E, et al: Therapeutic implications of adding the psychotropic drug escitalopram in the treatment of patients suffering from moderate-severe psoriasis and psychiatric comorbidity: a retrospective study. J Eur Acad Dermatol Venereol 2012; DOI: 10.1111/j.1468-3083.2012.04690.x.
14 Gupta MA, Guptat AK: The use of antidepressant drugs in dermatology. J Eur Acad Dermatol Venereol 2001;15:512–518.
15 Mitkov MV, Trowbridge RM, Lockshin BN, et al: Dermatologic side effects of psychotropic medications. Psychosomatics 2014;55:1–20.
16 Koo J, Gambla C: Cutaneous sensory disorder. Dermatol Clin 1996;14:497–502.
17 Gupta MA, Gupta AK: Cutaneous sensory disorder. Sem Cutan Med Surg 2013;32:110–118.
18 Bergdahl J, Anneroth G, Perris H: Cognitive therapy in the treatment of patients with resistant burning mouth syndrome: a controlled study. J Oral Pathol Med 1995;24:213–215.
19 Masheb RM, Kerns RD, Lozano C, et al: A randomized clinical trial for women with vulvodynia: Cognitive-behavioral therapy vs. supportive psychotherapy. Pain 2009;141:31–40.
20 Freudenmann RW, Lepping P: Delusional infestation. Clin Microbioly Rev 2009;22:690–732.
21 Heller MM, Wong JW, Lee ES, et al: Delusional infestations: clinical presentation, diagnosis and treatment. Int J Dermatol 2013;52:775–783.
22 Trabert W: 100 years of delusional parasitosis. Meta-analysis of 1,223 case reports. Psychopathology 1995;28:238–246.
23 Reichenberg JS, Magid M, Jesser CA, et al: Patients labeled with delusions of parasitosis compose a heterogeneous group: a retrospective study from a referral center. J Am Acad Dermatol 2013; 68:41–46, 6.e1–2.
24 Lepping P, Russell I, Freudenmann RW: Antipsychotic treatment of primary delusional parasitosis: systematic review. Br J Psychiatry 2007;191:198–205.
25 Heller MM, Koo JYM: Contemporary diagnosis and management in psychodermatology. Newton, Pennsylvania, Handbooks in Health Care Co., 2011.
26 Freudenmann RW, Lepping P: Second-generation antipsychotics in primary and secondary delusional parasitosis: outcome and efficacy. J Clin Psychopharmacol 2008;28:500–508.
27 Arnold LM, McElroy SL, Mutasim DF, et al: Characteristics of 34 adults with psychogenic excoriation. J Clin Psychiatry 1998;59:509–514.
28 Arnold LM, Auchenbach MB, McElroy SL: Psychogenic excoriation. Clinical features, proposed diagnostic criteria, epidemiology and approaches to treatment. CNS Drugs 2001;15:351–359.
29 Wilhelm S, Keuthen NJ, Deckersbach T, et al: Self-injurious skin picking: clinical characteristics and comorbidity. J Clin Psychiatry 1999;60:454–459.
30 Keuthen NJ, Deckersbach T, Wilhelm S, et al: The Skin Picking Impact Scale (SPIS): scale development and psychometric analyses. Psychosomatics 2001; 42:397–403.
31 Koblenzer CS: Dermatitis artefacta. Clinical features and approaches to treatment. Am J Clin Dermatol 2000;1: 47–55.
32 Sheppard NP, O'Loughlin S, Malone JP: Psychogenic skin disease: a review of 35 cases. Br J Psychiatry 1986;149:636–643.
33 Koblenzer CS: Neurotic excoriations and dermatitis artefacta. Dermatol Clin 1996;14:447–455.
34 Koblenzer CS: Psychosomatic concepts in dermatology. A dermatologist-psychoanalyst's viewpoint. Arch Dermatol 1983;119:501–512.
35 Christenson GA, Pyle RL, Mitchell JE: Estimated lifetime prevalence of trichotillomania in college students. J Clin Psychiatry 1991;52:415–417.
36 Rothbaum BO, Shaw L, Morris R, et al: Prevalence of trichotillomania in a college freshman population. J Clin Psychiatry 1993;54:72–73.
37 Cohen LJ, Stein DJ, Simeon D, et al: Clinical profile, comorbidity, and treatment history in 123 hair pullers: a survey study. J Clin Psychiatry 1995;56: 319–326.
38 Christenson GA, MacKenzie TB, Mitchell JE: Adult men and women with trichotillomania. A comparison of male and female characteristics. Psychosomatics 1994;35:142–149.

39 Walsh KH, McDougle CJ: Trichotillomania. Presentation, etiology, diagnosis and therapy. Am J Clin Dermatol 2001; 2:327–333.
40 Swedo SE, Leonard HL, Rapoport JL, et al: A double-blind comparison of clomipramine and desipramine in the treatment of trichotillomania (hair pulling). New Engl J Med 1989;321:497–501.
41 Morris SH, Zickgraf HF, Dingfelder HE, et al: Habit reversal training in trichotillomania: guide for the clinician. Expert Rev Neurother 2013;13:1069–1077.
42 Buhlmann U, Glaesmer H, Mewes R, et al: Updates on the prevalence of body dysmorphic disorder: a population-based survey. Psychiatry Res 2010;178: 171–175.
43 Koran LM, Abujaoude E, Large MD, et al: The prevalence of body dysmorphic disorder in the United States adult population. CNS Spectr 2008;13:316–322.
44 Conroy M, Menard W, Fleming-Ives K, et al: Prevalence and clinical characteristics of body dysmorphic disorder in an adult inpatient setting. Gen Hosp Psychiatry 2008;30:67–72.
45 Phillips KA, Menard W, Fay C, et al: Demographic characteristics, phenomenology, comorbidity, and family history in 200 individuals with body dysmorphic disorder. Psychosomatics 2005; 46:317–325.
46 Phillips KA, Kaye WH: The relationship of body dysmorphic disorder and eating disorders to obsessive-compulsive disorder. CNS Spectr 2007;12:347–358.
47 Phillips KA, Grant J, Siniscalchi J, et al: Surgical and nonpsychiatric medical treatment of patients with body dysmorphic disorder. Psychosomatics 2001;42: 504–510.
48 Veale D, Boocock A, Gournay K, et al: Body dysmorphic disorder. A survey of fifty cases. Br J Psychiatry 1996;169: 196–201.
49 Ipser JC, Sander C, Stein DJ: Pharmacotherapy and psychotherapy for body dysmorphic disorder. Cochrane Database Syst Rev 2009;1:CD005332.
50 Phillips KA, Hollander E: Treating body dysmorphic disorder with medication: evidence, misconceptions, and a suggested approach. Body Image 2008;5: 13–27.
51 Wilhelm S, Otto MW, Lohr B, et al: Cognitive behavior group therapy for body dysmorphic disorder: a case series. Behav Res Ther 1999;37:71–75.
52 Bjornsson AS, Didie ER, Phillips KA: Body dysmorphic disorder. Dialogues Clin Neurosci 2010;12:221–232.

Gabrielle Brown
515 Spruce Street
San Francisco, CA 94118 (USA)
E-Mail gebrown@email.arizona.edu

Balon R, Wise TN (eds): Clinical Challenges in the Biopsychosocial Interface. Update on Psychosomatics for the 21st Century. Adv Psychosom Med. Basel, Karger, 2015, vol 34, pp 135–142 (DOI: 10.1159/000369111)

Huntington's Disease: Looking Beyond the Movement Disorder

Mary K. Morreale

Department of Psychiatry and Behavioral Neurosciences, Wayne State University School of Medicine, Detroit, Mich., USA

Abstract

Although Huntington's disease is classically considered a motor disease, psychiatric, behavioral, and cognitive symptoms are often presenting signs of illness. Even in isolation, these comorbidities can lead to impairment in function and significant distress for patients and their families. Intended for treating psychiatrists, this review discusses the clinical presentation and treatment of Huntington's disease.

Introduction

Huntington's disease (HD) is an autosomal dominant neurodegenerative condition that is classically associated with chorea. Despite classification as a movement disorder, the presenting signs of illness are often unrelated. Although this chapter will discuss the motor indications of HD, the main focus will be on those areas pertinent to a treating psychiatrist, and specifically the cognitive, behavioral, and psychiatric manifestations of the disease.

Patients diagnosed with HD experience neuronal loss and gross atrophy in the caudate and cortex [1]. Symptomatic treatments exist, but there is no cure or mechanism to slow progression. The average survival after diagnosis, which in most cases occurs between the ages of 30 and 50, is 15–20 years [2]. Although individuals of any ethnicity can develop HD, the prevalence is highest in Northern Americans of Caucasian extraction, Europeans, and Australians, with 5.70 per 100,000 people affected [3].

HD is caused by expansion of CAG repeats in the huntingtin gene, which leads to abnormal lengthening of the huntingtin protein. In the general population, the huntingtin gene contains less than 27 repeats. Alleles containing 27–35 repeats do not cause HD but are capable of anticipation or expansion in offspring. While 36–39 repeats may or may not cause HD (reduced penetrance), a number greater than or equal to 40 unequivocally leads to symptoms by age 65 (fully penetrant). At the population level, larger numbers of repeats are associated with an earlier onset of significant motor symptoms and, less significantly, rapidity of progression [4]. There is no association, however, between the number of repeats and the development of psychiatric symptomatology [5]. For the individual diagnosed with HD, nothing can predict the age of onset, which symptoms may appear, how severe the illness will be, or the rate of clinical deterioration [6]. In addition, it is impossible to determine the course of illness based on the experience of affected relatives [6].

Despite the availability of predictive testing, less than 10% of those at risk chose to identify their genetic status [7]. Individuals who test positive but are disease free are considered to be in the pre-manifest phase of illness. Those with cognitive or psychiatric symptoms but no significant motor signs are in the prodromal phase. Manifest illness is diagnosed when significant motor symptoms appear. The Unified Huntington's Disease Rating Scale (UHDRS), which measures motor, cognitive, and psychiatric symptoms, is the most common clinical and research assessment utilized [8].

Functional decline can begin as early as the prodromal phase of illness. In a study examining 265 individuals during this period, approximately one-third reported some difficulty with activities of daily living [9]. The most common loss cited was in occupational performance (65.1%), followed by the ability to manage finances independently (between 35 and 49.2%, depending on the method of assessment), to drive safely (33.5%), and to supervise children (28.6%). Based on functional impairment, the Huntington's Disease Society of America (HDSA) divides manifest HD into three stages [7]. In the early stage of illness, the symptoms are minor, and deficits are minimal. Patients are able to drive, handle their finances, and live independently. As the disease progresses, greater impairment in voluntary movements develops, but the ability to dress, bathe, and feed oneself is unaffected. In the final stage of HD, individuals are unable to perform activities of daily living. Although movement is severely impacted in the end stage of illness and patients may be nonverbal, comprehension is not necessarily lost.

Juvenile HD will be mentioned briefly but will not be covered in the remainder of this review. Defined as disease diagnosed prior to age 20, this variant differs in many ways from the adult version. In most cases, the number of trinucleotide repeats is above 55, and clinical progression is much more rapid [7]. Juvenile HD occurs in less than 10% diagnosed, and the majority of patients inherit the mutation paternally [7]. The initial manifestations of illness are typically behavioral, and unlike the adult variant, motor symptoms begin with rigidity [7]. Declining school performance may indicate cognitive dysfunction, and attention deficit disorder is a common misdiagnosis [7]. Seizures are seen in 25% of children and adolescents diagnosed with HD and may be the first presenting sign of illness [7].

Motor Dysfunction

The motor symptoms of HD are dynamic and unique to the individual affected. More than 90% of patients develop chorea, which is often the first indication of motor illness [7, 8]. Chorea initially presents in the distal extremities but progresses to the proximal, axial, and facial musculature and, with time, increases in frequency and amplitude [7, 10]. In some patients, chorea plateaus and diminishes, while in others, worsening continues [7]. Dystonia and bradykinesia, which may be masked by comorbid chorea, develop in mid- to late-stage HD [7]. In advanced stages, rigidity is common [7, 10]. In the end stage of illness, nearly all movement-associated functions are affected, including finger dexterity, hand coordination, gait, speech, swallowing, and bowel and bladder control [7].

Effective pharmacotherapy for motor dysfunction depends on the type of abnormality present. Evidence suggests that increased dopamine release leads to chorea, while reductions cause bradykinesia [11]. In 2008, tetrabenazine became the first medication to be Food and Drug Administration approved for the treatment of HD. Indicated solely for chorea, tetrabenazine binds to the vesicular monoamine transporter, resulting in decreased reuptake of dopamine into synaptic vesicles. Although not Food and Drug Administration approved, additional treatments for chorea include typical antipsychotics and atypical agents that provide greater affinity for the D2 receptor (olanzapine and risperidone) [7, 12]. Despite the fact that all pharmacotherapies used to treat chorea potentially cause significant side effects, tetrabenazine is particularly troublesome, as it leads to initiation or exacerbation of depression in 20% of patients [7]. Regarding treatment of tetrabenazine-induced depression, only one case study exists, which reported success with reboxetine [13]. For the treatment of bradykinesia, small studies and case reports have found benefit with the dopaminergic agonists bromocriptine, levodopa, pramipexole, amantadine, and cabergoline [14, 15]. Benzodiazepines, baclofen, and botulinum toxin may be helpful for dystonia [7]. Once rigidity develops, the dose of tetrabenazine and antipsychotics should be reduced [7]. In addition, benzodiazepines, baclofen, and the dopamine agonist, cabergoline may be of value [7, 16].

Cognitive Dysfunction

Like motor dysfunction, cognitive decline has an unpredictable onset and course. Despite discussion in numerous articles, there is little agreement regarding symptomatology and progression [1]. What appears to be clear is that subclinical cognitive changes can occur 15 years prior to motor symptoms and may lead to early functional impairment, independent of other factors [1, 4, 7, 10]. In addition, cognitive decline is prevalent, with approximately 40% affected in the prodromal period and 75% affected as manifest disease nears [7, 17].

Although initially insidious, the cognitive decline tends to progress [18]. During the beginning of the HD prodrome, the most robust changes are seen in emotional recognition, processing speed, and both working and learning memory [6]. With time, impairments occur in additional areas, including smell identification, cued sequencing, attention, reaction time, and letter fluency [6]. Other domains affected include estimation of time, executive function, initiation and comprehension of conversation, and awareness of one's own feelings and actions [6].

Researchers emphasize the difference between cognitive dysfunction in HD compared with Alzheimer's disease and other neurodegenerative disorders and even suggest discrete criteria for diagnosis [19]. In HD, overall memory impairment and 'rapid forgetting' are not as pronounced [8]. Implicit memory, which involves coordination of movement in previously learned motor tasks, such as driving a car and chewing, may be affected, while memories of names and dates remain relatively intact [7].

There is no accepted battery of tests recommended to assess cognition in patients diagnosed with HD [6]. The UHDRS, mentioned above, contains three cognitive subtests, one of which evaluates the most sensitive indicator of cognitive function in HD, or the speed of processing [7]. The Mini-Mental Status Exam may detect longitudinal changes in cognition but lacks sensitivity [7]. In comparison, the Montreal Cognitive Assessment, which contains a more comprehensive evaluation of executive function, attention, and visuospatial abilities and relies less on intact verbal skills, may be a more sensitive instrument [20].

There is scant data related to the treatment of cognitive dysfunction. Several pharmacotherapies have been evaluated in small (n = 20–30) randomized placebo-controlled trials, but none has been proven to be particularly effective. No effect was seen with modafinil, atomoxetine, or donepezil, although modafinil increased alertness and atomoxetine led to self-reported enhancement of sustained attention [21–23]. Rivastigmine has been evaluated in two small trials, both showing a tendency for improvement [24, 25]. In studies of cognition as an ancillary measure, lamotrigine, fluoxetine, riluzole, amantadine, ketamine, and remacemide all failed to show benefit [26].

The HDSA suggests several behavioral strategies to help those patients who are cognitively compromised [7]. As estimation of time, initiation of activity, and attention may be impaired, distractions should be minimized, and extra time should be allowed for activities. Patients may need reminders of schedules, and calendars and clocks should be readily visible. In addition, a structured routine can be beneficial. Given the possibility of diminished insight, interventions to enhance adherence are vital.

Behavioral and Psychiatric Dysfunction

Changes in behavior and the development of psychiatric symptoms are quite common in HD and, similar to cognitive impairment, can present years prior to significant motor disease. Although these comorbid conditions can be the most distressing aspect of illness, they tend to be underdiagnosed and inadequately treated [27]. Perhaps part of the difficulty lies in studying these phenomena. First, assessment can be problematic, as symptoms do not always meet the threshold for formal diagnosis. Second, although multi-site studies are available, HD is a rare illness, and sample sizes are often small. Finally, establishing a control population is not always straightforward: should expansion-negative relatives be used, or members of the general population? Methodologies often differ, which makes comparison of information challenging.

Changes in personality are likely more common than concrete psychiatric diagnoses. HD patients can present with a 'dysexecutive or frontal lobe syndrome', which includes both disinhibited and deficit symptoms, possibly at the same time [7]. Disinhibited behaviors include impulsivity, perseveration, and irritability, whereas deficit symptoms consist of apathy, loss of spontaneity, indifference, and lack of insight. Regardless of origin, personality changes are difficult to manage and may respond to behavioral interventions more so than medications.

Perseveration can lead to fixation on a specific idea or task and is described as 'behavioral rigidity' [7]. This symptom can present in a manner similar to obsessive-compulsive disorder (OCD), although more so the obsessive criteria. Unfortunately, limited evidence is available regarding the treatment of perseveration, although, as in OCD, selective serotonin reuptake inhibitors (SSRIs) may be effective [7]. Per this author's experience, fluvoxamine has been a particularly effective agent. In addition, case studies have demonstrated improvement with the dopamine agonist amantadine [7].

The majority of patients diagnosed with HD experience irritability, and not surprisingly, this greatly concerns family members [7, 28]. The root of irritability may lie in many causes, including, but not limited to, depression, frustration, and confusion [7]. To minimize escalation toward violence, families should be encouraged to identify and minimize triggers, to redirect their loved one, and to maintain a calm and structured environment [7]. In potentially dangerous situations, the police may need to be summoned. Although no robust evidence exists to guide pharmacologic management of irritability, SSRIs may help if obsessive-compulsive or depressive symptoms are associated [7, 26]. Mood stabilizers can be prescribed as well and, in severe cases, antipsychotics or benzodiazepines [7, 26].

Apathy, which includes disinterest, amotivation, diminished goal-directed behavior, and emotional blunting, is extremely common as well, occurring in 34–76% of patients, depending on the stage of illness and the method of assessment [7, 29]. The prevalence and severity of apathy increase as HD progresses [29]. Apathy may be mistaken for depression but can be distinguished from a mood disorder diagnosis by the absence of neurovegetative symptoms [7]. Activating antidepressants may be helpful for apathy, but additional medications may be needed as well, including stimulants, amantadine, bromocriptine, and selegiline [7]. In this author's clinical experience, stimulants help somewhat with amotivation and may secondarily benefit difficulties with attention and initiation of activity. Antipsychotics and benzodiazepines may worsen apathy by further blunting emotion and cognition [7].

Collaborating investigators have studied discrete psychiatric symptoms during both prodromal and manifest illness. Compared with controls, individuals with prodromal HD (n = 589) display elevations in scales related to depression, obsessive-compulsiveness, anxiety, and psychoticism [30]. These symptoms are directly correlated to the severity of motor and cognitive impairments and inversely associated with overall function. In individuals (n = 1,941) with 'probable' or 'definite' manifest disease, 48.2% report treatment for past depression; 8.1%, for obsessive-compulsive disorder; and 5.2%, for psychosis [31]. Given the nature of retrospective reporting, it is impossible to know if full DSM criteria were met for the diagnoses specified.

Per Epping et al., clinically significant depression (Beck Depression Inventory score >13) is noted in 20–30% of gene-expanded individuals, which is slightly more frequent than in controls [32]. Depressive symptoms can occur at any time during prodromal HD and are not associated with proximity to genetic testing or the expected time to diagnosis [32]. Not surprisingly, gene-expanded females have a higher frequency of depression when compared with similar males, and the severity of symptoms contributes to increased cognitive impairment, perceived stress, and negative life experience [32–34]. Whereas unipolar depression is relatively common in HD, bipolarity is infrequently seen [7]. Irritability and impulsivity may look like symptoms of mania but tend to occur in the absence of additional criteria.

The rate of suicidal behavior in patients with HD is higher than in any other neurodegenerative disorder [35]. In the same 1,941 patients mentioned above, approximately 25% reported a history of suicidal ideation; 19%, of current suicidal ideation; and 9.5%, of at least one suicide attempt [31]. To put these data into perspective, in the general population, suicidal ideation exists in 3.3%, and a history of a suicide attempt exists in less than 1% [36]. Per Wetzel et al., no demographic, motor, or cognitive variables predict suicidal behavior, but there is a significant association with depression, anxiety, and aggression, as assessed by the UHDRS [31]. When looking at those with the most severe suicidal ideation, a past or current history of alcohol abuse becomes a predictive measure as well [31]. Suicidal risk increases during periods of functional loss, such as when work becomes too difficult or driving is no longer possible [31]. As the disease worsens and reductions in awareness occur, this risk decreases [31].

As stated earlier, although elevations in scales related to psychoticism occur in HD, chronic psychosis and schizophrenia are uncommon [7]. When psychotic symptoms do present, they tend to follow the diagnosis of manifest disease and develop in tandem with cognitive impairment, mood disorders, or delirium [37]. Per the HDSA, some HD patients suffer from resistant delusions, which are difficult to discern from perseveration [7]. As is the case with all delusional thinking, confrontation is rarely beneficial.

While elevations in anxiety levels are possible, there is little in the literature regarding the diagnosis and treatment of anxiety disorders. The probability of obsessive and compulsive symptoms, as assessed by the UHDRS, has been measured and shown to increase with disease severity, with a peak of 24% for obsessions and 12% for compulsions in advanced stages of illness [38]. The full criteria for OCD, however, are rarely met [38].

Unfortunately, scarce evidence exists regarding the treatment of psychiatric comorbidity in HD. In general, choosing a medication for a patient with HD is similar to doing so for any psychiatric patient, with the theoretical exception of a propensity toward increased side effects in the HD population. As with the use of antidepressants in all depressive illness, there are no concrete data to suggest the superiority of any one agent over another [7]. If the diagnostic criterion is met for mania, lithium should be avoided, as potential fluctuations in fluid intake can lead to toxicity [7]. It is important to distinguish mania from isolated irritability and impulsivity, as the latter do not typically respond to mood-stabilizing medications [7]. Expert consensus supports the use of SSRIs and clomipramine for obsessive-compulsive behaviors [39]. If psychosis is present, antipsychotics are indicated. As with psychotic illness in general, no particular agent is preferred [7]. If chorea exists, the high-potency typical agents may be of benefit, as they decrease movement via parkinsonism. In contrast, if the patient has either bradykinesia or rigidity, atypical antipsychotics are a better choice. Although there are only case studies regarding electroconvulsive therapy, evidence indicates improvement in mood and psychosis as well as decreased suicidality [40]. Interestingly, decreased cognition is not always the norm.

Conclusion

Although typically understood as a movement disorder, HD has significant cognitive, behavioral, and psychiatric comorbidity. Symptoms from any of these domains may present prior to motor abnormalities and alone can cause distress and functional impairment. The HDSA acknowledges that HD is more than a neurologic illness and necessitates that its Centers of Excellence provide psychiatric and psychological services.

Unfortunately, there are considerable limitations in the research related to the treatment of nonmotor manifestations of HD. Randomized placebo-controlled trials of medications have been small, and the bulk of information available comes from case studies and anecdotal evidence. Thankfully, there is no evidence to suggest that HD patients are less likely to benefit from psychiatric medications than non-HD populations. Hopefully, in the future, the work of collaborative investigators will help us to fine-tune our approach.

Behavioral interventions are a key component of managing patients with HD. As described above, the HDSA suggests several strategies to minimize both patient and family distress. Although there is no literature regarding psychotherapeutic strategies, psychoeducation, supportive therapy, cognitive-behavioral therapy, and family sessions should all be considered. In addition, all those affected by HD can potentially benefit from support groups, which are offered through multiple organizations.

In this author's opinion, it would be helpful for physicians, patients, and families if the diagnosis of manifest HD were expanded to reflect the significance of cognitive, behavioral, and psychiatric symptoms. The current standard, which only requires involuntary movement in the presence of a positive genetic test, minimizes the impact of these comorbid conditions. In a disease in which patients struggle with so many ambiguities, including which symptoms they will develop and how their illness might progress, an increase in diagnostic clarity could be a relief for all.

References

1 Papp KV, Kaplan RF, Snyder PJ: Biological markers of cognition in prodromal Huntington's disease: a review. Brain Cogn 2011;77:280–291.

2 Mestre T, Ferreira J, Coelho MM, Rosa M, Sampaio C: Therapeutic interventions for symptomatic treatment in Huntington's disease. Cochrane Database Syst Rev 2009;3:CD006456.

3 Pringsheim T, Wiltshire K, Day L, Dykeman J, Steeves T, Jette N: The incidence and prevalence of Huntington's disease: a systematic review and meta-analysis. Mov Disord 2012;27:1083–1091.

4 Novak MJ, Tabrizi SJ: Huntington's disease. BMJ 2010;340:c3109.

5 Vassos E, Panas M, Kladi A, Vassilopoulos D: Effect of CAG repeat length on psychiatric disorders in Huntington's disease. J Psychiatr Res 2008;42:544–549.

6 Paulsen JS: Cognitive impairment in Huntington disease: diagnosis and treatment. Curr Neurol Neurosci 2011;11:474–483.

7 Nance M, Paulsen JS, Rosenblatt A, Wheelock V, Huntington's Disease Society of America. A Physician's Guide to the Management of Huntington's Disease, ed. 3. New York, Huntington's Disease Society of America, 2013.

8 Ross CA, Aylward EH, Wild EJ, et al: Huntington disease: natural history, biomarkers and prospects for therapeutics. Nat Rev Neurol 2014;10:204–216.

9 Beglinger LJ, O'Rourke JJ, Wang C, et al: Earliest functional declines in Huntington disease. Psychiatry Res 2010;178:414–418.

10 Roos RA: Huntington's disease: a clinical review. Orphanet J Rare Dis 2010;5:40.

11 Chen JY, Wang EA, Cepeda C, Levine MS: Dopamine imbalance in Huntington's disease: a mechanism for the lack of behavioral flexibility. Front Neurosci 2013;7:114.

12 Kapur S, Seeman P: Does fast dissociation from the dopamine d(2) receptor explain the action of atypical antipsychotics?: A new hypothesis. AJP 2001;158:360–369.

13 Schreiber W, Krieg JC, Eichhorn T: Reversal of tetrabenazine induced depression by selective noradrenaline (norepinephrine) reuptake inhibition. J Neurol Neurosurg Psychiatry 1999;67:550.

14 White RF: Clinical Syndromes in Adult Neuropsychology: The Practitioner's Handbook. Amsterdam/New York, Elsevier, 1992.

15 Phillips W, Shannon KM, Barker RA: The current clinical management of Huntington's disease. Mov Disord 2008;23:1491–1504.

16 Martin B, Golden E, Keselman A, et al: Therapeutic perspectives for the treatment of Huntington's disease: treating the whole body. Histol Histopathol 2008;23:237–250.

17 Duff K, Paulsen J, Mills J, et al: Mild cognitive impairment in prediagnosed Huntington disease. Neurol 2010;75:500–507.

18 Paulsen JS, Langbehn DR, Stout JC, et al: Detection of Huntington's disease decades before diagnosis: the Predict-HD study. J Neurol Neurosurg Psychiatry 2008;79:874–880.

19 Peavy GM, Jacobson MW, Goldstein JL, et al: Cognitive and functional decline in Huntington's disease: dementia criteria revisited. Mov Disord 2010;25:1163–1169.

20 Mickes L, Jacobson M, Peavy G, et al: A comparison of two brief screening measures of cognitive impairment in Huntington's disease. Mov Disord 2010;25:2229–2233.

21 Beglinger LJ, Adams WH, Paulson H, et al: Randomized controlled trial of atomoxetine for cognitive dysfunction in early Huntington disease. J Clin Psychopharmacol 2009;29:484–487.

22 Cubo E, Shannon KM, Tracy D, et al: Effect of donepezil on motor and cognitive function in Huntington disease. Neurology 2006;67:1268–1271.

23 Blackwell AD, Paterson NS, Barker RA, Robbins TW, Sahakian BJ: The effects of modafinil on mood and cognition in Huntington's disease. Psychopharmacology (Berl) 2008;199:29–36.

24 de Tommaso M, Specchio N, Sciruicchio V, Difruscolo O, Specchio LM: Effects of rivastigmine on motor and cognitive impairment in Huntington's disease. Mov Disord 2004;19:1516–1518.

25 Rot U, Kobal J, Sever A, Pirtosek Z, Mesec A: Rivastigmine in the treatment of Huntington's disease. Eur J Neurol 2002;9:689–690.

26 Mestre TA, Ferreira JJ: An evidence-based approach in the treatment of Huntington's disease. Parkinsonism Relat Disord 2012;18:316–320.

27 Hubers AA, Reedeker N, Giltay EJ, Roos RA, van Duijn E, van der Mast RC: Suicidality in Huntington's disease. J Affect Disord 2012;136:550–557.

28 Pflanz S, Besson JA, Ebmeier KP, Simpson S: The clinical manifestation of mental disorder in Huntington's disease: a retrospective case record study of disease progression. Acta Psychiatr Scand 1991;83:53–60.

29 van Duijn E, Reedeker N, Giltay EJ, Roos RA, van der Mast RC: Correlates of apathy in Huntington's disease. J Neuropsychiatry Clin Neurosci 2010;22:287–294.

30 Duff K, Paulsen JS, Beglinger LJ, Langbehn DR, Stout JC, Predict-HD Investigators of the Huntington Study Group. Psychiatric symptoms in Huntington's disease before diagnosis: the predict-HD study. Biol Psychiatry 2007;62:1341–1346.

31 Wetzel HH, Gehl CR, Dellefave-Castillo L, et al: Suicidal ideation in Huntington disease: the role of comorbidity. Psychiatry Res 2011;188:372–376.

32 Epping EA, Mills JA, Beglinger LJ, et al: Characterization of depression in prodromal Huntington disease in the neurobiological predictors of HD (PREDICT-HD) study. J Psychiatric Res 2013;47:1423–1431.

33 Smith MM, Mills JA, Epping EA, Westervelt HJ, Paulsen JS, PREDICT-HD Investigators of the Huntington Study Group. Depressive symptom severity is related to poorer cognitive performance in prodromal Huntington disease. Neuropsychology 2012;26:664–669.

34 Downing N, Smith MM, Beglinger LJ, et al: Perceived stress in prodromal Huntington disease. Psychol Health 2012;27:196–209.

35 Harris EC, Barraclough B: Suicide as an outcome for mental disorders. A meta-analysis. Br J Psychiatry 1997;170:205–228.
36 Kessler RC, Berglund P, Borges G, Nock M, Wang PS: Trends in suicide ideation, plans, gestures, and attempts in the United States, 1990–1992 to 2001–2003. JAMA 2005;293:2487–2495.
37 Nagel M, Rumpf HJ, Kasten M: Acute psychosis in a verified Huntington disease gene carrier with subtle motor signs: psychiatric criteria should be considered for the diagnosis. Gen Hosp Psychiatry 2014;36:361.e3–e4.
38 Beglinger LJ, Langbehn DR, Duff K, et al: Probability of obsessive and compulsive symptoms in Huntington's disease. Biol Psychiatry 2007;61:415–418.
39 Anderson K, Craufurd D, Edmondson MC, et al: An international survey-based algorithm for the pharmacologic treatment of obsessive-compulsive behaviors in Huntington's disease. PLoS Curr 2011;3:RRN1261.
40 Cusin C, Franco FB, Fernandez-Robles C, DuBois CM, Welch CA: Rapid improvement of depression and psychotic symptoms in Huntington's disease: a retrospective chart review of seven patients treated with electroconvulsive therapy. Gen Hosp Psychiatry 2013;35:678.e3–e5.

Mary K. Morreale, MD
Department of Psychiatry
3901 Chrysler Service Dr.
Detroit, MI 48201 (USA)
E-Mail mmorreale@med.wayne.edu

Balon R, Wise TN (eds): Clinical Challenges in the Biopsychosocial Interface. Update on Psychosomatics for the 21st Century. Adv Psychosom Med. Basel, Karger, 2015, vol 34, pp 143–157 (DOI: 10.1159/000369113)

Joint Hypermobility, Anxiety and Psychosomatics: Two and a Half Decades of Progress Toward a New Phenotype

Antoni Bulbena[a, b] • Guillem Pailhez[a, b] • Andrea Bulbena-Cabré[a, e] • Nuria Mallorquí-Bagué[a, c] • Carolina Baeza-Velasco[d]

[a]Departament de Psiquiatria i Medicina Legal Universidad Autónoma de Barcelona, Bellaterra Barcelona, [b]Unidad de Ansiedad, Institut de Neuropsiquiatria i Addiccions (INAD), Hospital del Mar, Parc de Salut Mar, Barcelona, [c]Unidad de Psiquiatria y Psicología, Hospital Universitario Quirón Dexeus, Barcelona, Spain; [d]Institut de Psychologie, Université Paris Descartes, Sorbonne Paris Cité, France; [e]Department of Psychiatry, Metropolitan Hospital Center, New York Medical College, New York, N.Y., USA

Abstract

The strong association between a heritable collagen condition and anxiety was an unexpected finding that we first described in 1988 at the Hospital del Mar in Barcelona. Since then, several clinical and nonclinical studies have been carried out. In this paper, after summarizing the concept and diagnosis of joint hypermobility (hyperlaxity), we review case-control studies in both directions (anxiety in joint hypermobility and joint hypermobility in anxiety disorders) as well as studies on nonclinical samples, review papers and one incidence study. The collected evidence tends to confirm the strength of the association described two and a half decades ago. The common mechanisms that are involved in this association include genetics, autonomic nervous system dysfunctions and interoceptive and exteroceptive processes. Considering clinical and nonclinical data, pathophysiological mechanisms and the presented nosological status, we suggest a new Neuroconnective phenotype, which around a common core Anxiety-Collagen hyperlaxity, includes five dimensions: behavioral, psychopathology, somatic symptoms, somatosensory symptoms, and somatic illnesses. It is envisaged that new descriptions of anxiety disorders and of some psychosomatic conditions will emerge and that different nosological approaches will be required. The Neuroconnective model is a proposal that is under study and may be useful for clinical practice.

History of Link Joint Laxity – Anxiety

The relationship between a heritable collagen condition and anxiety was an unexpected finding that we first described in 1988 at the Hospital del Mar in Barcelona [1]. It really was a clinical observation, rather than a pathophysiological reasoning.

While working at the psychiatric outpatient clinic, we repeatedly found a particular rubber stamp in the medical records of most of our patients suffering from anxiety: 'Hiperlaxitud

Articular'. That stamp was put there by the rheumatologist JC Duró, who was using it to systematically collect criteria for the Joint Hypermobility Syndrome (JHS) that had been described and studied by his mentor, Prof. Rotés. The reiterated coincidence of the two conditions, anxiety and the collagen condition, prompted us to study this association in more detail.

This observation prompted us to send a letter containing preliminary results to *The Lancet* [1], and soon after, we carried out the first case-control study.

Considering the high prevalence of mood disorders in patients suffering from collagenosis, psychiatrists have begun to associate collagen conditions with autoimmune illnesses, such as systemic lupus erythematosus or rheumatoid arthritis, whereas structural collagen disorders (mainly heritable) seemed to be less in mind due to the lack of knowledge of the psychiatric status of these patients.

However, scattered observations pointed in this new direction. In 1957, rheumatologist J. Rotés observed a remarkable degree of nervous tension suffered by patients with hypermobility [2]. To a certain extent, there were some indirect references about the relationship between 'visceroptosis' and anxiety/phobias in the classical psychosomatic literature [3]. On the other hand, in 1980, Carlsson and Rundgren [4] found higher hypermobility scores in alcoholic patients compared to controls. Although not mentioned, the case group might have consisted of a high percentage of patients with anxiety.

What is Joint Laxity (Hypermobility) Syndrome

In order to clarify the terminology throughout this paper, we shall indistinctly use joint laxity (the original name) and joint hypermobility (JH; the given name). Although the second is more often used in English publications, it in fact refers to a rather unspecific consequence (increased mobility), whereas hyperlaxity more correctly refers to the intrinsic mechanism (increased laxity of fibers).

The condition was described for the first time about 60 years ago, when it was properly identified and associated with pathology of the musculoskeletal system [2]. The original name proposed by Rotés was 'joint laxity' (Laxité Articulaire), and it was published in a French journal *(Revue du Rhumatisme)*. In 1964, Carter and Wilkinson, also using the term 'joint laxity', published a relevant paper in which they proposed diagnostic criteria [5]. In 1973, after an epidemiological study by Beighton et al. [6], who used both 'joint laxity' and 'joint mobility', the syndrome gained general interest in rheumatology and, by then, was renamed JH and began to be studied in a broader way as a separate entity [7]. Later on, the seminal work of Rodney Grahame was very important for the revisiting of JHS by rheumatologists. Grahame has published three editions of the Beighton book [8] as well as other books and has boosted clinical research on this topic [9, 10]. Another prominent author who has provided insightful clinical descriptions of JHS is Dr. J. Bravo [11].

JHS has an estimated prevalence in the general population of 10–20%. It is more frequent in females (3:1), and it is one of the connective tissue hereditary disorders that also include other conditions such as Ehlers-Danlos syndrome (EDS), Marfan syndrome and osteogenesis imperfecta [8]. In fact, it does overlap with EDS type III. JHS has an autosomal dominant pattern, and twin studies showed that genetics, rather than environmental factors such as training, accounts for at least 70% of the phenotype variance. Joint hypermobility is characterized by an extended range of motion of the joints, increased distensibility of joints in passive movements and hypermobility in active movement in the absence of another rheumatologic disease.

JHS is more common in childhood and tends to decline with age. The prevalence is higher in women, and there are probably ethnic differences, which suggests genetic variations. JHS is also associated with musculoskeletal dysfunctions, possibly resulting from a glycoprotein deficiency and genetic alterations affecting the formation of collagen, which would explain the tissue looseness, prolapsed organs, visceroptoses, pneumothorax and vulnerability to trauma in these patients.

Clinical features of JHS can be articular or extra-articular and are always related to the connective tissue. Arthralgia, lumbalgia, soft-tissue rheumatism (e.g., epicondylitis, tenosynovitis, and bursitis), recurrent dislocations, childhood scoliosis, or rheumatoid arthritis are some common articular features [11, 12]. On the other hand, hernias, varicose veins, 'easy bruising', hypertrophic scars and keloids, uterine or rectal prolapse, spontaneous pneumothorax, fibromyalgia, dysautonomia and other conditions linked to panic disorders (PDs) such as asthma, mitral valve prolapse (MVP), thyroid dysfunction or irritable bowel syndrome, are some of the best-known, extra-articular features of JHS [12, 13].

The Diagnosis of Joint Hypermobility (Hyperlaxity)

Several sets of criteria show minimal variations from the original disease proposed by Rotés, although new self-assessment questionnaires have been recently added to the assessment methods of JHS [14, 15]. A review paper of all available criteria showed a high degree of agreement among all of them [16], but a more comprehensive set of 10 criteria that were obtained by cluster analysis was also proposed. However, the most often used are the 'Beighton criteria', which is a nine-point clinical scale by which subjects with a score ≥4 are considered as having JH. The condition is characterized through the examination of five body areas, each one receiving a separate score of hyperextension: fifth fingers, thumbs, elbows, knees and trunk.

In 2010, Grahame [17] developed the Brighton criteria to replace the Beighton criteria for JHS. According to these criteria, the diagnosis of the syndrome is made by taking into account the Beighton score as well as some other clinical manifestations associated with hypermobility. As expected, the correlation between them is very high, but they are seldom used outside of rheumatology. The main sets of criteria are shown in table 1.

The clinical assessment of the Joint Laxity Syndrome is not difficult, but examiners should be trained in order to ensure the reliability of the exam. Our group has developed a 2-day training course that includes a support CD [18].

Clinical Studies

The first case-control study on the association between joint hypermobility and anxiety disorders was published in 1993 [19]. Patients were recruited from an outpatient rheumatology clinic, and the final study included 114 JHS cases and 59 controls. A high prevalence of anxiety disorders within the JH group (70%) was found compared to the control group (20%), with PD/agoraphobia (PD/A) (OR 4.12) and simple phobia (OR 3.03) showing the most significant correlations. MVP was only found in subjects with JH, and those patients were more likely (OR 2.95) to suffer from anxiety disorders compared to subjects without MVP; however, the association did not reach statistical significance.

Later, we carried out the reverse case-control study, that is to say, we blindly assessed joint hypermobility among anxiety patients compared to controls, who were carefully matched by age and gender, in a general teaching hospital [20]. The sample included 99 newly diagnosed patients with PD and/or agoraphobia and 163 controls who were recruited from the psychiatric (n = 99) and medical clinics (n = 64). The prevalence of JH was significantly higher (70%) in the PD/A group compared to the psychiatric (10%) and medical

Table 1. Hypermobility criteria, description of Beighton, and Hospital del Mar and Brighton criteria, with suggested cut-off points

Beighton criteria

1. Passive dorsiflexion of the little fingers beyond 90° (one point for each hand).
2. Passive apposition of the thumbs to the flexor aspects of the forearm (one point for each thumb).
3. Hyperextension of the elbows beyond 10° (one point for each elbow).
4. Hyperextension of the knee beyond 10° (one point for each knee).
5. Forward flexion of the trunk with knees fully extended so that the palms of the hands rest flat on the floor (one point).

A general score of 4/5 in the Beighton system, which is the usual cut-off point in clinical practice, is proposed in order to diagnose a case.

Hospital del Mar Criteria

Upper extremities

1. Passive apposition of the thumb to the flexor aspect of the forearm at a distance of less than 21 mm.
2. The passive dorsiflexion of the fifth finger is 90° or more.
3. The active hyperextension of the elbow is 10° or more.
4. External rotation of the shoulder up to more than 85°.

Lower extremities; supine position

5. The passive hip abduction can be taken to an angle of 85° or more.
6. Hypermobility of the rotula.
7. Hypermobility of the ankle and foot.
8. Dorsal flexion of the toe of 90° or more.

Lower extremities; prone position

9. Hyperflexion of the knee.
10. Ecchymoses.

Bulbena et al. [16] propose to consider males with a score of 3/4 probable cases of joint hypermobility and women with a score of 4/5 probable cases of joint hypermobility. For age, it is suggested that patients older than 40 with a score of 3/4 probable cases of joint hypermobility and that patients younger than 40 years with a score of 4/5 probable cases of joint hypermobility be considered. A general score of 3/4 in the Hospital del Mar system, which is the usual cut-off point in clinical practice, is proposed.

Brighton Criteria

Major criteria

1. A Beighton score of 4/9 or more (either currently or historically).
2. *Arthralgia* for longer than 3 months in 4 or more joints.

Minor criteria

1. *Beighton* score of 1, 2 or 3 (0, 1, 2 or 3 *if aged 50 years or older*).
2. *Arthralgia* in 1–3 joints, *lumbalgia* for more than 3 months, spondylosis or spondylolysis/spondylolisthesis.
3. *Dislocation/subluxation* in more than one joint or in one joint on more than one occasion.
4. *Soft tissue rheumatism* in three or more lesions (e.g., epicondylitis, tenosynovitis, bursitis).
5. *Marfanoid Habitus* (tall, slim, span/height ratio >1.03, upper/lower segment ratio <0.89, arachnodactily).
6. *Abnormal skin:* striae, hyperextensibility, thin skin or papyraceous scarring.
7. *Eye signs*: drooping eyelids or antimongoloid slant.
8. *Varicose veins, hernia or uterine/rectal prolapse.*

BJHS is diagnosed if the patient presents 2 major criteria, 1 major and 2 minor criteria, or 4 minor criteria. Two minor criteria are enough when there is a first-degree relative who is clearly diagnosed with the syndrome. BJHS is excluded by the presence of Marfan or Ehlers-Danlos syndrome. The 1st major and 1st minor criteria exclude each other, as do the 2nd major and 2nd minor criteria.

controls (12%). In this study, patients with PD/A were 17 times more likely to suffer from JH.

Lumley et al. [21] evaluated the psychosocial functioning of patients suffering from EDS (JHS is considered EDS type III). The patients were selected from an outpatient research clinic, and the results showed that the EDS type III group had higher anxiety, depression, and interpersonal sensitivity scores as well as higher scores for the symptomatology checklist and pain scales.

Other lines of research studied possible specific somatotype characteristics in patients with PD/A [22]. Patients with panic and/or agoraphobia from an outpatient mental health clinic were compared to psychiatric and medical controls matched by age and gender. Within the entire sample, the asthenic somatotype was associated with higher JH scores. Interestingly, the prevalence of an asthenic somatotype was at the same time significantly higher in the panic/agoraphobia group (33.3%) compared to the psychiatric (19.2%) and medical (18.7%) controls. The authors finally concluded that the relationship between PDs and asthenic somatotype might be mediated through JHS. These results were confirmed by another study carried out by the same group in 2014 [23]. This study included 60 patients with PD/A and 60 controls and found that an ectomorphic somatotype was independently related to JH status [OR 3.25, 95% CI 1.35–7.8, p = 0.008].

Nevertheless, some studies failed to find a significant correlation between PD and JH. The study by Benjamin et al. was carried out in Israel on 101 patients with PD and on 39 controls [24]. The authors also attempted to examine the possible association between reactivity to carbon dioxide and JH. The rate of JH did not differ between the cases and controls or between JH and carbon dioxide responses. However, they used the crude number of hyperlax joints instead of the scoring method, which carries the cut-off point to the extreme of the distribution and therefore is not fully comparable to other studies. On the other hand, the instruments used to assess anxiety in these patients (the self-rating scale of the National Institute of Mental Health, DSM IV panic symptoms scores and 100-mm visual analogue scales of anxiety) are uncommon and could explain the results of the study.

Gulpek et al. designed a study to test the association between JHS and PD and to determine whether MVP accounted for or changed this association [25]. The sample consisted of 115 subjects who were divided into 3 groups. The first group (n = 42) included patients with PD and MVP, the second group (n = 35) consisted of patients with PD without MVP, and the third group (n = 38) had patients with MVP and no psychiatric diagnosis. No significant differences were found in prevalence or severity of JH between the groups according to the Beighton criteria scoring. However, JH was present in 59.5% of PD patients with MVP and in 52.6% of the control subjects. Compared to other studies, the prevalence of JH in the control group was never found to be as high as in this study. Since the prevalence of JH was higher in patients with PD and MVP (59.5%), the authors suggested that MVP affects the prevalence of JH in PD. The prevalence of PD was also higher in the JH group compared to the controls.

Another research group from Turkey studied the relationship between thorax deformity, anxiety and joint hypermobility. Fifty-two males with thorax deformity and 40 healthy controls from a general outpatient medical clinic were selected to participate in the study [26]. Twenty patients (40%) from the cases group met criteria for JH, and those subjects had significantly higher anxiety scale scores, particularly for PD. All of the cases (with and without JH) had higher anxiety scores compared to the controls.

Ercolani and his team designed a study to assess the psychological features of the JHS [27]. They recruited 30 JH subjects and 2 control groups: 25 healthy subjects and 30 fibromyalgic patients. The JH group showed significant psychological distress and increased frequency and intensity of somatic symptoms compared to both control groups.

Garcia-Campayo designed a case-control study to assess the association between JHS, PD and fibromyalgia [28]. The sample included 220 patients and was divided into 4 different groups. The first group included newly diagnosed PD patients; the second group included patients with psychiatric diagnosis other than anxiety; the third group included patients with fibromyalgia; and the last group consisted of healthy controls. This study also confirmed the higher prevalence of JH in the PD group (61.8%) as well as an intermediate prevalence (25.4%) in fibromyalgia patients. There was a significant correlation between the Beighton criteria (JH) and panic anxiety scale scores.

One recent study provided insight into the importance of autonomic symptoms, such as the hypermobility type of EDS [29]. This group included 80 patients with EDS JH, as well as eleven patients with classical EDS, 7 with vascular EDS, 38 with fibromyalgia and 43 healthy controls. The total autonomic symptom burden was higher in EDS JH (57.9 ± 21.57) than in the other groups but was comparable to the fibromyalgia group (53.8 ± 19.85). They concluded that joint hypermobility and neuropathy might play a role in the development of autonomic symptoms.

In the same line of research, another study described the life experience of EDS JH patients and the impact of the symptoms on daily functioning [30]. The most frequent physical symptoms were joint pain (99%), hypermobility (99%) and limb pain (91%). They also reported a high frequency of other conditions such as chronic fatigue (82%), anxiety (73%), depression (69%) and fibromyalgia (42%). These studies are summarized in table 2.

Nonclinical Studies

Multiple nonclinical studies have assessed the relationship between these two variables in the general population. Our group recruited 1,305 subjects from the general population and found that patients suffering from JH were significantly more likely to suffer from PD (OR 8.19; 95% CI 3.41–19.67), agoraphobia (OR 5.89; 95% CI 2.98–11.66) and social phobia (OR 7.79; 95% CI 2.44–24.85) [31]. Concerning other anxiety conditions, no increased risk was found for simple phobia alone, obsessive-compulsive disorder alone, generalized anxiety disorder alone, dysthymic disorder alone or major depression alone when panic and agoraphobia were excluded. Therefore, the authors concluded that the features of JHS should be used as routine screening.

The same group recruited patients from the medical department of a large auditing and consulting firm of legal services in Barcelona and studied the possible relationship between anxiety and JH in this group of nonclinical subjects [32]. Males and females with JHS showed significantly higher trait anxiety scores (median scores 11, $p < 0.05$; and 17, $p < 0.001$, respectively) than nonhypermobile subjects; however, the difference in state anxiety was not significant for any gender. Both trait and state anxiety showed modest but significant correlations with JHS (Spearman's rho, 0.10–0.16; $p < 0.05$). This was the first article that showed higher anxiety levels in nonclinical subjects with JHS.

Some studies assessed the relationship between JH and fears. Our group designed a cross-sectional study to compare cultural fears in subjects with and without joint hypermobility [33]. The sample was recruited from a rural town, and JH was assessed using Beighton's criteria. The mean scores of the fear survey were higher in the JH group, and significant differences were found between groups, reinforcing the hypothesis that the intensity of fears is greater in subjects with JH. These results showed that the association between JH and phobic anxiety might represent a susceptibility factor for these anxiety conditions.

In the same line of research, another study was designed to see if the relationship between fears and JH was influenced by chocolate consumption

Table 2. Characteristics of clinical and non-clinical studies on the association between joint hypermobility and anxiety

Study (author/ year/country)	Design	Setting	Sample	Variables studied	Main results
Clinical studies					
Bulbena* [1], 1988 [19], 1993 Spain	Case control	Rheumatology outpatient clinic	114 JH 59 controls	Anxiety: HAD-A EPQ, SCID III JH: Beighton	Significant association between JH and PD/A [OR 10.7 (4.8–23.8)] and simple phobia [OR 5.8 (2.0–16.20)]. No association with GAD [OR 2.5 (0.6–9.4)] JH patient with MVP, did not present with more anxiety
Martin-Santos* [20], 1998 Spain	Case control	Outpatient psychiatric and medical clinic	99 newly diagnosed PD/A 99 psychiatric controls 64 medical controls	Anxiety: HAM A/D, SCID III JH: Beighton Other: ECHO	JH found in 67.7% of patients with anxiety [OR 18.6 (8.6–40.5)] (10.1% in psychiatric control and 12.5% in medical control).
Lumley [21], 1994 USA	Case control	Outpatient research clinic	21 EDS III/JH 20 controls (other EDS)	Anxiety: HAM-A JH: EDS subtypes	EDS III (JH) higher scores for anxiety, depression and interpersonal sensitivity and greater scores for symptomatology and pain
Bulbena* [22], 1996 Spain	Case control	Outpatient mental/ medical clinic	99 PD/A 99 psychiatric controls 64 medical controls	Anxiety JH: Beighton Other: *Quetelet index*	Significant correlation between asthenic somatotype and PD/A [OR 2.23] PD/A and asthenic somatotype may be medication through JH
Pailhez* [23], 2014 Spain	Case control	Outpatient clinic	60 PD/A 60 controls	Anxiety: JH: Other: somatotype, sociodemographic	Ectomorphic somatotype was independently related to JH status [OR = 3.25, 95% CI 1.35–7.8, p = 0.008]
Benjamin [24], 2001 Israel	Case control	Anxiety out-patient clinic	101 PD/A 30 healthy controls	Anxiety: NIMH, PSS, VAS 100 mm JH: Beighton	JH = in both groups No association between carbon dioxide response and JH
Gulpek [25], 2004 Turkey	Case control	Outpatient psychiatric clinic	36 PD/A 42 PD/A + MVP 38 MVP	Anxiety: SCID IV JH: Beighton Other: ECHO	JH = 3 groups PD/A higher JH MVP may affect JH prevalence in PD
Gulsum [26], 2007 Turkey	Case control	Outpatient clinic	52 thorax deformity 40 controls	Anxiety: SCID, HAM-A JH: Beighton Other: thorax diameter	21 patients with TD had JH + (40%) JH group had higher anxiety scores (especially PD). TD group had higher anxiety scores (JH + and –)
Ercolani [27], 2008 Italy	Case control	General outpatient medical clinic	JH 30 30 control fibromyalgia 25 healthy control	Anxiety: DSM IV JH: Beighton Others: SCL-90-R, IBQ, SQ, FSF	JH group showed psychological distress and increased frequency and intensity of somatic symptoms
Garcia-Campayo [28], 2010 Spain	Case control	Primary care clinic	55 PD/A 55 psychiatric controls 55 fibromyalgia controls 55 healthy control	Anxiety: PAS, STAI JH: Beighton Other: SPPI	Prevalence of JH in PD was higher than in controls Prevalence of JH in PD was 61.8% Significant correlation between PAS scores and Beighton criteria
De Wandele [29], 2014 Belgium	Case control	Outpatient clinic	80 EDS-JH 11 classic EDS 7 vascular EDS 38 fibromyalgia 43 controls	Anxiety: HADS JH: GHQ Others: ASP, QOL, SF 36, GHQ, fatigue checklist, Baecke physical activity	The total autonomic symptom burden was higher in EDS-HT (57.9 ± 21.57) than in the other groups but was comparable to FM (53.8 ± 19.85)

Table 2. Continued

Study (author/ year/country)	Design	Setting	Sample	Variables studied	Main results
Murray [30], 2013 USA	Cross-sectional	Outpatient clinic	466 adults with EDS JH	237 online survey	High frequency of chronic fatigue (82%), anxiety (73%), depression (69%), and fibromyalgia (42%) among EDS JH
Nonclinical studies					
Bulbena* [31], 2004 Spain	Cross-sectional	General population	1,305 subjects	Anxiety: JH: Beighton MVP	Significant association between JH and PD/A [OR 10.7 (4.8–23.8)] and simple phobia [OR 5.8 (2.0–16.20]. JH patient with MVP did not present with more anxiety
Bulbena* [32], 2004 Spain	Cross-sectional	Medical department of an auditing consultancy	526 subjects	Anxiety: STAI JH: Hospital del Mar	Males and females with JHS had significantly higher trait anxiety scores (median scores 11, $p < 0.05$; and 17, $p < 0.001$, respectively). Both trait and state anxiety showed significant correlations with JHS (Spearman's rho, 0.10–0.16; $p < 0.05$)
Bulbena* [33], 2006 Spain	Cross-sectional	General population	1,305 subjects	Anxiety: FSS JH: Beighton	JH group had higher fear scores and higher intensity of fears. The association of JH and phobic anxiety might represent a susceptibility factor for these anxiety conditions
Pailhez* [34], 2011 Spain	Cross-sectional	High school students	150 subjects	Anxiety: FSS JH: Hackim and Grahame Others: chocolate rate	Higher fear scores in JH Frequency of chocolate intake higher in JH
Baeza-Velasco* [35], 2009 France	Cross-sectional	Internet survey of tall subjects (>180-cm females and >190-cm males)	158 subjects	Anxiety: LSAS JH: Beighton	High rate of JH and social phobia in tall subjects JH greater social phobia symptoms
Baeza-Velasco* [36], 2010 Chile	Case control	University students	50 JH 50 control	Anxiety: HADS, LSAS JH:	JH group had higher use of antidepressants and anxiolytics compared to the controls. They also exhibited a greater anxiety background, anxiety symptoms and psychosomatic complaints
Baeza-Velasco* [37], 2011 France	Cross-sectional	University students	365 subjects	Anxiety: HADS, LSAS JH: Beighton	JH was associated with higher levels of somatosensory amplification as well was higher scores for depression and general anxiety females
Bulbena* [38], 2011 Spain	Cohort study	General population	137 subjects, followed 15 years	Anxiety: SCID, STAI, ASI, FSS JH: Beighton, Hospital del Mar Other: GHQ 28	JH RR: PD/A: 22 (5-109); Social phobia: 6.5 (1.7–24.2) Simple phobia: 3.3 (1.1–9.6); GAD: 2.9 (0.97–8.6) JH score higher on the social dysfunction subscale and other use of anxiolytics Concordance between the Beighton and Brighton (Kappa = 0.91) and Hospital del Mar (Kappa = 0.61) scales
Baeza-Velasco* [39], 2014 France	Cross-sectional	College students	305 females	Anxiety: STAI JH: self-administered JH Other: alcohol, cigarettes	More tobacco and alcohol if JHS JH higher scores on state anxiety

Table 2. Continued

Study (author/ year/country)	Design	Setting	Sample	Variables studied	Main results
Eccles [40], 2012 UK	Cross-sectional	General population	72 healthy volunteers	Anxiety: BAI JH: Beighton Other: Brain MRI, PBPQ	Amygdala volume greater in JH JH higher scores in interoceptive sensitivity and anxiety JH linked to brain center implicated with emotions and physiological responses

(*) Although most papers came from the same research group, but there is no study duplication. Only Bulbena et al. [31] and Bulbena et al. [33] extracted results from the same sample, but they dealt with different variables.
HADS = hospital anxiety and depression scale; ASI = anxiety severity index; EPQ = Eysenck personality questionnaires; SCID = structured clinical interview for DSM; HAM = Hamilton anxiety and depression scale; ECHO = echocardiogram; NIMH = self-rating scale of mental symptoms; PSS = panic symptom scale checklist; VAS = visual analog scale of anxiety; SCL-90 = symptom checklist 90 R; IBQ = illness behavior questionnaire; SQ = symptom questionnaire; FSF = function symptoms frequency; PAS = panic and agoraphobia scale; STAI = state trait anxiety inventory; SPPI = standardized polyvalent psychiatric interview; LSAS = Liebowitz social anxiety scale; ASP = autonomic symptom profile; QOL = quality of life scale; SF-96 = checklist of individual strength; FSS = fear survey schedule; GHQ = general health questionnaire; BAI = Beck anxiety inventory; SSAS = somatosensory amplification scale; PBPQ = Porges body perception questionnaire.

[34]. Significant differences were found in the severity of fears between the groups with and without hypermobility (7.6 vs. 11; $p = 0.001$), reinforcing the hypothesis that the intensity of fears is greater in subjects with hypermobility. Only the frequency of chocolate intake was significantly higher among subjects with hypermobility (31.2 vs. 51.2%; $p = 0.038$) and could correspond to self-treatment of the syndrome.

The relationship between social phobia and height was studied in a cross-sectional study that explored the frequency of social phobia as well as of a heritable disorder of the connective tissue (HDCT) in tall people [35]. One hundred and fifty-eight female subjects with heights greater than 180 cm and male subjects with heights greater than 190 cm were included in the study. Social phobia and HDCT were highly prevalent in tall subjects, and JHS was associated with a greater prevalence of social phobia symptoms.

The association between anxiety disorders and JHS was also assessed in a sample of university students from Chile [36]. Fifty university students with JH and 50 controls were selected to participate in this case-control study. The JH group had higher use of antidepressants and anxiolytics compared to the controls, and they exhibited greater anxiety background, anxiety symptoms and psychosomatic complaints.

A similar study was carried out by Baeza-Velasco et al. on a group of undergraduates in a French university [37]. The aim of this study was to explore the JHS in university students and to assess a possible relationship between this collagen condition and certain psychological variables. Three hundred and sixty-five undergraduates from the French university were included in the study, and the researchers found that JH was present in almost 40% of the sample and was associated with higher levels of somatosensory amplification as well as with higher scores for depression and general anxiety in females.

The first incidence study designed to assess whether JHS is a risk factor for developing anxiety disorders was carried out in a 15-year prospective follow-up study by our group [38]. One hundred and fifty-eight individuals without anxiety problems were recruited from a rural town in Spain. JH at baseline was found in 21.1% of the sample, and we found a higher cumulative incidence of panic/agoraphobia disorder in the JH group (41.4%) compared to the control group (1.9%), representing a relative risk of 22.3 [95% CI 4.6–108.7, $p < 0.0001$]. The incidence of simple phobia and social phobia was also significantly higher in the JH group [RR = 6.52, 95% CI 1.7–24.2, $p < 0.001$; and RR = 3.31, 95% CI 1.1–9.6, $p = 0.02$, respectively].

Joint hypermobility has also been assessed in relation to psychoactive substances. Baeza-Velasco [39] designed a cross-sectional study on college students to assess the use of alcohol and tobacco. The odds of being assessed to have JH were greater in those who consumed tobacco and alcohol. Furthermore, women with JH had higher levels of state anxiety and used emotion-focused coping (i.e., efforts to regulate affect) more than any other coping strategies to deal with stress.

The first structural neuroimaging study on this association was published in 2012 and evaluated regional cerebral grey matter in regards to hypermobility status in 72 healthy volunteers [40]. Interestingly, bilateral amygdala volume was higher in the hypermobile group, and their findings linked hypermobility to the structural integrity of a brain center implicated in normal and abnormal emotions and physiological responses. These studies are summarized in table 2.

Reviews

In the last years, several reviews have pointed out and confirmed the association between anxiety disorder and collagen laxity. Garcia-Campayo et al. summarized the articles about the association between JHS and anxiety disorders that were published from their inception to October 2010 [41]. This group reviewed the articles published about JHS and anxiety as well as genetic studies and hypothesized an etiologic explanation for such an association. The most relevant conclusions of the study were that JHS is more prevalent in patients with PA/A and that patients with JHS present a greater prevalence of PD/A. They also found an association between JHS severity and the severity of anxiety symptoms. The authors finally concluded that MVP might play a secondary role in the association of these two variables.

Sanches et al. [42] published the first systematic review on the clinical association between JH and anxiety disorders. This group included articles up to December 2011, and the final study included 17 articles. They found that most of the studies tended to support an association between JH and anxiety disorders, with PD/A being the anxiety disorder most commonly associated with JH. The authors highlighted the need for more research on different anxiety disorders as well as the need of a multidisciplinary approach for the treatment of those patients.

A British group has recently published a systematic review including a meta-analysis, although they used the unspecific title of 'psychological distress' [43]. They included studies that evaluated the prevalence and incidence of 'psychological' conditions for people diagnosed with JHS. The final study included 14 papers and 3,957 participants: 1,006 people with and 2,951 controls without BJHS. The results indicated that people with JH had a higher probability of demonstrating agoraphobia ($p < 0.05$), anxiety (OR 4.39, 95% CI 1.92–10.40), depression (OR 4.10, 95% CI 1.79–9.41) and PDs (OR 6.72, 95% CI 2.22–20.35) than those without JHS ($P < 0.005$). JH was also associated with significantly greater perception of fear and more intense fear ($p < 0.05$). The authors concluded that people with JH commonly exhibit a range of symptoms related to anxiety and depression, and they pointed out that considerable emotional symptoms accompany JHS.

Finally, Moreno-Peral et al. [44] have just published a systematic review to assess the available evidence on risk factors associated with the onset of PD and Generalized Anxiety Disorder in cohort studies of the general population. PD was associated with age, female gender, few economic resources, smoking and alcohol problems, the number of physical diseases suffered and the JHS.

Psychosomatic Mechanisms Involved

Once the link between anxiety and the Joint Laxity Syndrome is established and their association achieves validity and clinical utility, their common etiological and pathophysiological mechanisms should be identified. Concerning the etiology and the origin of this 'new' revealed condition, so far, only a common genetic linkage has been partially proven. The fact that both conditions (anxiety disorders and joint hyperlaxity syndrome) are highly heritable provides high likelihood for a genetic etiological pathway. In our first genetic study, using pedigree analysis, we found a duplication in chromosome 15 (15q24-q26 named 'DUP25') that appeared to be present in subjects with both conditions. Although replication studies by other research groups failed to confirm this particular duplication, recent studies of the same chromosome showed complex mental and somatic clinical conditions as well as relevant clues for both anxiety (among other features) and morphological anomalies, either in deletion studies [45] or in supernumerary chromosome marker studies [46]. Furthermore, heritability is very often found in both types of patients; it is estimated to be at least 40% in anxiety patients [47], whereas 65% of hypermobile subjects have at least one first-degree relative who suffers from the same condition, albeit it often goes unnoticed.

In regards to the possible pathophysiology of the link between JHS and anxiety, there are two main sources of evidence. First is 'dysautonomia', which is a 'blanket term'-type of disorder that has been related to both conditions. This controversial but successful concept collects a combination of autonomic disorders and, very often, only collections of anxiety symptoms that are simply named differently [48]. On the other hand, the JHS has been repeatedly related to dysautonomia [49, 50].

The second source of evidence for common mechanisms is body awareness, particularly interoception processing. Working together with Prof. Critchley and his group at the Brighton & Sussex Universities, we confirmed a significant correlation between the state anxiety score and joint hypermobility [51]. Interoceptive accuracy was associated with both state anxiety and hypermobility and was formally shown to mediate the relationship between these two conditions. Hypermobile participants, when compared to non-hypermobile individuals, displayed heightened neural reactivity to sad and angry scenes in the brain regions implicated in anxiety states, notably the insular cortex. These findings highlight the dependence of the emotional state on bodily context and increase our understanding of the mechanisms through which vulnerability to anxiety disorders arises in people bearing a heritable variant of collagen.

Toward a New Psychosomatic Phenotype: The Neuroconnective Phenotype

Although there is increasing evidence for somatic comorbidity in the major psychiatric conditions, actual psychiatric classifications do not yet include specific psychiatric illnesses associated with medical conditions other than organic dementias and secondary psychiatric conditions. Apparently two main factors concur for this. First, present nosologies only include two conditions if there is a causal direction between them, for instance, organic brain disorder (dementia) with mental symptoms. Along these lines, concepts like vascular depression or even vascular psychiatry are emerging. The reasoning behind this point of view is quite straightforward because it implies the search for etiology and therefore for treatment.

Second, little evidence has shown specific somatic signs or conditions for the description of the present psychiatric illnesses, which has reduced psychiatrists' expectancies to find a coexistence of both, other than the secondary psychosomatic comorbidity. There are already examples of such comorbid situations, like diabetes and schizophrenia, which some have considered part of the same illness [52]. However, the most studied and developed comorbid condition is the JHS in anxiety patients.

When talking about phenotypes in psychiatry, authors tend to include only behavioral and psychopathological traits, which again, represents a bias against somatic or body characteristics. During the first part of the 20th century, one classic part of the clinical assessment that was neglected was the somatotype (i.e., Leptosomatic, Pyknic, Athletic) due to the contributions of Sheldon and Kretschmer. Nevertheless, currently, somatotype is being used in areas of medicine other than psychiatry, notably in Sports Medicine. Our group carried out several studies assessing somatotype in psychiatric samples, and we replicated the findings of the associations between ectomorphic features and anxiety and joint hypermobility twice [22, 23].

However, at the moment, there is no clear nosological place for these coexistent clinical situations. Therefore, there is a need to develop clinical phenotypes containing both psychopathological and somatic features or even proper psychiatric and somatic conditions.

The new phenotype will be built around the core of the association between anxiety disorders (particularly, panic, agoraphobia and social phobia) and the Joint Hypermobility (or better, Hyperlaxity) Syndrome.

The proposed name 'Neuroconnective' for this new phenotype is both comprehensive and specific. It covers the neural component along with the connective dimension of the new phenotype. The prefix *neuro-* refers to the neural basis of the syndrome, which includes the dysfunctional Autonomic Nervous System and enhanced 'body awareness', including interoception, proprioception and exteroception. Furthermore, as a kind of homage, we would like to consider that the *neuro-* prefix also recalls the concept of neurosis, which was a comprehensive category that included both mental and extensive physical symptoms at the same level during the 19th century. 'Connective' refers to the relevant value of the HDCT and to the 'connectivity' between systems, i.e., mind and body.

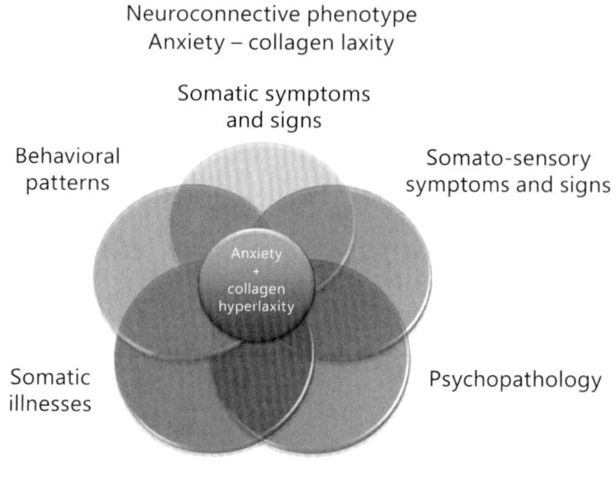

Fig. 1. Diagram of the neuroconnective phenotype with the five components surrounding the core anxiety – collagen laxity.

Therefore, on the basis of the collected genetic, neurophysiological, neuroimaging and most clinical data, several dimensions could be organized in this Neuroconnective model.

The Neuroconnective model is shown in figure 1, in which, around a common core Anxiety-Collagen hyperlaxity, it includes five dimensions: behavioral, psychopathology, somatic symptoms, somatosensory symptoms, and somatic illnesses, with minor overlap.

Two components appear in the core. The first is anxiety and includes any lifetime presence of panic, agoraphobia, or specific and social phobia. Generalized anxiety should be considered when it has reached great severity or when it is a residual state of any of the previous disorders. The second component of the core is the Joint Hyperlaxity (hypermobility) Syndrome, which could also be classified as EDS type III among the hereditary disorders of the connective tissue.

There is a common characteristic of the components of this core, as very often both go unnoticed and undiagnosed. Failure and delay in initial treatment for patients with anxiety disorders is much higher and longer than in mood disorders [53]. On the other hand, the diagnosis of the JHS is very often neglected, unless there are articular complaints, such as pain, or collateral manifestations, such as sprains or repeated twisted joints.

Each of the following five dimensions includes features that may be present at different degrees and with individual variations. In the content of each dimension, we have included patterns, clinical symptoms, signs and illnesses that appear in these patients. We summarize the main characteristics of each dimension without going into detail because this will be dealt with in a separate paper.

Behavioral dimensions are patterns of defensive mechanisms that are often identifiable at the extreme of a continuous axis. They include active flight or fight (hypervisibility), passive flight or fight (hypovisibility), trophotropism (increased appetite, sleep, social withdrawal, and rest), ergotropism (decreased appetite, weight, but increased activity and aggressiveness), over control (ritualism, compulsions), addictions (alcohol and other nonchemical), restriction (avoidance of spaces, people, activities or delayed use of time, i.e., procrastination) and dependency (of people, spaces, activities).

Somatic symptoms include dysautonomia, asthenic somatotype, dark or 'blue' sclera, 'easy bruising' (especially in women), eczemas, esophageal dyskinesia, sprains and dislocations, visceroptosis, prolapses, allergies, dyspareunia, and hypertrophic scars or keloids.

The somatosensory symptoms include increased olfactory sensitivity (especially for negative odors), difficulties with eye contact and sensitivity to some luminous stimuli, dizziness (unsteadiness), sighing, dyspnea, dysphagia or choking, palpitations, urologic and vaginal pains (dynias), joint pain (especially cervical or lumbar) and intolerances or enhanced sensitivities to weather, drugs (particularly psychotropic), chemicals, heat or cold.

Psychopathology includes increased exteroception (e.g., meteorosensibility), increased interoception (visceral-body), increased and distorted proprioception, depersonalization, high loss sensitivity, anticipatory anxiety, high positive confrontation (high ability to deal with real acute problems), fear of annihilation or neutralization, fear of rejection, abandonment or neglect, amplification or exaggeration, denial, or avoidance. This dimension could include fears and phobias, including fear of medication (side effects or addiction) and fear of illness or hypochondriasis, and mood disorders (depression and hypomanic states).

Finally, somatic illness includes irritable bowel, dysfunctional esophagus, multiple chemical sensitivity, dizziness or unsteadiness (central vestibular pattern), chronic fatigue, fibromyalgia, glossodynia, vulvodynia, hypothyroidism, asthma, migraines, temporomandibular dysfunction, intolerances to food and drug hypersensitivity.

Some clinical models, particularly the 'Spectrum project' developed by Cassano [54], also propose the inclusion of maladaptive behavioral traits and temperamental traits with features described in the DSM. However, none of these models include the somatic features or conditions included in the Neuroconnective model of illness that is proposed in this paper.

Conclusions

The well-established association between a collagen condition and anxiety has opened new methods for clinical and basic research. Most probably, new forms of psychosomatic conditions will emerge and different nosological approaches will be required. The Neuroconnective model is a proposal that is being studied and may be useful in clinical practice. Nevertheless, new basic and clinical research on this reviewed association is mandatory because it might open new ways for assessing, understanding and treating patients.

References

1 Bulbena A, Duró JC, Mateo A, et al: Joint hypermobility syndrome and anxiety disorders. Lancet 1988;2:694.
2 Rotés-Querol J, Argany A: La laxité articulaire comme facteur des altérations de l'appareil locomoteur. Rev Rhum Mal Osteoartic 1957;24:535–539.
3 Flanders Dunbar H: Mind and Body: Psychosomatic Medicine. Boston, Random House, 1955.
4 Carlsson C, Rundgren A: Hypermobility of the joints in women alcoholics. J Stud Alcohol 1980;41:78–81.
5 Carter C, Wilkinson J: Persistent joint laxity and congenital dislocation of the hip. J Bone Joint Surg Br 1964;46:40–45.
6 Beighton P, Solomon L, Soskolne CL: Articular mobility in an African population. Ann Rheum Dis 1973;32:413–418.
7 Beighton P, Grahame R, Bird H: Hypermobility of Joints, ed 1. London, Springer London, 1983.
8 Beighton P, Grahame R, Bird H: Hypermobility of Joints, ed 3. London, Springer, 1999.
9 Grahame R: Hypermobility: an important but often neglected area within rheumatology. Nat Clin Pract Rheumatol 2008;4:524.
10 Hakim AJ, Kerr R, Grahame R: Hypermobility, Fibromyalgia, and Chronic Pain. London, Elsevier Health Sciences UK, 2010.
11 Bravo J, Wolff H: Clinical study of hereditary disorders of connective tissues in a Chilean population: joint hypermobility syndrome and vascular Ehlers-Danlos syndrome. Arthritis Rheum 2006;54:515–523.
12 Kerr RM, Grahame R: Hypermobility Syndrome: Diagnosis and Management for Physiotherapists. London, Butterworks, 2003.
13 Mishra MB, Ryan P, Atkinson P, et al: Extra-articular features of benign joint hypermobility syndrome. Rheumatology 1996;35:861–866.
14 Hakim AJ, Grahame R: A simple questionnaire to detect hypermobility: an adjunct to the assessment of patients with diffuse musculoskeletal pain. Int J Clin Pract 2003;57:163–166.
15 Bulbena A, Mallorquí-Bagué N, Pailhez G, et al: Self-reported screening questionnaire for the assessment of Joint Hypermobility Syndrome (SQ-CH), a collagen condition, in Spanish population. Eur J Psychiatry 2014;28:17–26.
16 Bulbena A, Duró JC, Porta M, et al: Clinical assessment of hypermobility of joints: assembling criteria. J Rheumatol 1992;19:115–122.
17 Grahame R, Bird HA, Child A, et al: The revised (Brighton 1998) criteria for the diagnosis of benign joint hypermobility syndrome. J Rheumatol 2000;27:1777–1779.
18 Bulbena A, Benito P: Joint Hyperlaxity: Definition and Clinical Assessment. Interactive CD Training Software. Almirall Prodesfarma, 2006.
19 Bulbena A, Duró JC, Porta M, et al: Anxiety disorder in the joint hypermobility syndrome. Psychiatry Res 1993;43:59.
20 Martín-Santos R, Bulbena A, Porta M, et al: Association between joint hypermobility syndrome and panic disorder (PD). Am J Psychiatry 1998;155:1578–1583.
21 Lumley MA, Jordan M, Rubenstein R, et al: Psychosocial functioning in the Ehlers-Danlos syndrome. Am J Med Genet 1994;53:149–152.
22 Bulbena A, Martín-Santos R, Porta M, et al: Somatotype in panic patients. Anxiety 1996;2:80–85.
23 Pailhez G, Rosado S, Baeza-Velasco C, et al: Ectomorphic somatotype and joint hypermobility are linked in panic and agoraphobic patients: a case-control study. Int J Psychiatry Clin Pract 2014;18:112–117.
24 Benjamin J, Zen-Bion IZ, Dannon P, et al: Lack of association between joint hyperlaxity and, I: panic disorder, and II: reactivity to carbon dioxide in health volunteers. Hum Psychopharmacol Clin Esp 2001;16:189–192.
25 Gulpek D, Bayraktar E, Akbay SP, et al: Joint hypermobility syndrome and mitral valve prolapse in panic disorder. Prog Neuropsychopharmacol Biol Psychiatry 2004;28:969–973.
26 Gülsun M, Yilmaz, MB, Pinar M, et al: Thorax deformity, joint hypermobility and anxiety disorders. Saudi Med J 2007;28:1840–1844.
27 Ercolani M, Galvani M, Franchini C, et al: Benign joint hypermobility syndrome: psychological features and psychopathological symptoms in a sample pain-free at evaluation. Percept Mot Skills 2008;107:246–256.
28 Garcia-Campayo J, Asso E, Alda M, et al: Association between joint hypermobility syndrome and panic disorder: a case-control study. Psychosomatics 2010;51:55–61.
29 De Wandele I, Calders P, Peersman W, et al: Autonomic symptom burden in the hypermobility type of Ehlers-Danlos syndrome: a comparative study with two other EDS types, fibromyalgia, and healthy controls. Semin Arthritis Rheum 2014;44:353–361.
30 Murray B, Yashar BM, Uhlmann WR, et al: Ehlers-Danlos syndrome, hypermobility type: a characterization of the patients' lived experience. Am J Med Genet A 2013;161A:2981–2988.

31 Bulbena A, Gago J, Martín-Santos R, et al: Anxiety disorder and joint laxity: a definitive link. Neurol Psychiatry Brain Res 2004;11:137–140.
32 Bulbena A, Agulló A, Pailhez G, et al: Is joint hypermobility related to anxiety in a non-clinical population also? Psychosomatics 2004;45:432–437.
33 Bulbena A, Gago J, Sperry L, et al: The relationship between frequency and intensity of fears and a collagen condition. Depress Anxiety 2006;23:412–417.
34 Pailhez G, Rosado S, Bulbena Cabré A, et al: Joint hypermobility, fears and chocolate consumption. J Nerv Ment Dis 2011;199:903–906.
35 Baeza-Velasco C, Bulbena A: Ansiedad social y alteración de colágeno en personas de gran estatura. C Med Psicosom 2009;89/90:40–46.
36 Baeza-Velasco C, Bulbena A, Bravo J: Sintomatología ansiosa y sindrome de hiperlaxitud articular en un grupo de universitarios chilenos. Ansiedad y Estrés 2010;16:1–12.
37 Baeza-Velasco C, Gély-Nargeot MC, Bulbena A, et al: Association between psychopathological factors and joint hypermobility syndrome in a group of undergraduates from a French University. Int J Psychiatry Med 2011;41:187–201.
38 Bulbena A, Gago J, Pailhez G, et al: Joint hypermobility syndrome is a risk factor trait for anxiety disorders: a 15-year follow-up cohort study. Gen Hosp Psychiatry 2011;33:363–370.
39 Baeza-Velasco C, Stoebner-Delbarre A, Cousson-Gélie F, et al: Increased tobacco and alcohol use among women with joint hypermobility: a way to cope with anxiety? Rheumatol Int 2014; DOI: 10.1007/s00296-014-3053-8.
40 Eccles JA, Beacher FD, Gray MA, et al: Brain structure and joint hypermobility: relevance to the expression of psychiatric symptoms. Br J Psychiatry 2012;200: 508–509.
41 Garcia-Campayo J, Asso E, Alda M: Joint hypermobility and anxiety: the state of the art. Curr Psychiatry Rep 2011;13: 18–25.
42 Sanches S, Osório F, Udina M, et al: Anxiety and joint hypermobility association: a systematic review. Rev Bras Psiquiatr 2012;34(suppl 1):S53–S60.
43 Smith T, Easton V, Bacon H, et al: The relationship between benign joint hypermobility syndrome and psychological distress: a systematic review and meta-analysis. Rheumatology 2014;53: 114–122.
44 Moreno-Peral P, Conejo-Cerón S, Motrico E, et al: Risk factors for the onset of panic and generalised anxiety disorders in the general adult population: a systematic review of cohort studies. J Affect Disord 2014;168C:337–348.
45 Palumbo O, Palumbo P, Palladino T, et al: An emerging phenotype of interstitial 15q25.2 microdeletions: clinical report and review. Am J Med Genet Part A 2012;158A:3182–3189.
46 Kleefstra T, de Leeuw N, Wolf R, et al: Phenotypic spectrum of 20 novel patients with molecularly defined supernumerary marker chromosomes 15 and a review of the literature. Am J Med Genet Part A 2010;152A:2221–2229.
47 Hettema JM, Neale MC, Kendler KS: A review and meta-analysis of the genetic epidemiology of anxiety disorders. Am J Psychiatry 2001;158:1568–1578.
48 Bulbena A, Pailhez G, Gago J: 'Connective tissue' between panic disorder and dysautonomia. Am J Med 2004;116: 783–784.
49 Gazit Y, Nahir AM, Grahame R, et al: Dysautonomia in the joint hypermobility syndrome. Am J Med 2003;115:33–40.
50 Kanjwal K, Saeed B, Karabin B, et al: Comparative clinical profile of postural orthostatic tachycardia patients with and without joint hypermobility syndrome. Indian Pacing Electrophysiol J 2010;10:173–178.
51 Mallorquí N, Bulbena A, Pailhez G, et al: Mind body interactions in anxiety and related conditions. Harvard Review of Psychiatry 2014; in press.
52 Lin PI, Shuldiner AR: Rethinking the genetic basis for comorbidity of schizophrenia and type 2 diabetes. Schizophr Res 2010;123:234–243.
53 Wang PS, Berglund P, Olfson M, et al: Failure and delay in initial treatment contact after first onset of mental disorders in the National Comorbidity Survey Replication. Arch Gen Psychiatry 2005; 62:603–613.
54 Shear MK, Frank E, Rucci P, et al: Panic-agoraphobic spectrum: reliability and validity of assessment instruments. J Psychiatr Res 2001;35:59–66.

Antoni Bulbena
Departament de Psiquiatria i Medicina Legal, Medical School Building M
Universidad Autónoma de Barcelona, Campus Bellaterra
ES–08193 Barcelona (Spain)
E-Mail abulbena@gmail.com

Author Index

Subject Index